Functional Neurological Disorder

Editors

DAVID L. PEREZ
SARA A. FINKELSTEIN

NEUROLOGIC CLINICS

www.neurologic.theclinics.com

Consulting Editor
RANDOLPH W. EVANS

November 2023 • Volume 41 • Number 4

ELSEVIER

1600 John F. Kennedy Boulevard • Suite 1800 • Philadelphia, Pennsylvania, 19103-2899

http://www.theclinics.com

NEUROLOGIC CLINICS Volume 41, Number 4
November 2023 ISSN 0733-8619, ISBN-13: 978-0-323-93839-6

Editor: Stacy Eastman
Developmental Editor: Varun Gopal

Neurologic Clinics (ISSN 0733-8619) is published quarterly by Elsevier Inc., 360 Park Avenue South, New York, NY 10010–1710. Months of issue are February, May, August, and November. Periodicals postage paid at New York, NY, and additional mailing offices. Subscription prices are $353.00 per year for US individuals, $809.00 per year for US institutions, $100.00 per year for US students, $433.00 per year for Canadian individuals, $980.00 per year for Canadian institutions, $489.00 per year for international individuals, $980.00 per year for international institutions, $210.00 for foreign students/residents, and $100.00 for Canadian students/residents. To receive student/resident rate, orders must be accompanied by name of affiliated institution, date of term, and the *signature* of program/residency coordinator on institution letterhead. Orders will be billed at individual rate until proof of status is received. Foreign air speed delivery is included in all *Clinics* subscription prices. All prices are subject to change without notice. **POSTMASTER:** Send address changes to *Neurologic Clinics*, Elsevier Health Sciences Division, Subscription Customer Service, 3251 Riverport Lane, Maryland Heights, MO 63043. **Customer Service: Telephone: 1-800-654-2452 (U.S. and Canada); 314-447-8871 (outside U.S. and Canada). Fax: 314-447-8029. E-mail: journalscustomerservice-usa@elsevier.com (for print support); journalsonlinesupport-usa@elsevier.com (for online support).**

Reprints. For copies of 100 or more of articles in this publication, please contact the Commercial Reprints Department, Elsevier Inc., 360 Park Avenue South, New York, New York, 10010-1710; Tel.: +1-212-633-3874; Fax: +1-212-633-3820, and E-mail: reprints@elsevier.com.

Neurologic Clinics is also published in Spanish by Nueva Editorial Interamericana S.A., Mexico City, Mexico.

Neurologic Clinics is covered in *Current Contents/Clinical Medicine, MEDLINE/PubMed (Index Medicus), EMBASE/Excerpta Medica, and PsycINFO, and ISI/BIOMED.*

Contributors

CONSULTING EDITOR

RANDOLPH W. EVANS, MD
Clinical Professor, Department of Neurology, Baylor College of Medicine, Houston, Texas, USA

EDITORS

DAVID L. PEREZ, MD, MMSc
Functional Neurological Disorder Unit, Division of Cognitive Behavioral Neurology, Department of Neurology, Division of Neuropsychiatry, Department of Psychiatry, Massachusetts General Hospital, Harvard Medical School, Boston, Massachusetts, USA

SARA A. FINKELSTEIN, MD, MSc, FRCPC
Instructor in Neurology, Functional Neurological Disorder Unit, Division of Cognitive Behavioral Neurology, Department of Neurology, Division of Comprehensive Neurology, Massachusetts General Hospital, Instructor, Harvard Medical School, Boston, Massachusetts, USA

AUTHORS

CAITLIN ADAMS, MD
Division of Behavioral Neurology, Functional Neurological Disorder Unit, Departments of Neurology and Psychiatry, Massachusetts General Hospital, Harvard Medical School, Boston, Massachusetts, USA

SELMA AYBEK, MD
Neurology, Faculty of Science and Medicine, Fribourg University, Fribourg, Switzerland

JANET BAKER, LACST, MSc, PhD
Adjunct Associate Professor, Flinders University, Adelaide, South Australia

GASTON BASLET, MD
Chief of Neuropsychiatry, Division of Neuropsychiatry, Department of Psychiatry, Brigham and Women's Hospital, Associate Professor, Harvard Medical School, Boston, Massachusetts, USA

VERÓNICA CABREIRA, MD
Centre for Clinical Brain Sciences, University of Edinburgh, Edinburgh, United Kingdom

ALAN CARSON, MBChB, MPhil, MD, FRCPsych, FRCP
Department of Clinical Neurosciences, Centre for Clinical Brain Sciences, University of Edinburgh, Royal Infirmary of Edinburgh, Edinburgh, United Kingdom

ILARIA DI VICO, MD
Movement Disorders Division, Department of Neurosciences, Neurology Unit, Biomedicine and Movement Sciences, University of Verona, Verona, Italy

BARBARA A. DWORETZKY, MD
Chief of Epilepsy Division, Department of Neurology, Brigham and Women's Hospital, Professor, Harvard Medical School, Boston, Massachusetts, USA

MARK J. EDWARDS, MBBS, PhD
Institute of Psychiatry, Psychology and Neuroscience, King's College London, United Kingdom

SARA A. FINKELSTEIN, MD, MSc, FRCPC
Instructor in Neurology, Functional Neurological Disorder Unit, Division of Cognitive Behavioral Neurology, Department of Neurology, Division of Comprehensive Neurology, Massachusetts General Hospital, Instructor, Harvard Medical School, Boston, Massachusetts, USA

JENNIFER L. FREEBURN, MS, CCC-SLP
Department of Speech, Language, and Swallowing Disorders, Massachusetts General Hospital, Boston, Massachusetts, USA

ELLEN GODENA, LICSW
Functional Neurological Disorder Unit, Division of Cognitive Behavioral Neurology, Massachusetts General Hospital, Harvard Medical School, Boston, Massachusetts, USA

WESLEY T. KERR, MD, PhD
Clinical Instructor, Department of Neurology, University of Michigan, Ann Arbor, Michigan, USA

KASIA KOZLOWSKA, MBBS, FRANZCP, PhD
Children's Hospital Westmead Clinical School, Faculty of Medicine and Health, University of Sydney, Westmead Institute for Medical Research, Westmead, Australia

MACKENZIE P. LERARIO, MD, NYS, CRPA/CPS-p
Fordham Graduate School of Social Service, New York, New York, USA; Greenburgh Pride, Greenburgh, New York, USA

SARAH C. LIDSTONE, MD, PhD, FRCPC
Integrated Movement Disorders Program, Toronto Rehabilitation Institute, University Health Network, University of Toronto, Toronto, Canada

JULIE MacLEAN, OTR/L
Functional Neurological Disorder Unit and Research Group, Department of Neurology, Department of Occupational Therapy, Massachusetts General Hospital, Boston, Massachusetts, USA

JULIE MAGGIO, PT
Functional Neurological Disorder Unit, Division of Cognitive Behavioral Neurology, Harvard Medical School, Department of Physical Therapy, Massachusetts General Hospital, Boston, Massachusetts, USA

TINA MASCHI, PhD, LCSW
Fordham Graduate School of Social Service, New York, New York, USA; Greenburgh Pride, Greenburgh, New York, USA

LAURA McWHIRTER, PhD
Centre for Clinical Brain Sciences, University of Edinburgh, Edinburgh, United Kingdom

TRACEY MILLIGAN, MD
Department of Neurology, Westchester Medical Center Health Network, New York Medical College, Valhalla, New York, USA

DANIEL MILLSTEIN, PhD
Functional Neurological Disorder Unit, Division of Cognitive Behavioral Neurology, Massachusetts General Hospital, Harvard Medical School, Boston, Massachusetts, USA

M. ANGELA O'NEAL, MD
Chief of General Neurology, Assistant Professor, Harvard Medical School, Boston, Massachusetts, USA

DAVID L. PEREZ, MD, MMSc
Functional Neurological Disorder Unit, Division of Cognitive Behavioral Neurology, Department of Neurology, Division of Neuropsychiatry, Department of Psychiatry, Massachusetts General Hospital, Harvard Medical School, Boston, Massachusetts, USA

GINGER POLICH, MD, MS
Department of Physical Medicine and Rehabilitation, Spaulding Rehabilitation Hospital, Brigham and Women's Hospital, Harvard Medical School, Boston, Massachusetts, USA

STOYAN POPKIROV, PD, MD
Department of Neurology, University Hospital Knappschaftskrankenhaus Bochum, Bochum, Germany

JESSICA RANFORD, MS, OTR/L
Functional Neurological Disorder Unit and Research Group, Department of Neurology, Department of Occupational Therapy, Massachusetts General Hospital, Boston, Massachusetts, USA

WINFRIED RIEF, PhD
Departments of Clinical Psychology and Psychotherapy, Philipps-University Marburg, Marburg, Germany

NICOLE ROSENDALE, MD
Department of Neurology, Weill Institute for Neurosciences, University of California, San Francisco, San Francisco, California, USA

KAROLINE S. SAUER
Department of Clinical Psychology, Psychotherapy, and Experimental Psychopathology, Johannes Gutenberg-University of Mainz, Mainz, Germany

ANEETA SAXENA, MD
Division of Behavioral Neurology, Functional Neurological Disorder Unit, Department of Neurology, Massachusetts General Hospital, Harvard Medical School, Boston, Massachusetts, USA

TEREZA SERRANOVÁ, MD, PhD
Department of Neurology and Centre of Clinical Neuroscience, General University Hospital and First Faculty of Medicine, Charles University, Prague, Czech Republic

JEFFREY P. STAAB, MD, MS
Professor and Chair, Department of Psychiatry and Psychology, Consultant, Departments of Psychiatry and Psychology and Otorhinolaryngology–Head and Neck Surgery, Mayo Clinic, Rochester, Minnesota, USA

JON STONE, MBChB, FRCP, PhD
Consultant Neurologist and Honorary Professor of Neurology, Department of Clinical Neurosciences, Centre for Clinical Brain Sciences, University of Edinburgh, Royal Infirmary of Edinburgh, Edinburgh, United Kingdom

MICHELE TINAZZI, MD, PhD
Professor, Movement Disorders Division, Department of Neurosciences, Neurology Unit, Biomedicine and Movement Sciences, University of Verona, Verona, Italy

JACK TURBAN, MD, MHS
Division of Child and Adolescent Psychiatry, University of California, San Francisco, San Francisco, California, USA

JEFF L. WAUGH, MD, PhD
Department of Pediatrics, UT Southwestern Medical School, Dallas, Texas, USA

MICHAEL WITTHÖFT, PhD
Department of Clinical Psychology, Psychotherapy, and Experimental Psychopathology, Johannes Gutenberg-University of Mainz, Mainz, Germany

Contents

The idea that a neurologist would do an 'FND clinic' or that functional neurological disorder (FND) could be a subspecialty of neurology would have been outlandish even 20 years ago but has become a reality in many places around the world. In this personal review, I reflect on 25 years of being a neurologist with an interest in FND, initially as a research fellow and later as a consultant/attending. I review lessons in relation to the diagnosis and management of FND in the hope that they may assist neurologists embarking on a similar career or other health professionals whose roles overlap.

 Video content accompanies this article at http://www.neurologic. theclinics.com.

Functional movement disorder (FMD) is a common, potentially reversible source of disability in neurology. Over the last two decades, there have been major advances in our understanding of the clinical picture, diagnosis, and management of this condition. Motor presentation is heterogeneous and several non-motor symptoms (e.g., pain, fatigue) are part of the clinical spectrum. The diagnosis should be made by neurologists or neuropsychiatrists based on the presence of positive signs of inconsistency and incongruence with neurological diseases. Promising evidence has accumulated for the efficacy of physiotherapy, psychotherapy, or both in the management of FMD, for a majority of patients.

Diagnosis of functional seizures, also known as psychogenic nonepileptic seizures, starts with a clinical interview and description of the seizures. A targeted approach to this evaluation can provide valuable information to gauge the likelihood of functional seizures as compared with other similar conditions including but not limited to epileptic seizures. This review focuses on the use of patient and witness descriptions and seizure videos to identify patients with probable functional seizures. Particular emphasis is given to recognizing the limitations of the available data and the influence of health-care provider expertise on diagnostic accuracy.

Functional cognitive disorder is an increasingly common cause of referral to the memory clinic. As a substantial source of disability, clinicians involved in the management of patients with cognitive complaints need to familiarize themselves with this important differential diagnosis. Our approach focuses on the identification of positive features of internal inconsistency (historical and clinical clues alongside patterns of performance) instead of an exclusionary approach. Although effective treatments are desperately needed, promising therapies include metacognitive retraining and cognitive-behavioral therapy modalities. Future research should focus on a better understanding of disease trajectories and outcomes as well as the development of evidence-based interventions.

Historically, formal training for speech-language therapists (SLTs) in the area of functional speech and voice disorders (FSVD) has been limited, as has the body of empirical research in this content area. Recent efforts in the field have codified expert opinions on best practices for diagnosing and treating FSVD and have begun to demonstrate positive treatment outcomes. To provide comprehensive interventions for these complex conditions at the intersection of neurology, psychiatry, and other medical specialties, the SLT must not only build knowledge of diagnostic strategies and components of symptomatic treatment in FSVD but also embrace behavior change techniques and counseling strategies.

Persistent postural-perceptual dizziness (PPPD) is a functional neuro-otologic (vestibular) disorder manifesting dizziness, unsteadiness, or nonspinning vertigo lasting 3 months or more and exacerbated by upright posture, active or passive motion, and complex visual stimuli. PPPD is the most common cause of chronic vestibular symptoms. Early pathophysiologic models of PPPD emphasized the adverse effects of anxiety on postural control and spatial orientation. More recent concepts added predictive processing of sensory inputs and alterations in motion perception. Herein, a third-generation model incorporates prioritization of postural stability over fluid locomotion to explain symptoms, physiologic and neuroimaging data, and effects of current treatments.

Functional neurological disorder (FND) is a "rule-in" diagnosis, characterized by positive examination signs or semiological features. Similar to other clinical diagnoses, providers should ideally see robustly present features, including if possible the identification of multiple features consistent with FND for the diagnosis to be made with a high degree of certainty. Diagnostic pitfalls need to be guarded against and vary depending on FND symptom subtype and the specific patient presentation. This perspective article aims to review pitfalls based on an FND symptom subtype, as well as discuss differential diagnostic considerations with respect to both neurologic and psychiatric entities.

Functional neurological disorder (FND) is a neuropsychiatric condition. In this field, prospective psychotherapy trials and consensus recommendations for physiotherapy, occupational therapy, and speech language therapy have been published. However, significant clinical complexities remain. "Rule in" signs – while critical for making a positive diagnosis – do not equate to a personalized treatment plan in many instances. Here, we propose that the neuropsychiatric assessment and real-time development of a work-in-progress biopsychosocial clinical formulation aids the development of a patient-centered outpatient treatment plan. This precision medicine approach is based on the literature, expert opinions and our clinical experience working in an interdisciplinary FND service.

Occupational therapy (OT) is an important treatment modality for patients with paroxysmal functional neurological disorder (FND) symptoms. In our clinical experience, an outpatient, OT-based sensory modulation treatment can address sensory processing difficulties often endorsed by patients with paroxysmal motor FND and functional seizures. This article aims to describe in detail the goals and treatment strategies for occupational therapists to replicate this approach. This article is also an important first step in aiding the development and execution of clinical trials to further evaluate the effectiveness of sensory-based treatment in patients with FND.

Functional neurological disorder (FND) is a common condition for which neurology residents often receive little to no formal teaching. Using a question-and-answer format, this article puts forward a case for why an FND curriculum is needed and aims to provide guidance on possible curricular content including medical knowledge, clinical skills, communication, and team-based collaboration. The authors also discuss methods for teaching and evaluating this knowledge and associated clinical skills, linking this to current Accreditation Council for Graduate Medical Education neurology

Setting up Functional Neurological Disorder Treatment Services: Questions and Answers   729

Sara A. Finkelstein, Alan Carson, Mark J. Edwards, Kasia Kozlowska,
Sarah C. Lidstone, David L. Perez, Ginger Polich, Jon Stone, and Selma Aybek

Functional neurological disorder (FND) is commonly encountered across
outpatient and inpatient medical settings. Given the potential for a high
burden of disability in some patients and mounting evidence for the efficacy of FND-specific multidisciplinary treatment services, expanding clinical services for this population is a necessity. In this perspective article,
we discuss considerations for creating FND services, including the types
of services that exist, how to start, how to identify appropriate referrals,
and how to develop and monitor individualized treatment plans. In addition, we discuss how this effort can be done sustainably – balancing patient needs with limited healthcare resources.

Somatic Symptom Disorder and Health Anxiety: Assessment and Management   745

Karoline S. Sauer, Michael Witthöft, and Winfried Rief

The fifth edition of the Diagnostic and Statistical Manual of Mental Disorders (DSM-5) Somatic Symptom Disorder (SSD) and Illness Anxiety Disorder (IAD) replaced the diagnostic entities of the fourth edition of the
Diagnostic and Statistical Manual of Mental Disorders (DSM-IV) somatoform disorders and hypochondriasis. SSD turns away from specifying
the presence or absence of a medical condition for presented symptoms
and instead focuses on excessive symptom-related affects, cognitions,
and behaviors. People with pathological health anxiety can be diagnosed
with SSD or IAD, depending on the intensity of accompanying somatic
symptoms. Cognitive-behavioral therapy shows the best empirical evidence for an effective treatment of SSD and IAD.

Functional Neurological Disorder Among Sexual and Gender Minority People   759

Mackenzie P. Lerario, Nicole Rosendale, Jeff L. Waugh, Jack Turban, and
Tina Maschi

Sexual and gender minority (SGM) people can face unique stressors and
structural discrimination that result in higher rates of neuropsychiatric
symptoms, such as depression, anxiety, and suicidality. Although more
rigorous studies are needed, emerging data suggest a possible higher
prevalence of functional neurological disorder and other brain-mind-
body conditions in SGM people. Representation and iterative feedback
from affected community members is critical to the process of developing
affirming environments. More research is needed to explore the relevance
of functional neurological disorder in SGM people within a biopsychosocial
framework.

NEUROLOGIC CLINICS

ISSUES OF RELATED INTEREST

Neurosurgery Clinics
https://www.neurosurgery.theclinics.com/
Neuroimaging Clinics
https://www.neuroimaging.theclinics.com/
Psychiatric Clinics
https://www.psych.theclinics.com/
Child and Adolescent Psychiatric Clinics
https://www.childpsych.theclinics.com/

THE CLINICS ARE AVAILABLE ONLINE!
Access your subscription at:
www.theclinics.com

Preface

Functional Neurological Disorder

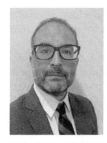
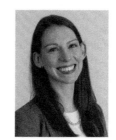

David L. Perez, MD, MMSc   Sara A. Finkelstein, MD, MSc
Editors

For the field of functional neurological disorder (FND), a sentiment of renewal and progress abounds. Historically neglected by neurology and psychiatry,[1] and at times wrongly confused with malingering,[2] the field of FND is now rapidly growing and helping to close the gap between two specialties for the same organ (ie, the brain).[3] The transformations and progress in the field of FND have been catalyzed by a diagnostic approach emphasizing rule-in signs and semiologic features that are specific for the diagnosis.[4,5] Improved diagnostic specificity has led to a boom of research, expanding the therapeutic toolkit and advancing our understanding of mechanisms and etiologies for this condition. Large multisite clinical trials have been completed, and others are underway.[6,7]

We enthusiastically took on this *Neurologic Clinics* issue on FND with the aim of broadly disseminating expert knowledge. To begin, this issue features Jon Stone, who shares with readers an immensely rich and thoughtful set of lessons learned as a practicing neurologist with 25 years of experience building and refining an FND specialty practice. Thereafter, the next five articles cover the full range of FND presentations, including functional movement disorder, functional seizures, functional cognitive disorder, functional speech/voice disorders, and persistent postural-perceptual dizziness. In doing so, practical and up-to-date contributions were received from an international panel of authors spanning the United States (Jeffrey Staab, Wesley Kerr, Jennifer Freeburn), United Kingdom (Alan Carson, Laura McWhirter, Verónica Cabreira), Czech Republic (Tereza Serranová), Italy (Michele Tinazzi, Ilaria Di Vico), and Australia (Janet Baker).

Next, Sara Finkelstein and Stoyan Popkirov bring to the readers' attention common diagnostic pitfalls of FND, including both neurologic and psychiatric differential diagnostic considerations. Thereafter, David Perez (with contributions from Sara Finkelstein, Caitlin Adams, and Aneeta Saxena) details the use of the neuropsychiatric assessment and biopsychosocial formulation to develop a patient-centered, precision medicine approach to clinical care in FND. While treatment is covered in this issue

Neurol Clin 41 (2023) xiii–xv
https://doi.org/10.1016/j.ncl.2023.05.004
0733-8619/23/© 2023 Published by Elsevier Inc.

across several articles, Jessica Ranford and Julie MacLean wrote an occupational therapy–focused article on how to assess and manage sensory processing difficulties in patients with FND. We hope that this article will spur clinical trial research at the intersection of sensory processing and functional neurological symptoms. Two articles in question-and-answer format follow, discussing FND education and clinical program development. The former, led by Sara Finkelstein and M. Angela O'Neal, along with input from a multidisciplinary group of coauthors (Gaston Baslet, Barbara Dworetzky, Ellen Godena, Julie Maggio, Daniel Millstein, Tracey Milligan, and David Perez) discusses the "why" and "how" regarding the development and implementation of an expanded curriculum on FND during neurology training. The latter, led by Sara Finkelstein, brings together an international panel of coauthors to discuss opportunities and challenges that frequently occur when initiating FND clinical care pathways. In addition to benefiting from contributions by those that have also lent expertise elsewhere in this issue, this article includes insights from Selma Aybek, Mark Edwards, Kasia Kozlowska, Sarah Lidstone, and Ginger Polich.

Our issue ends with two articles addressing gaps in the field. The first covers other functional somatic symptoms and pathologic health anxiety, written by Karoline Sauer, Michael Witthöft, and Winfried Rief. The second covers the timely and under-researched topic of sexual and gender–minority people with FND, a piece led by Mackenzie Lerario—with contributions from Nicole Rosendale, Jeff Waugh, Jack Turban, and Tina Maschi.

In closing, we are grateful to all the coauthors for generously sharing their expertise with readers. We would also like to thank the patients and various patient-advocacy groups for the many insights they have provided us over the years. Enjoy the issue!

David L. Perez, MD, MMSc
Functional Neurological Disorder Unit
Division of Behavioral Neurology
Department of Neurology
Division of Neuropsychiatry
Department of Psychiatry
Massachusetts General Hospital
Harvard Medical School
Boston, MA, USA

Sara A. Finkelstein, MD, MSc
Functional Neurological Disorder Unit
Division of Behavioral Neurology
Division of Comprehensive Neurology
Department of Neurology
Massachusetts General Hospital
Harvard Medical School
Boston, MA, USA

E-mail addresses:
dlperez@nmr.mgh.harvard.edu (D.L. Perez)
safinkelstein@mgh.harvard.edu (S.A. Finkelstein)

REFERENCES

1. Fend M, Williams L, Carson AJ, et al. The Arc de Siècle: functional neurological disorder during the 'forgotten' years of the 20th century. Brain 2020;143(4):1278–84. https://doi.org/10.1093/brain/awaa037.
2. Edwards MJ, Yogarajah M, Stone J. Why functional neurological disorder is not feigning or malingering. Nat Rev Neurol 2023;19:246–56. https://doi.org/10.1038/s41582-022-00765-z.
3. Finkelstein SA, Adams C, Tuttle M, et al. Neuropsychiatric treatment approaches for functional neurological disorder: a how to guide. Semin Neurol 2022;42(2):204–24. https://doi.org/10.1055/S-0042-1742773.
4. Aybek S, Perez DL. Diagnosis and management of functional neurological disorder. BMJ 2022;376:o64. https://doi.org/10.1136/BMJ.O64.
5. Hallett M, Aybek S, Dworetzky BA, et al. Functional neurological disorder: new subtypes and shared mechanisms. Lancet Neurol 2022;21(6):537–50. https://doi.org/10.1016/S1474-4422(21)00422-1.
6. Goldstein LH, Robinson EJ, Mellers JDC, et al. Cognitive behavioural therapy for adults with dissociative seizures (CODES): a pragmatic, multicentre, randomised controlled trial. Lancet Psychiatry 2020;7(6):491–505. https://doi.org/10.1016/S2215-0366(20)30128-0.
7. Nielsen G, Stone J, Buszewicz M, et al. Physio4FMD: protocol for a multicentre randomised controlled trial of specialist physiotherapy for functional motor disorder. BMC Neurol 2019;19(1):242. https://doi.org/10.1186/s12883-019-1461-9.

Lessons from a Neurologist After 25 Years of Functional Neurological Disorder Subspeciality Practice

Jon Stone, MB ChB, FRCP, PhD*

KEYWORDS

- Functional neurological disorder • Neurology • Misdiagnosis • Lessons
- Management • Diagnosis • Conversion disorder

KEY POINTS

- Functional neurological disorder (FND) is a rewarding new subspeciality of neurology which relies on clinical skills, communication, and wide general neurology knowledge.
- Diagnostic pitfalls include overweighting a history of psychological comorbidity, and failing to consider other neurological comorbidity including prodromal states of neurodegenerative disease.
- Management pitfalls include insufficient time for assessment, making premature assumptions about prognosis, and forgetting that sometimes all someone may be looking for is 'peace of mind'.
- FND is a multidisciplinary and interdisciplinary endeavor. Find colleagues locally or online to do it with.

FUNCTIONAL NEUROLOGICAL DISORDER NEUROLOGY IN THE LATE TWENTIETH AND EARLY TWENTY-FIRST CENTURY

It was during several junior jobs in Neurology in various parts of the United Kingdom in the 1990s that I met my first patients with functional neurological disorder (FND). A man who owned a stately home and had a functional hemiparesis in the middle of the night after hitting his head and having a panic attack. A student with functional paraplegia discharged home with no treatment. There were many patients with functional seizures who were misdiagnosed with epilepsy and taken to intensive care, or conversely treated as feigners with an approach that makes me shiver now, thinking about it.

Centre for Clinical Brain Sciences, University of Edinburgh, Edinburgh, UK
* Department Clinical Neurosciences, Royal Infirmary of Edinburgh, Edinburgh EH16 4SA, United Kingdom.
E-mail address: Jon.Stone@ed.ac.uk

Neurol Clin 41 (2023) 569–582
https://doi.org/10.1016/j.ncl.2023.02.001
0733-8619/23/© 2023 Elsevier Inc. All rights reserved.

neurologic.theclinics.com

At that time, FND was very much in a state of neglect. There was no mention of it in neurology textbooks or training where its presence had been declining steadily for 100 years.[1] Patients with FND were generally told that there was 'nothing neurologically wrong', that it was 'good news' because the scans were normal, and often told they were in the wrong department. At neurology 'grand rounds', FND appeared much more than now, usually as a 'mystery case'. With hindsight, this was mainly because awareness of FND clinical features was poor, and it was usually treated as a diagnosis of exclusion. Once the patient left the room, discomfort at the diagnosis often found its expression in clinicians laughing about the fact that there was 'nothing wrong' or labeling the condition 'bogus'.[2] One of my seniors, seeing my interest in this problem as a young trainee, became concerned that I might be committing some kind of career suicide.

It would be wrong to present a blanket caricature. Most neurologists were doing what they could without any training or research to guide them.[3] There was often talk of helping the patient to 'save face'. This was well meant but is a concept that is only necessary if a patient has something to be shamefaced about, such as the nature of their condition, or because they were considered to be feigning, at least in part. The most senior neurologist in the department often took responsibility for people with FND, partly because others were concerned about making the diagnosis. One neurologist I know who worked in a continental European country told me that only the head of the neurology department was *allowed* to make the diagnosis.

THE BENEFITS OF BEING AN FND NEUROLOGIST

FND has many qualities that lend itself to being a subspeciality in Neurology. It is common in neurological practice, and many neurologists do not feel competent dealing with it,[4] both issues that can make the new FND neurologist popular with their peers.

Diagnostically, it requires familiarity with the whole range of neurology to maintain wariness of comorbidity or misdiagnosis, discussed below. It is a specialty that emphasizes bedside diagnostic and communication skills that are being eroded or devalued in many other subspecialties by advances in genetics and neuroimaging.

From a treatment perspective, the FND neurologist may often have the pleasure of being able to give answers to a patient who has been looking for them for a long time. FND is a disorder where it is usually possible to inject some hope into the situation, and if not that, then at least peace of mind, or an improved understanding of a long-term condition. It also gives a home to neurologists who also are interested in psychiatry and the philosophical aspects of neuroscience–why do we have dualism of brain and mind? Is there really a 'hard' problem of consciousness? How do we separate a person from their illness when it is happening in their brain?

THE DOWNSIDES OF BEING AN FND NEUROLOGIST

Many conditions in neurological practice are potentially draining for a neurologist to work with because they are untreatable and produce so much misery for everyone concerned. FND can be all of those things, but also highly treatable to the point of joy in some cases. Approaching FND with as wide an angle as possible is important. I see clinicians getting frustrated that they cannot get all their FND patients better when that was an unreasonable starting point. FND treatments have a low "number needed to treat" but are still not yet that good, and the barriers to recovery for some are huge.

People with FND often overflow with symptoms and distress and need time to be seen properly (see below). But that process requires patience and does not suit everyone. It is undoubtedly challenging to attempt to put yourself in the shoes of many FND patients and can be time-consuming to communicate and provide management.

Neurologists often do not receive formal psychiatric training, and even when they do, often feel unprepared for the psychiatric aspects of their role which encompass not just FND but most neurological conditions.[5]

THE IMPORTANCE OF CONSULTATION LENGTH, FOLLOW-UP, AND CONTINUING GENERAL NEUROLOGY

In many health service settings, neurologists only have 30 minutes to see a new patient. This is clearly insufficient for most people with FND and at least an hour is recommended. Some important territory can be covered in 30 minutes but not that well. You would not expect a neurosurgeon to take out someone's pituitary adenoma in the same time it takes to remove a lumbar disk. The surgeon could do it quickly, but it is not a good idea and the patient is more likely to have a bad outcome. Neurologists have been weak at defending the importance of consultation length in creating better outcomes for patients. When I began training, my seniors were considered heroic to see 40 patients in a morning. It was necessary at the time–but not something to be coveted.

Follow-up slots in neurology services are scarce and under pressure from hospital managers and others who often prefer to count new patients. Few neurologists would diagnose someone with multiple sclerosis (MS) or Parkinson's disease and not arrange any follow-up for them. Without a follow-up appointment, an FND neurologist will have no opportunity to gain feedback about the effectiveness of their initial diagnosis and communication strategy. The first appointment in some ways is the easy one. The patient is often delighted to be heard and given a diagnosis. At subsequent appointments, the reality of the day-to-day symptoms, the lack of 'quick fixes', and barriers to treatment must be confronted.

For some patients, an onward referral to treatment services is not appropriate at the first visit. You may still be establishing trust (see Case 10 below) or there may be investigations that need to be completed (see Cases 4 and 5). The first follow-up appointment, ideally a few weeks after the first one and after the patient has had a chance to see your letter and read relevant self-help educational material, is a chance to gauge factors including diagnostic confidence and "motivation for change". Careful triage using factors like this enables best use of therapy services, prevents patients 'going through the motions' who will probably not benefit from treatment, or need more time to understand what is happening.

Diagnostic Lessons

In a previous article, developed together with Markus Reuber and Alan Carson, we discussed common issues of diagnosis and misdiagnosis in FND.[6] Whereas the obsession in the past has always been not to miss a recognized/structural neurological condition in a patient labeled as having FND, we highlighted in that article how commonly people with FND are misdiagnosed as having other neurological conditions.

Studies in this area tend to suggest that the latter occurs more than the former. For example, in our cohort study of 3781 new neurology outpatients across Scotland, there were 4/1144 patients misdiagnosed with a functional disorder,[7] whereas there were 10/2378 who had a functional disorder that had been incorrectly classified as another neurological condition.[8] The proportions (0.4%) are similar, but because the functional disorder category was smaller, there were twice as many people with diagnostic errors in the latter category. A synthesis of studies on the misdiagnosis of FND and MS came to similar conclusions.[9] A recent study of 107 patients misdiagnosed with autoimmune encephalitis found that FND was the leading missed initial diagnosis.[10]

The following highlight common pitfalls in the diagnosis of FND and are all anonymized but based on actual cases.

Case 1. Psychological comorbidity or stress should not be used to diagnose functional neurological disorder

A 63-year-old woman was referred with acute left hemiparesis at the moment she found out that her brother had died. She was tearful with a variable hemiparesis but no documentation of positive features of FND. A CT head scan was normal and FND diagnosed.

An MRI showed a new *brainstem infarct*.

Stress can trigger stroke and heart attack. Stress is so ubiquitous that it is not difficult to find a 'stress' narrative in most people if you look hard enough. Do not use the presence of 'stress' to make a diagnosis but do use it to consider in the formulation once you have made a clinical diagnosis.

Case 2. Functional neurological disorder can happen with no psychological comorbidity

A 54-year-old man presented with a 3-year history of back pain and gait difficulties. He came from work to the appointment and presented a straightforward history with no comorbid psychiatric disorder or psychological risk factors.

Examination showed clear evidence of a *functional gait disorder* with abnormal flexion movements when walking forwards, but normal backward walking and running. FND-focused physiotherapy resolved his problems within 18 months.

Studies of psychiatric comorbidity in FND show that it is common but that there is a minority without it or where it is at a subdiagnostic threshold level common in neurology patients generally. Similarly, prior stress or maltreatment is between two and four times more common in FND than healthy controls, but anywhere between 30% and 70% have not had those experiences when asked.[11]

Case 3. Avoid making a functional neurological disorder diagnosis without positive clinical evidence or just because a neurological presentation looks 'bizarre'

An 11-year-old presented with difficulty walking and some dystonia of her feet. Her clinicians noticed that her gait was variable and would often be much better in the morning. She had a normal MRI, lumbar puncture, and routine blood tests. She and her family agreed with an FND diagnosis, but treatment failed to improve the situation.

Several years later, she was found to have variable generalized dystonia with neck extension, a tendency to walk on tiptoes, with a tendency for knee extension and hyperlordosis.

The gait was unusual but there were no positive features of FND. A trial of levodopa produced a complete and long-lasting resolution of her disability. She had a mutation in the GCH1 gene known to be associated with *dopa-responsive dystonia*.

The diagnosis here was missed because of emphasis on a weak diagnostic feature, variability, taken on its own without any clear-cut diagnostic features of FND. It can be tempting to diagnose a functional disorder without them, but I have learned to step back and ask myself–am I really seeing typical features of FND here?

A similar issue arises in patients where the clinical presentation is really unusual. Very few presentations of FND are 'bizarre.' FND acquired that reputation because clinicians were unfamiliar with the typical ways in which it presents. If a presentation is obviously outside the normal range for FND then think carefully about other unusual diagnoses, for example: the stiffness and jerkiness of stiff person syndrome; unusual hyperkinetic events in frontal lobe epilepsy; and combinations of psychiatric, behavioral change, and faciobrachial dystonic seizures in LGI1 autoimmune encephalitis. **Box 1** has a list of diagnoses that are particularly likely to catch out the unwary neurologist diagnosing FND.

Case 4. Other neurological conditions are commonly comorbid with functional neurological disorder. Have a low threshold for investigations

A 44-year-old woman presented with right leg weakness. She had a typical dragging gait with her hip externally rotated and a positive Hoover's sign and hip abductor sign. She had been experiencing fatigue and impaired concentration for several months and had a history of irritable bowel syndrome and migraine. There were no clinical features of an additional neurological condition such as abnormal reflexes or upgoing plantar response.

An MRI scan of brain and spine done at the first visit showed typical changes of multiple sclerosis meeting McDonald Criteria. At follow-up, the clinical features of FND had improved and the course of her illness followed one quite typical for *relapsing-remitting MS*.

FND can be comorbid with MS at any point in the condition, but in my experience, it is more common in the early stages of the disorder, which is partly supported by the existing literature.[9] Subtle changes in motor and sensory function caused by demyelination are an understandable trigger for secondary functional disorders.

In someone with a functional hemiparesis, I have learned to do MRI brain and whole spine on most occasions at the first visit if not already done. I have a low threshold for brain MRI scanning in patients with functional seizures, where we know the frequency of structural abnormalities is higher than expected.[12] It is important to find an L5 radiculopathy or low-grade excess of possible demyelinating lesions at the first visit. Telling someone that the results are likely to be normal for age or show incidental abnormalities reduces anxiety while waiting for results.

Box 1
Some neurological conditions that are especially likely to be mistaken for functional neurological disorder

- Frontal lobe epilepsy
- Epilepsia partialis continua
- Epileptic seizures triggered by stress or that are 'self-induced' (eg, as may be in the case of epilepsy with a specific trigger such as hyperventilation)
- Autoimmune encephalitis
- Stiff person syndrome
- Frontotemporal dementia
- Apraxic disorders of limbs and speech
- Dystonic gait–may be better running or backward
- Vestibular disorders–running may be better than walking
- Paroxysmal dyskinesia
- Periodic paralysis

Also, look hard for common neurological comorbidities. Migraine is exceptionally prevalent in FND and often worth treating in its own right. Treatable nerve entrapment syndromes like meralgia paraesthetica, carpal tunnel syndrome, and ulnar nerve irritation often explain why FND symptoms are in a certain location.

Case 5. Comorbid degenerative neurological conditions may take some time to present and may not be detectable at initial presentation with functional neurological disorder

A 37-year-old man presented with an intermittent tremor in the right hand and weakness in the right leg, both of which had textbook features of FND. He had no features of additional neurological conditions, including a careful screen for any prodromal features of Parkinson's disease.

On follow-up over 3 years, he developed reduced blink rate, reduced arm swing, small handwriting, and REM sleep behavior disorder. An Ioflupane Dopamine Transporter Scan showed asymmetrical, side-appropriate, changes in keeping with *Parkinsonian syndrome.* The patient responded to levodopa. Over time, the features of FND improved and features of Parkinson's disease became more obvious.

This story is perhaps the commonest comorbidity pitfall in FND practice. Studies show how commonly FND can occur in the prodrome of Parkinson's disease,[13] and that patients with Parkinson's disease are much more likely to experience functional symptoms and disorders than individuals with Alzheimer's disease.[14]

I have also met two patients who presented with definite FND-related leg weakness, who developed motor neuron disease (amyotrophic lateral sclerosis) between 2 and 3 years later. Other disorders I have seen emerge over time in someone with an initial FND diagnosis include frontotemporal dementia, spinocerebellar ataxia, genetic prion disease, Wilson disease, and progressive supranuclear palsy. The initial diagnosis of FND in all of these cases was correct in my view, it just turned out to be incomplete, similar to anxiety presenting as a prodromal symptom in Parkinson's disease. In most of these cases, FND symptoms responded to initial treatment, at least to a degree, before being superseded by symptoms of another progressive neurological condition.

This is an issue that may encourage neurologists to follow-up their FND patients more, although such scenarios do remain relatively rare, except Parkinson's disease. Our prospective follow-up study of 107 patients with functional limb weakness over 14 years only found 1 patient who had been misdiagnosed with hindsight (multiple sclerosis).[15] There were, however, three patients with neurodegenerative diseases (Huntington's disease, Parkinson's disease, and idiopathic cerebellar degeneration) where the disorders did not explain FND but where this prodromal disease state was probably relevant.

Case 6. Functional neurological disorder signs do not have 100% specificity

A 78-year-old woman presented with progressive left hemiparesis. Her academic daughter contacted the FND neurologist wondering if her mother might have FND because her mobility appeared so variable, and imaging had only shown age-related atrophy. She had a strongly positive Hoover's sign.

The overall clinical and imaging picture was compatible with the *corticobasal syndrome,* with progressive apraxia, that had produced a false positive Hoover's sign, which was present, but misleading.

Most neurological signs need to be put together with other clinical features to produce a likely diagnosis. It is dangerous to rely solely on one physical sign. Hoover's sign would be expected in apraxia where there is an explicit deficit of planned and sequenced voluntary movement but preservation of automatic motor function.[16] No FND clinical sign is 100% reliable.

Case 7. Think about psychiatric differential diagnosis too

A 63-year-old retired business executive presented with progressive loss of mobility, limb aching, and reduced speech and a diagnosis of FND. He denied feeling depressed but did very little.

There were no positive diagnostic features of FND, apart from some give-way weakness. Over time it became clear that he had a *severe major depression*. He did not respond to antidepressants or psychotherapy but following a course of electroconvulsive therapy made a good recovery back to independent living with improved mood and normal mobility.

Primary psychiatric disorders may present in a bodily way. Catatonia is perhaps the most extreme example of that. I have also seen severe obsessive compulsive disorder presenting with an akinetic mute state and recurrent (denied) alcohol intoxication presenting as unexplained "blackouts."

Case 8. Feigning is rare but does occur and you do need to look out for it

A 32-year-old man presented with a persistently abducted thumb after a work-related injury. He had a personal injury claim but said he would 'do anything' to recover. He had FND-focused treatment including physiotherapy and an attempt at therapeutic sedation without success.

Subsequent footage emerged of him using his hand normally while playing a games console online which he said he could not do. His legal case collapsed on the basis that he was *feigning,* and he did not return for follow-up.

Factitious disorder and malingering (the latter not a disorder) hang like specters over FND, especially for neurologists. I meet several patients a year where there is evidence for this, mostly in medicolegal, rather than usual, clinical practice. Evidence has been assembled as to why FND is usually *not* malingering from historical, clinical, and neuroscience accounts/studies.[17] When looking for feigned symptoms, the main evidence should usually come from lying, or a major discrepancy between reported and observed function. Do not be timid about asking about litigation as this has a massive potential influence on treatment, even in patients with genuine symptoms. Be especially wary of symptoms that are rare in your usual FND practice like this patient's unusual thumb abduction.

Management Lessons

Whoever makes the diagnosis of FND, usually a neurologist, has a crucial role in laying the groundwork so that the patient is ready for therapy, if appropriate. Ideally, the patient will have a good understanding and confidence in why the diagnosis of FND has been made, understand why physical or psychological rehabilitation is being suggested to improve FND symptoms, and have goals that motivate them to engage with therapy. But what happens when things do not go so smoothly? I can only address a handful of issues here and also recommend this article.[18]

Case 9. Give everyone a fair chance even if things look unpromising

A 58-year-old man presented with 20 years of poor mobility, including pain, left-sided weakness, seizures, and fatigue. He had recurrent depression and was on high doses of opioids and gabapentin. He was dissociated and hard to communicate with so appeared to have difficulty engaging with his diagnosis and suggested treatment.

He had his opioids and gabapentin slowly weaned and stopped. By the third visit, he was much brighter, and his wife and physiotherapist said that he was improving. After a year, he was volunteering in a men's charity project. He was still symptomatic but doing much more than anyone had hoped would be possible initially.

It is tempting to use clinical experience to think that you can guess the outcome of the intervention. But I am constantly surprised by patients I fear will not do well, who do much better than I anticipated, and vice versa. This clinical experience is mirrored in data from prognostic studies which show how difficult it is to predict an individual outcome. In a recent re-analysis of 3781 neurology outpatients over 1 year, even machine learning using every available data point at baseline could not predict the outcome at 1 year.[19] Prognostic studies in FND have found repeatable factors such as agreement with diagnosis, short duration, and less comorbidity to be better, but that still does not mean those things necessarily apply at an individual level.[20]

Case 10. Sometimes it takes time to help people understand their diagnosis

A 34-year-old woman with frequent functional seizures and right-sided weakness returned to the clinic for follow-up. She had been generally satisfied with the consultation but was not able to repeat back anything about her diagnosis or the rationale for treatment.

It took two more visits to get to the point where she had some confidence about what was wrong and could explain it. She was not in disagreement with the original diagnosis, but it turned out that she was repeatedly thinking that if it was FND that must mean it was 'her fault' and so she just needed to 'push through' and it would 'go away'. By the fourth visit, she was finally in a place where she felt that she could accept that this had happened to her, was not her fault, and that therapy might help her. With hindsight, I wondered if I should have referred her earlier, but the patient said that she would not have been ready.

It should not be forgotten just how difficult it is to understand FND and some people need time to do so. Sometimes it appears that a patient disagrees with the diagnosis when they are having more complex issues of self-blame, trust with health professionals, or having trouble communicating that they are not ready for treatment.

Case 11. Look for health anxiety and address it explicitly if present

A 38-year-old man presented with intense global headache, dizziness, and impaired cognition. He was distraught in the clinic holding his head in his hands. He admitted that he was terrified that something awful was happening inside his body and worried that he would not wake up. The experience brought back teenage memories of the sudden death of his father from a heart attack.

He was given an explanation of the mechanisms of headache and persistent postural perceptual dizziness (PPPD), but later visits indicated that he remained very worried and was spending a lot of time researching his symptoms online and presenting to the emergency department. We had a more direct conversation about health anxiety–that it is a really distressing and familiar issue. The patient had an internal battle in his head between a rational explanation of what was wrong, and terrifying thoughts of death and illness.

Pathological health anxiety describes persistent worry and anxiety about medical conditions like cancer or multiple sclerosis which typically is recognized as irrational by the sufferer, at least part of the time. It is not the same as someone with FND who has not had a good explanation of their diagnosis, having a strong view that they have another condition, or feeling gloomy about their outlook.

In health anxiety, reassurance from health professionals is actively unhelpful as it leads to only a temporary reduction of distress which is then sought again. Instead, it must be confronted as a condition in its own right that can respond well to therapy. Health anxiety is an important but, in its severe form, not that common issue, alongside FND, which, if addressed well, can lead to large rewards. Most people I meet with health anxiety also have functional symptoms or disorders which still benefit from explanation. Health anxiety will often respond to a consistent approach between medical professionals involved and psychological therapy which is well described.[21]

Case 12. Do not overdiagnose functional neurological disorder when an additional label may not be helpful

A 14-year-old young man presented with widespread joint pain, fatigue, anxiety, and difficulty attending school. He was referred because his left leg was a little heavier than the right and had been told that he had FND. His gait was normal and there was a mild Hoover's sign, but leg weakness was really a minor issue in comparison to his fatigue and pain.

At assessment, it was explained that the additional label of FND was not helpful here. He did have some mild functional leg weakness. However, the focus should remain on pain, fatigue, and anxiety through the help he was already receiving from a pain management program.

I notice increasingly, as FND gains better awareness, that it is becoming more misused as a term for all functional disorders or added, often prematurely, to long lists of other diagnoses. Signposting people with paralysis, tremor, and seizures to an FND label makes sense, but diagnostic labels can also be harmful, especially in a health care system where many health professionals do not feel confident about FND.

When I first started writing articles about FND, I used the term functional neurological symptoms. It was patient advocates who taught me that 'symptoms' is not good enough to describe a situation where someone has seizures or has been in a wheelchair for 10 years. We should, however, be willing to describe functional neurological "symptoms" rather than "disorder" if symptoms are milder (eg, mild sensory symptoms alone), but also recognize when a 'disorder' diagnosis is more appropriate.

This issue also arises when setting boundaries around referrals to a neurologist-led FND clinic. Be careful not to become a destination for patients with *all* functional disorders such as chronic pain syndromes or irritable bowel syndrome, that are outside neurology expertise, even if familiarity is required (see the additional article on FND pathways elsewhere in this volume of Neurologic Clinics).[22]

Case 13. Be willing to agree to disagree

A 35-year-old woman presented with tremor, pain, limb weakness, and seizures in combination with orthostatic intolerance. She could not sit upright without collapsing and having a several-minute duration episode of loss of awareness with eyes closed. There were multiple features of FND present and no additional neurological diagnoses. She had had extensive investigations to rule out spontaneous intracranial hypotension (SIH) and a normal tilt table test. The patient was convinced that the symptoms were those of SIH and that a surgeon in another country would be able to diagnose and remedy the situation.

The patient recognized that I was listening and believed how disabled she was, but it proved impossible to find common ground for agreement about a way forward. I suggested we had little to lose by trying rehabilitation for orthostatic intolerance with a focus on FND, on the basis that she had been deconditioned to an upright position. For the patient, it was not possible to engage with that possibility. We had to 'agree to disagree' about the diagnosis and management, but I left the door open for further discussion.

Case 14. Do not just diagnose, formulate!

An 18-year-old woman presented with severe FND including seizures, lower leg weakness, and dystonia in the context of persistent fatigue that had been present since she was 12. She had such bad 'brain fog' and sensory sensitivity that she no longer did any reading or writing and had stopped school at 14, despite being an A-grade student. Her parents, desperate to help, were keeping things as quiet and as dark as possible. The patient described a constant sense of 'fight or flight' and was frequently tearful but did not feel that she had 'anything to be worried about'.

In this severe scenario, we acknowledged some diagnostic labels were appropriate but also that the situation required a more detailed formulation of how she had arrived at this situation. We agreed that her body had 'shut down', in response to infectious illness and school/sporting expectations. She now agreed that it made sense to help desensitize her nervous system, very slowly through rehabilitation. Recovery slowly occurred and led to university.

Neurologists are generally taught to diagnose and not to formulate, which is a skill routinely learned by psychiatrists and psychologists. In FND, most things work better if you can learn a little about what someone else on the team might do. Stay within your professional boundaries, but trying some formulation of predisposing, precipitating, and perpetuating factors with patients can be productive. Make suggestions to patients, but ideally collaborate on building a formulation that everyone can agree on. Discuss how treatment might logically approach that formulation.

Case 15. Knowing when 'peace of mind' is enough

A 61-year-old woman with a 20-year history of fatigue, chronic pain, and seizures had been through a pain management program but did not understand why her left side was weak. Her husband, also her carer, was frightened by the seizures.

At follow-up, it became clear that they were not looking for or expecting any change, but were pleased to understand that the neurological symptoms had an explanation and were common. They said they were grateful for some 'peace of mind' which had been missing before the consultation.

Sometimes 'peace of mind' is an important and main outcome for the FND neurologist. Do not underestimate its importance to patients and carers.

THE IMPORTANCE OF A TEAM AND MENTORSHIP

One essential lesson for an FND neurologist is to have a team to share patients with, both formally and informally. FND is a multidisciplinary activity and difficult to do as a lone practitioner. It works best, and is most rewarding, when you are learning from other colleagues, and able to do "a little" of what they do and vice versa. Colleagues in a team are vital to discuss difficult patients and to generally provide support and a sounding board, especially if a consultation has been unusually challenging. A team meeting can accomplish this, but it may be important to have individuals with whom you can have more private conversations where frank views can be aired and tested.

For me, doing research on FND for 25 years has been a tremendous way to help me personally through difficult clinical situations, but I have also been fortunate to have colleagues with whom I can relax and share difficult patient scenarios. Consider whether you should have a formally identified mentor to guide you in your career. No one is too old for such an approach or immune from developing 'burnout' working with what can be an emotionally demanding group of patients. Encourage visitors to your clinics to feedback on anything they might have done differently, whatever their seniority.

DO WE NEED FND NEUROLOGISTS AND IS IT SUSTAINABLE BEING ONE?

Yes. In 2021, the European Academy of Neurology announced that FND and Neuropsychiatry would become one of 19 core areas for training.[23] In 2022, the UK

Table 1
Some lessons from the functional neurological disorder clinic

General	Diagnostic	Management
Fight for enough time to see patients properly	Psychological comorbidity should not be used to diagnose FND and may be absent	Give all patients a fair chance, even if the prognosis looks unpromising
Follow-up patients and learn from them	Avoid diagnosing FND without positive evidence	Some people need time to gain confidence in an FND diagnosis
Develop triage skills to enhance the outcome of therapy	Avoid diagnosing FND because a presentation is unfamiliar or 'bizarre'	Treat pathological health anxiety specifically when present
Learn some of the skills possessed by multidisciplinary colleagues	Consider comorbid other neurological conditions, including prodromal states of neurodegenerative disorders	Do not overdiagnose FND if another problem is dominant. Functional neurological symptoms may be more appropriate than FND in some
Cultivate colleagues/friends to support/mentor you	FND signs, especially in isolation, do not have 100% specificity	Be willing to agree to disagree with a patient who has strong views
FND is a new and legitimate subspecialty of Neurology	Think about psychiatric differential diagnosis	Do not just diagnose, formulate too
	Feigning is rare but look out for it	Providing 'peace of mind' about the diagnosis alone may be a valid outcome

neurology curriculum introduced FND and Neuropsychiatry as one of eight core topics in training.[24]

We will continue to need movement disorder and epilepsy specialists with FND expertise. We also need psychiatrists with subspecialty expertise in neurology and FND. But there is also room for a neurologist who covers multiple types of FND clinically,[25] for training requirements coming from these new curricula, and for doing research.

I hope the diagnostic and management lessons I have raised in this article are of some assistance to neurologists and other health professionals working with people who have FND (**Table 1**).

After 25 years, I still find it rewarding and fascinating seeing and trying to help people with FND. It is an area of medicine that has its roots in so many diverse areas of human physiology and experience that, even at the start of my career, I always doubted I would ever truly 'get to the bottom of it'. The huge advances in the field mean that I am less in the dark than I was when I started. But I also know there is much to learn and that the diversity of FND and the unique way it presents in every patient is one of the things that continue to make it rewarding.

CLINICS CARE POINTS

- Fight for enough time to see your FND patients and provide follow up.
- Be vigilant for hidden neurological and psychiatric comorbidity and be willing to revise or update an FND diagnosis.
- Learn to triage patients for therapy based on their agreement and readiness for the treatment.
- Become familiar with elements of multidisciplinary therapy and discuss them with your FND patients as part of getting them 'ready' for therapy.
- Learn psychological formulation skills and grow a multidisciplinary team to work with and learn from.

DISCLOSURE

Professor J. Stone reports: honoraria from UptoDate for articles on FND; Personal fees from Expert Witness Work involving personal injury and negligence cases, some of which relate to patients with FND. J. Stone runs a self-help website, www.neurosymptoms.org, for patients with FND, is secretary of FND Society and medical adviser to several FND charities.

ACKNOWLEDGMENTS

Special thanks to my neurology colleague, Ingrid Hoeritzauer, for detailed comments and suggestions to this article, as well as my neuropsychiatry colleagues Alan Carson and Laura McWhirter and past and present members of our FND research group (FRG) at the University of Edinburgh. I am supported by an National Research Scotland Career Fellowship.

REFERENCES

1. Stone J, Hewett R, Carson A, et al. The 'disappearance'of hysteria: historical mystery or illusion? J R Soc Med 2008;101(1):12–8.

2. Tolchin B, Baslet G, Dworetzky B. Psychogenic seizures and medical humor: Jokes as a damaging defense. Epilepsy Behav 2016;64:26–8.
3. Fend M, Williams L, Carson AJ, et al. The Arc de Siècle: functional neurological disorder during the 'forgotten' years of the 20th century. Brain 2020;143(4): 1278–84.
4. Carson A.J., Stone J., Warlow C., et al., Patients whom neurologists find difficult to help, J Neurol Neurosurg Psychiatr, 75 (12), 2004, 1776-11778.
5. Shalev D, Jacoby N. Modernizing Psychiatry Training for Neurologists—From Off-Service to In-Service. JAMA Neurol 2022;79(2):113.
6. Stone J, Reuber M, Carson A. Functional symptoms in neurology: mimics and chameleons. Practical Neurol 2013;13(2):104–13.
7. Stone J, Carson A, Duncan R, et al. Symptoms "unexplained by organic disease" in 1144 new neurology out-patients: how often does the diagnosis change at follow-up? Brain 2009;132(10):2878–88.
8. Walzl D, Carson AJ, Stone J. The misdiagnosis of functional disorders as other neurological conditions. J Neurol 2019;266(8):2018–26.
9. Walzl D, Solomon AJ, Stone J. Functional neurological disorder and multiple sclerosis: a systematic review of misdiagnosis and clinical overlap. J Neurol 2022; 269(2):654–63.
10. Flanagan E.P., Geschwind M.D., Lopez-Chiriboga A.S., et al., Autoimmune encephalitis misdiagnosis in adults, JAMA Neurol, 80(1), 2023, 30-39.
11. Ludwig L, Pasman JA, Nicholson T, et al. Stressful life events and maltreatment in conversion (functional neurological) disorder: systematic review and meta-analysis of case-control studies. Lancet Psychiatr 2018;5(4):307–20.
12. Reuber M, Qurishi A, Bauer J, et al. Are there physical risk factors for psychogenic non-epileptic seizures in patients with epilepsy? Seizure 2003;12(8): 561–7.
13. Wissel BD, Dwivedi AK, Merola A, et al. Functional neurological disorders in Parkinson disease. J Neurol Neurosurg Psychiatr 2018;89(6):566–71.
14. Onofrj M, Russo M, Carrarini C, et al. Functional neurological disorder and somatic symptom disorder in Parkinson's disease. J Neurol Sci 2022;433:120017.
15. Gelauff JM, Carson A, Ludwig L, et al. The prognosis of functional limb weakness: a 14-year case-control study. Brain 2019;142(7):2137–48.
16. Ercoli T, Stone J. False Positive Hoover's Sign in Apraxia. Mov Disord Clin Pract 2020;7(5):567–8.
17. Edwards MJ, Yogarajah M, Stone J. Why functional neurological disorder is not feigning or malingering. Nat Rev Neurol 2023;19:246–56.
18. Adams C, Anderson J, Madva EN, et al. You've made the diagnosis of functional neurological disorder: now what? Practical Neurol 2018;18(4):323–30.
19. Shipston-Sharman O, Popkirov S, Hansen CH, et al. Prognosis in functional and recognised pathophysiological neurological disorders - a shared basis. J Psychosom Res 2022;152:110681.
20. Gelauff J, Stone J. Prognosis of functional neurologic disorders. Handb Clin Neurol 2016;139:523–41.
21. Cooper K, Gregory JD, Walker I, et al. Cognitive Behaviour Therapy for Health Anxiety: A Systematic Review and Meta-Analysis. Behav Cognit Psychother 2017;45(2):110–23.
22. Finkelstein SA, Carson A, Edwards MJ, et al. Setting up functional neurological disorder treatment services: questions and answers. Neurol Clin 2023; In Press.

23. European Academy of Neurology. European Training Requirements for Neurology. 2021. Available at: https://www.ean.org/learn/career-development/european-curricula.

24. Joint Royal Colleges of Physicians Training Board. Curriculum for Neurology Training. 2022. Available at: https://www.jrcptb.org.uk/specialties/neurology.

25. Hallett M, Aybek S, Dworetzky BA, et al. Functional neurological disorder: new subtypes and shared mechanisms. Lancet Neurol 2022;21(6):537–50.

Functional Movement Disorder

Assessment and Treatment

Tereza Serranová, MD, PhD[a,*], Ilaria Di Vico, MD[b],
Michele Tinazzi, MD, PhD[b]

KEYWORDS

- Functional motor disorder • Functional neurological disorder • Inconsistency
- Incongruence • Electrophysiology • Non-motor symptoms • Physiotherapy

KEY POINTS

- Functional movement disorder (FMD) is a rule-in diagnosis based on the demonstration of inconsistency and incompatibility with other neurologic diseases.
- If needed, electrophysiology can support the diagnosis of functional tremor and myoclonus in diagnostically challenging cases.
- Psychological abnormalities are not necessary or sufficient for the diagnosis of FMD.
- Neurologic assessment, delivery of positive diagnosis, and education are part of the treatment.
- Individualized treatment should involve physiotherapy, psychotherapy, or both in most patients.

 Video content accompanies this article at http://www.neurologic.theclinics. com.

INTRODUCTION

Functional movement disorder (FMD) is common in clinical practice, accounting typically for 3% to 6% of referrals to specialized movement disorder services[1,2] and around 10% of admissions to acute stroke services.[3] FMD is associated with high disability and impaired quality of life compared with that seen in people with Parkinson disease.[4] FMD is characterized by abnormal motor control manifesting with hyperkinetic (eg, tremor, dystonia, myoclonus) and hypokinetic movements (eg, parkinsonism), as

[a] Department of Neurology and Centre of Clinical Neuroscience, General University Hospital and First Faculty of Medicine, Charles University, Kateřinská 30, 12 800, Prague, Czech Republic;
[b] Movement Disorders Division, Department of Neurosciences, Neurology Unit, Biomedicine and Movement Sciences, University of Verona, Piazzale L. A. Scuro 10, 37124, Verona, VR, Italy
* Corresponding author.
E-mail address: tereza.serranova@vfn.cz

Neurol Clin 41 (2023) 583–603
https://doi.org/10.1016/j.ncl.2023.02.002
neurologic.theclinics.com
0733-8619/23/© 2023 Elsevier Inc. All rights reserved.

well as weakness, which can be significantly altered by distraction, beliefs, and expectations, and are clinically incongruent/incompatible with movement disorders known to be caused by other neurologic diseases.[5] The clinical spectrum of FMD is heterogeneous in terms of motor symptom presentations. In accordance with the current neurobiological models proposing a unified (transdiagnostic) pathophysiology of the full range of functional symptoms across different domains, numerous functional motor, sensory, cognitive symptoms, and functional seizures, as well as other somatic symptoms, often coexist.[6,7] People with FMD have a high prevalence of non-motor symptoms such as pain, fatigue, bladder and bowel problems, along with psychological symptoms (eg, depression and anxiety) that all have a major impact on their health-related quality of life.[8]

Importantly, increasing scientific interest in FMD has recently shaped a new understanding of underlying mechanisms, diagnosis, diagnostic explanation, and treatment.[9] In the context of a biopsychosocial model of FMD pathophysiology, new avenues for treatment have been traced, including novel awareness of the role of multidisciplinary rehabilitation. Recent advances notwithstanding, the unmet need of evidence-based recommendations and several gaps in health care systems limit current clinical practice,[10] with diagnosis remaining delayed or missed, prognosis sometimes unfavorable, and symptoms potentially disabling in the long term.[11]

TERMINOLOGY AND NOSOLOGIC CLASSIFICATION

FMD is not an officially recognized term/diagnostic category in the current classification systems. For the purposes of this review, the authors include functional limb weakness under the umbrella of FMD. The authors have also avoided use of the term "organic" in opposition to the term "functional" to avoid perpetuating dualistic thinking.

FMD is classified as a functional neurological symptom disorder (conversion disorder) with abnormal movements or weakness in the Diagnostic and Statistical Manual of Mental Disorders, 5th Edition (DSM-5) and as a motor dissociative (conversion) disorder in the Psychiatry section of the International Classification of Diseases, 10th Edition (ICD-10).[12,13] The revised ICD-11 also introduced the term "functional" in their diagnostic labels, and several FMD subtypes are also included in the Neurology section.[13] Yet, the revised ICD-11 classification remains unsatisfactory, as the whole phenotypic range of FMD is not consistently represented in the Neurology section and other functional somatic symptoms, such as pain and fatigue, commonly present in people with FMD, are currently classified separately (**Table 1**). This diagnostic division, which is also present in the DSM-5, has important impact/implications on the organization of specialized services: people with FMD often need to seek help for associated symptoms in different outpatient services, and complex specialized care is not available. A preliminary revision to the DSM-5 diagnostic criteria allowing for an etiologically neutral specifier noting the presence of other prominent non-sensorimotor somatic symptoms has been proposed.[14] The identification of FMD patients with prominent pain or fatigue would allow clinicians to consider guiding individuals toward interdisciplinary brain-mind-body treatment programs that may be potentially more suitable for initial management than physical therapy alone.

EPIDEMIOLOGY

Functional neurological disorder (FND) and related conditions represent the second most common reason to see a neurologist after headache.[1] FMD has an incidence of 4 to 5/100,000 per year and women represent around 75% of FMD patients, with mean age at onset of 40 years.[15]

Table 1
Diagnostic division of coexistent functional neurological and somatic symptoms

	Motor Symptoms	Non-Motor Symptoms (Pain and Fatigue)
DSM-5	*Somatic Symptom and Related Disorders* "Motor functional neurological symptom (conversion) disorder with abnormal movements or weakness"	*Somatic Symptom and Related Disorders* Associated pain or fatigue is labeled as "somatic symptom disorder"
ICD-10	*Psychiatry (F)* "Motor dissociative (conversion) disorder" (F.44.4)	*Psychiatry (F)* "Persistent somatoform pain disorder" (F45.4) *Musculoskeletal (M)* "Fibromyalgia" (M79.7) *Symptoms, signs and abnormal clinical and laboratory findings, not elsewhere classified (R)* "Chronic fatigue syndrome" (R53.82)
ICD-11	*Diseases of the nervous system (08)* "Functional parkinsonism" (8A00.3) "Functional dystonia" (8A02.3) "Functional tremor" (8A04.4) *Mental, behavioral or neurodevelopmental disorders (06)* "Dissociative neurologic symptom disorder with movement disturbance (6B60.81), gait disturbance (6B60.7), with paresis or weakness (6B60.6)"	*Symptoms, signs or clinical findings, not elsewhere classified (21)* "Chronic widespread pain (MG30.01) "Fatigue" (MG22)
Gupta and Lang criteria	*Psychogenic movement disorders*	-
Fahn and Williams criteria	*Psychogenic movement disorders*	-
Shill and Gerber criteria	*Psychogenic movement disorders*	Excessive pain or fatigue are specified as primary criteria

Abbreviations: DSM-5, Diagnostic and Statistical Manual of Mental Disorders, 5th Edition; ICD-10 and 11, International Classification of Diseases, 10th and 11th Edition—Chapter/Section, "Diagnostic Label," (Code).

CLINICAL ASPECTS AND DIAGNOSIS OF FUNCTIONAL MOVEMENT DISORDER

The diagnosis of FMD is clinical and, in some instances, can be corroborated by neurophysiological findings if needed. It is a rule-in diagnosis based on the demonstration of positive signs of internal inconsistency and incongruence/incompatibility with other neurologic conditions (**Box 1**).[5,12] In particular, demonstration of distractibility is useful as it is a sign of both inconsistency and incongruence. So far, 37 bedside clinical tests for the diagnosis of FMD with some form of validation have been reported in a recent review (which we refer to for complete information).[9] Overall, given the high overall specificity (64%–100%), these signs should be used routinely in clinical practice. However, their sensitivity is highly variable, ranging from 9% to 100%; thus, they should not be used in isolation. Some signs, including the well-validated Hoover's sign, have also been found in other neurologic diseases, highlighting the need for a direct comparison with different clinical groups presenting with abnormal motor control and/or pain compromising patient compliance and providing updated estimates of false positive results.[16] In addition, most studies have based their validation on a single evaluation without blinding in small cohorts

---

Box 1
Inconsistency and incongruence

Inconsistency is characterized by variability of motor symptoms over time, selective disability, and alteration by distraction (distractibility), expectations, or illness beliefs. A careful clinical observation over long periods of time and during the performance of multiple tasks may be necessary to detect signs of distractibility, variability, and selectivity of motor symptoms.

- *Variability* refers to changes in movement pattern (eg, phenotype, frequency, body location) or severity over time.
- *Selectivity of impairment* refers to a mismatch between the objectively observed impairment in a function during different tasks (eg, severely paralyzed leg during strength and voluntary movement assessments vs preserved ability to walk).
- *Distractibility* refers to significant improvement of the abnormal motor function when the patient is volitionally performing a competitive task. Regardless of motor phenotype, competitive complex tasks, either motor or cognitive (eg, using mental arithmetical) can be used to divert attention away from the affected body part. Conversely, when the attention is focused on the affected body part, the symptoms usually become more prominent. Besides *suppression or disappearance* of functional motor symptoms during correct task performance, a *poor task performance* with persisting abnormal movements is also suggestive of functional etiology. In some cases, the abnormal movement may persist even with the attention diverted away (eg, in cases of non-distractible functional tremor or dystonia).
- *Changes in motor symptoms due to expectations or illness beliefs* can be elicited using suggestion and non-physiological maneuvers (eg, triggering motor symptoms by application of a vibrating tuning fork to the limb, or inducing myoclonic jerk when the tendon hammer is stopped just short of the tendon).

Incongruence involves a combination of symptoms and signs that are not seen in other neurologic disorders; the pattern itself is incompatible with anatomic and physiologic principles. FMD often presents with bizarre, mixed movements, difficult to classify and precipitated paroxysms. However, to be certain that abnormal movement patterns do not manifest or progress according to the wide phenotypic range of other known movement disorders requires extensive expertise in movement disorder.

Distractibility and suggestibility are signs of both inconsistency and incongruency in most phenotypes.

The exception is tics, which also change over time and are suppressible with complex tasks, and pain associated with weakness, which can also be distractible.

and validation of diagnostic utility in larger cohorts is thus needed for most of the tests, as suggested by the discrepancy between studies documenting prevalence of convergence spasm in FMD (initially reported high prevalence of convergence spasm in FMD [n = 13][17] which was not confirmed in larger cohort of consecutive FMD patients [n = 101][18]). Phenotype-specific tests useful for the diagnosis of FMD are presented in **Table 2** (tests with validation[9,19,20]) and **Table 3** (tests recommended by experts).

Besides signs of inconsistency and incongruence of abnormal movements, the impairment of explicit motor control during the examination is also characteristic for FMD, whereas automatic/spontaneous movements during transfers in the room, getting dressed/undressed, and so forth are normal (see Video 3, Case 1 and Video 6, Case 2). Expressive behavior (also called the huffing and puffing sign) including disproportionate effort, grimacing, vocalizations and crying, heavy breathing, and breath-holding seems to be rather specific to FMD.[19,21]

When both inconsistency and incongruence signs are present, the diagnosis of clinically definite FMD can be made in the absence of an additional psychiatric disturbance or multiple somatizations, which were required for the same level of diagnostic certainty in the original Fahn and Williams criteria.[5,22] Similarly, the diagnosis of functional neurological symptom disorder according to the DSM-5 criteria no longer requires the identification of an associated psychological stressor.[12] Importantly, the presence of psychiatric comorbidities, psychological factors (ie, adverse life experiences, mental health conditions), involvement in litigation, or a potential secondary gain should not bias the diagnostic process as these can also be present in other neurologic diseases.[23,24]

Features of inconsistency and incongruence can also be found in the history. These features are not diagnostic of FMD, but they can be helpful clues in the diagnostic process.[5] Patients often describe sudden onset and rapid progression of symptoms, which might be triggered by a physical event/trauma.[25,26] Unlike the slowly progressive course of most neurodegenerative movement disorders, FMD can rapidly progress to severe symptoms. Phenomenology may change over time, one phenotype may change into another or new manifestations may be acquired. Patients also may report marked variability in symptom severity often associated with fatigue and pain in day-to-day life or complete remissions and sudden recurrences.[26] A mismatch between observed impairment and the self-reported limitations during activities of daily living can also be regarded as inconsistency. Response to placebo or suggestion has become part of the diagnostic criteria for a documented FMD.[5,22] However, a recent study did not find stronger placebo responses in patients with FMD compared with healthy controls. It has been argued that occasional dramatic placebo responses may occur because functional neurologic symptoms are inherently more modifiable than those due to structural brain disease.[27]

FUNCTIONAL MOVEMENT DISORDER PHENOTYPES

The clinical presentation of FMD is very heterogeneous. FMD may present with any type of abnormal movement, often with mixed manifestations combining movements of different types and functional weakness. Mixed FMD (23.1%), tremor (21.6%), and weakness (18.1%) were the most common phenotypes in a recent meta-analysis including a large population of FMD patients (n = 4905).[15] Increased startle or startle-like movements and precipitated paroxysmal movements are frequent in patients with FMD.[5]

Table 2
Validated bedside tests and reliable positive signs informing the diagnosis of a functional movement disorder

	Tests/Signs	Other Motor Disorders	Functional Movement Disorder
Tremor	*Entrainment test* Tapping with the less affected limb at different frequencies (1, 3, 5 Hz)	No changes in tremor frequency and amplitude	Tremor suppression Shift in tremor frequency/pure entrainment—tremor frequency changes/matches tapping frequency Inaccurate tapping
	Weight load 0.5–1 kg weight load attached to the affected limb	Decrease in tremor amplitude	Increase in amplitude, shift in frequency
	Ballistic movements with the less affected limb	No pause/interruption in the tremor	Pause in the tremor
Weakness	*Muscle strength examination*	Consistent weakness, compatible with recognized neurologic conditions	Give-way weakness: sudden loss of resistance after initial good strength Co-contraction (no movement at the joint due to co-contraction of the agonist and antagonist muscles)
	Pronator drift sign in upper limb weakness	Present	Absent, but may see drift without pronation
	Hoover's sign in proximal/hip extension weakness. (The effect of contralateral hip flexion on hip extensors weakness in the affected limb)	Negative Hoover's sign (false positive in pain, cortical neglect, and parietal lesion)	Positive Hoover's sign: improvement in hip extensor strength during voluntary hip flexion in the contralateral less affected leg
	Spinal injuries center test in paraplegia: knees are passively lifted by the examiner, sole of feet touching the bed	Negative: the leg falls back on the bed	Positive: the weaker leg remains in this position

	Sternocleidomastoideus sign assessment of head rotation strength in patients with hemiparesis	Negative: asymmetric weakness of head rotation when turning away from the affected arm and leg	Positive: asymmetric weakness of head rotation when turning toward the affected arm and leg
	Hip abductor sign in unilateral leg weakness	Negative: no changes in leg abduction when asked to abduct both legs against resistance	Positive: improvement in the weaker leg abduction strength when asked to abduct both legs against resistance
Gait Disorder	*Monoplegic leg dragging*	Absent	Present: the weaker leg is externally rotated and dragged
Postural Instability	*Romberg test*	Positive in sensory ataxia. Negative in central ataxia.	Distractible abnormal performance: excessive truncal sways without falling that improves with competitive tasks (eg, graphesthesia)
	Shoulder-touch/tap test applicable in the presence of a positive pull test: shoulders are tapped with downwards but no backwards force applied	No abnormal postural response	Exaggerated postural response: taking ≥3 steps to recover or falling if not caught by the examiner

Note: Presented tests/signs have been validated in at least two clinical and/or neurophysiological studies except for hip abductor sign and postural instability tests which have been validated in a single study.
Data from Refs[8,18,19].

Table 3
Expert recommendations/non-validated bedside tests and positive signs

	Tests/Signs	Other Motor Disorders	Functional Movement Disorder
Gait Disorder	Straight walking + performing a dual task	May cause slower speed	Abnormal gait pattern is suppressed or significantly improved with distraction (eg, base narrowing in unstable gait, disappearance of abnormal posturing in dystonia, normal activation of weak muscles)
	Running	Consistent presentation, improvement of gait pattern and limb posturing in foot dystonia or distal paresis	Significant variability when performing these tasks or inability to perform them
	Walking backwards	Consistent presentation, improvement of gait pattern in foot dystonia or distal paresis	
	Weight shifting from side to side, skating	Consistent presentation	
	Tandem gait	Inability to perform tandem gait without side steps in	
Dystonia	Evaluation of abnormal limb posturing during different tasks	Mobile dystonia movements/postures are typically initiated or worsened by voluntary action and are associated with overflow of muscular activity. Sensory trick can be present.	Fixed/paroxysmal dystonia Abnormal posturing with typical patterns (often associated with pain) Hand dystonia: wrist/3–5 fingers flexion sparing 1–2 fingers (pincer function) Foot dystonia: foot plantar flexion and inversion Cranial dystonia: unilateral tonic lip and/or jaw deviation, ipsilateral platysma involvement. Cervical dystonia: fixed laterocollis, ipsilateral shoulder elevation, contralateral shoulder depression
	Evaluation of muscle tone	Increased muscle tone Owing to coactivation of agonist-antagonist muscles (less applicable to hand dystonia)	Resistance against passive movement Can be distractible with competitive tasks

Myoclonus	*Entrainment test in frequent rhythmic myoclonic jerks (see tremor)*	No changes in frequency or amplitude	Myoclonus suppression Entrainment Inaccurate tapping/task performance
	Stimulus-sensitive myoclonus assessment stopping the hammer without touching the tendon	Myoclonus does not occur	Stimulus-sensitive myoclonus can be triggered
	Repetitive stimuli	No habituation of stimulus-sensitive myoclonus	Habituation of stimulus-sensitive myoclonus
Parkinsonism	*Bradykinesia*	Decrement in speed and amplitude during repetitive movements	Excessive slowness without decremental amplitude
	Muscle tone	Rigidity	Paratonia: variable resistance against passive movement without cogwheel rigidity
	Evaluation of tremor	Non-distractible, non-variable resting/re-emergent tremor	See functional tremor
	Pull test	Small balance correcting steps (>2 abnormal); in moderate/severe cases absence of postural response	Excessive postural response truncal sway without falling or falling passively backwards in the presence of an otherwise good balance performance

Functional Weakness

Functional weakness is characterized by variability in severity over time and discordant performance in different tasks during a single examination session (Video 1).[28,29] Functional weakness often presents with a non-pyramidal distribution and/or as collapsing or give-way weakness.[19] Commonly used rule-in signs for functional leg weakness include Hoover's sign and hip abductor sign.

Functional Tremor

Functional tremor is characterized by variability of frequency, characteristic response to externally cued rhythmic movements (entrain to the cued frequency), and distractibility (Video 2). These are the key features that distinguish functional tremor from tremor associated with other movement disorders, which presents with a stable frequency, and is not distractible by competitive motor or cognitive tasks.[30,31]

Functional Dystonia

Although dystonia as a manifestation of other neurologic disorders is typically mobile and tends to be action-induced, patients with functional dystonia typically present with fixed abnormal postures (Video 3).[32] Functional dystonia is often less distractible than other abnormal functional movements. There is no specific diagnostic test for functional dystonia. Functional dystonia is commonly accompanied by severe pain, and there is an overlap with complex regional pain syndrome type 1.[33,34] Recent work showed that a combination of sudden onset, fixed dystonia, and acute peripheral trauma is highly sensitive and specific for functional dystonia.[35]

Functional Myoclonus/Jerks

Myoclonus should be a simple, sudden, and brief involuntary movement. Functional myoclonus is usually variable in duration and distribution of jerks, often with multiple components over time.[36] Functional myoclonus may be distractible and it may also entrain to externally cued rhythmic movements (Video 4).[37] Functional stimulus-sensitive reflex myoclonus is characterized by latencies that are variable and similar to voluntary reaction time.[36] Palatal myoclonus and the so-called propriospinal myoclonus—characterized by repetitive, usually arrhythmic fixed pattern flexion movements of the trunk, hips, and knees—are often of functional neurological origin (see Video 7).[38,39]

Functional Gait and Postural Instability

Most functional gait disorders look bizarre and incongruent with other known gait disorders.[40] Balance during examination is often better than subjective report, and compensatory strategies sometimes tend to be counterproductive. Several gait patterns have been identified as common and typical for a functional neurological etiology.[21] These include dragging of a leg behind the body, excessive slowness with an exaggerated delay in gait initiation, walking on ice pattern with decreased stride length and height along with stiff knees and ankles, gait with uneconomic postures, gait with sudden knee buckling, robotic, tremulous, or unsteady gait characterized by crossed legs and sudden side steps (Video 5).[19] However, relying on the phenotype exclusively is problematic, and for a clinically established diagnosis, multiple tests including straight walking, performing a dual-task, running or walking backwards, and/or walking with eyes closed are usually needed to identify improvement or marked change in gait pattern (ie, positive signs of distractibility/inconsistency and incongruence) (Video 6).[40]

Other Phenotypes

Functional facial and eye movement abnormalities are a common presentation of FMD.[18,41] Functional tic-like movements can manifest either alone or in overlap with tic disorder. Given their similarities such as action monitoring and attentional allocation, the diagnosis is often challenging (Video 7).[42,43] In contrast to a primary tic disorder, functional tic-like movements and behaviors are characterized by female prevalence, a short period of time to have a peak of severity in the majority of patients, a very high frequency of complex movements and vocalizations, and a lack of response to tic-suppressing medications.[44] Although a minority of patients who are adolescents and young adults seem to have a preexisting primary tic disorder, exposure to tic-related social media content was recently found in almost 60%, suggesting an important role of social modeling. In addition to tics, other types of paroxysmal functional movements can be seen and can be similarly challenging to diagnose.[45]

Comorbid Conditions

Psychiatric comorbidities such as mood and anxiety disorders, post-traumatic stress disorder, personality disorders, and dissociation are commonly reported in patients with FMD.[11,46,47] However, a high frequency of psychiatric comorbidities is also found in other neurologic disorders.[23]

FND and other medical/neurologic conditions are often coexistent. Functional neurologic symptoms are present in up to 12% of other neurologic disorders across neurologic subspecialties.[48] Recent studies reported frequent functional neurologic symptoms in Parkinson disease (including the prodromal phase) and multiple sclerosis may also be associated with functional neurologic symptoms.[49,50] Non-motor symptoms could also result from other treatable neurologic disorders, such as restless legs syndrome, periodic limb movement syndrome, and obstructive sleep apnea, which should be recognized and treated.[51]

ELECTROPHYSIOLOGY

Electrophysiological studies can identify features of FMD that can be useful for the diagnosis, specifically in tremor and myoclonus that are not possible to obtain from the physical examination in diagnostically challenging cases.[52] Electrophysiological recordings of electromyographic activity and movement using accelerometers can demonstrate inconsistency in parameters that are difficult to assess by the naked eye, such as latencies, variability, and change in frequency. Electrophysiology can also document incongruencies, that is, the clinically unobservable phenomena that are present in FMD but not in other neurologic disorders such as the premotor potential, also called the bereitschaftspotential, which precedes functional movements and can be obtained using the electroencephalography back-averaging technique.[52] The fact that the electrophysiological characterization of tremor and myoclonus can provide valuable information has been reflected in the revised diagnostic criteria for FMD with a new category of laboratory, that is, electrophysiologically supported definite FMD.[5]

Typical electrophysiological findings in tremor and myoclonus of functional neurologic and other origins are summarized in **Tables 4** and **5**. Functional tremor is highly variable in its presentation. Several studies have shown that one single electrophysiological test alone (including the entrainment test or ballistic task) does not reach a satisfactory combination of sensitivity and specificity,[20,53,54] whereas a battery of electrophysiological tests provided excellent diagnostic accuracy in distinguishing functional and other forms of tremor.[20] Functional myoclonus is electrophysiologically

Table 4
Electrophysiological assessment of tremor

Test	Variable Assessed	Other Neurologic Tremor	Functional Tremor
Assessment of rest, posture, or action tremor	Frequency	Characteristic, minimal variability	High variability
	Amplitude	Low variability	High variability
	Coactivation antagonists	No	A tonic discharge of antagonist muscles 300 ms before the tremor onset
	Coherence between affected limbs	No coherence (except for orthostatic tremor)	Significant coherence
Weight loading 0.5–1 kg	Amplitude	Decrease	Increase
Contralateral competitive motor task effect on tremor	Tapping/rhythmic movements 1, 3, and 5 Hz	No interference	1. Entrainment 2. Shift in frequency 3. Tremor suppression
	Ballistic movement	No interference	Tremor interruption

Table 5
Electrophysiological assessment of myoclonus

Test	Variable Assessed	Epileptic Myoclonus	Non-Epileptic Myoclonus	Functional Myoclonus
Poly-EMG	EMG burst length	30–50 ms	>50 ms	>100 ms
	Antagonist muscle relationship	Synchronous	Variable	Variable
	EMG pattern	Stereotyped/low temporal variability	Stereotyped/low temporal variability	Temporal variability
EEG back-averaging	EEG correlates to the movement	Change in voltage preceding the jerk by 20 ms	None	Bereitschaftspotential: slow negativity preceding the jerk by 1–2 s

Abbreviations: EEG, electroencephalography; EMG, electromyography; Poly-EMG, polymyography.

characterized by longer burst duration, variation in muscle recruitment order, variation in burst duration and/or amplitude, and stimulus sensitive and startle-like jerks' onset latencies generally greater than 100 ms in electromyography recordings. Premovement potential on the back-averaging is present in 47% to 86% of patients with FMD. Recently published data on combining premovement potential with event-related desynchronization demonstrated excellent diagnostic accuracy (sensitivity 80%, specificity 100%).[20,52] Despite these developments, the evidence for diagnostic accuracy of available neurophysiological tests in differentiating between different movement disorders is limited for most of the electrophysiological features of myoclonus including synchronicity and regularity of burst pattern recordings, burst duration, and recruitment pattern.[20]

Treatment

FMD management is a process that begins with a comprehensive appraisal of the whole set of motor, non-motor, and comorbid manifestations, so that, where possible, an integrated multidisciplinary approach can be started.[55] The crucial step of management is providing a positive diagnosis, when the neurologist is called to correctly explain the condition, demonstrate positive signs on examination, and convey the perspective of potential recovery. There are several elements in the assessment of various aspects of FMD (**Box 2**) and approaches to communicating the diagnosis (**Box 3**) that can be therapeutic [55]; however, education is generally not considered a definitive treatment when used in isolation.[56]

Given the high complexity of FMD, a biopsychosocial-informed triage of patients into dedicated treatment services depending on their symptoms and comorbidities is essential for a patient-centered treatment plan. Once again, the neurologist or neuropsychiatrist should lay the foundation of the process, ideally relying on the potential collaboration of psychiatrists, other mental health professionals, speech and language therapists, physiotherapists, and occupational therapists.

Physical rehabilitation is the mainstay of FMD treatment. Specialized physiotherapy has been shown to improve motor aspects of the disease, quality of life, along with physical and social functioning in two randomized controlled trials (RCTs)[57,58] and several observational and cohort studies. How to better deliver rehabilitation (inpatient or outpatient setting) and the choice of optimal candidates is not well established. A protocol of 5-days of outpatient rehabilitation showed good outcomes in up to 70% of patients and a moderate-to-large size effect with sustained benefit up to 6-months follow-up,[57,58] excluding patients with severe pain, fatigue, and psychiatric illnesses. New evidence of the effect of physiotherapy followed by a self-management plan or

---

Box 2
Assessment as treatment in functional movement disorder

- Asking about *the whole range of symptoms* (motor, sensory, cognitive symptoms, pain, fatigue, psychological)

- Asking about symptom *fluctuations*

- Asking about *dissociation and panic*

- *Asking about beliefs and expectations* regarding the condition and potential for improvement

- *Avoiding overemphasis on the role of psychological stressors* at first encounter, although a biopsychosocial-informed interview can be helpful in developing a patient-centered treatment plan

---

Box 3
Delivery of the diagnosis and explanation

- *Naming the condition (delivering positive diagnosis)* is a crucial first step.

- *Favoring the explanation of how* (mechanisms of FMD, ie, malfunctioning of brain network communication) instead of why (etiology is complex and heterogeneous) avoids unnecessary overemphasis on psychological stressors as causative factors.

- *Using analogies*, such as a "hardware vs software" problem, makes communication more effective.

- *Demonstration of positive signs* (eg, Hoover's sign, distractibility of tremor) and explanation of the impact of abnormal attention helps patients understand that FMD is genuine, common, and a potentially reversible disorder.

- *Providing additional explanation and education* (for patients and their relatives, eg, www. neurosymptoms.org) can improve acceptance of diagnosis and readiness for treatment.

12-week telemedicine on physical fatigue has recently emerged, although needs to be confirmed in further studies.[59,60]

Consensus recommendations based on the evidence and expert opinion provide a description of the general approach and specific strategies for different motor phenotypes.[61] The general approach reported in **Box 4** consists of education with the demonstration that normal movement can occur and an explanation of the impact of abnormal attention, movement retraining, and self-management strategies. Movement retraining consists in building up the components of the movement using automatic symptom-free movements reemerging with diverted attention. Another key component is changing maladaptive behaviors related to symptoms. Occupational therapy (OT) is an integral part of multidisciplinary rehabilitation for physical and mental health problems in patients with FMD. Recently, recommendations for OT in FND have been published, identifying core OT interventions in a biopsychosocial-informed practical rehabilitation of symptoms supporting patients' independence and self-management strategies.[62,63]

Box 4
General principles of specialized physiotherapy for functional movement disorder

- *Education:* to reinforce information about the condition and the full range of symptoms, introducing the role of physiotherapy to regain motor control.

- *Exploration of unhelpful thoughts and behaviors:* to prevent patients' expectations of abnormal movements to further influence motor output.

- *Exploration of how symptoms affect movement and posture as well as demonstration of positive signs:* to engage patients in diagnosis and treatment and encourage them to regain normal movements.

- *Retraining movements using strategies for attention redirection:* to minimize self-focused attention while increasing external focus, fostering automatically generated movements. (This can be achieved through distractive maneuvers during meaningful tasks: eg, arithmetical exercises, finger tapping, or hand pronation-supination while walking.)

- *Avoidance of walking aids, splints, and orthoses*: to prevent interference from adaptive behaviors.

- *Encourage and set self-management plan:* to improve mobility, endurance, and function in daily life, reducing symptom relapses.

Psychological interventions, traditionally considered the only treatment of choice for FND, are still often recommended to patients with FND, with more robust evidence for cognitive behavioral therapy (CBT), and some evidence for psychodynamic approaches.[64] Psychological therapy for FND is centered on exploring relationships between physical symptoms and linking thoughts, emotions, and behaviors. Moreover, another critical point is the identification of predisposing, precipitating, and perpetuating factors.[65] In a mixed cohort of patients with FND, self-guided CBT plus usual care showed a subjective improvement at 3 months versus usual care alone, also improving anxiety and somatic symptom burden.[66] Patients' selection characteristics to guide treatment modality remains to be determined, but a key factor for achieving a positive outcome seems to be acceptance of the impact of psychological factors on symptoms.[64]

Evidence from RCTs has suggested the efficacy of emerging techniques such as *neuromodulation* (eg, transcranial magnetic stimulation [TMS])[67] and *hypnosis*.[68] However, single-pulse TMS paradigms used in several studies were unlikely to cause neuromodulatory changes in the brain; rather, a cognitive behavioral effect can be assumed.[69] Reliable evidence is still lacking for a clear neuroanatomical target from imaging studies, such as the left dorsolateral prefrontal cortex targeted by TMS in depression.[70] RCTs examining *chemodenervation with botulinum neurotoxin injection* in FMD have not provided evidence for its efficacy in chronic jerky and tremulous FMD,[71] or functional dystonia,[71,72] compared with placebo. Other techniques that require further validation are *therapeutic sedation*[73] and approaches using *virtual reality*.[74]

Psychiatric comorbidity should be screened for, including a careful assessment of current and past depression, anxiety, trauma-related symptoms, self-injurious behaviors, or mental health treatment, and referral to a specialist should be made in selected cases.[75] In addition, taking a detailed social history can help identify perpetuating factors (eg, unstable housing, major financial difficulties), that if concurrently addressed can help improve clinical outcomes.

Despite new treatment options for FMD, cases of refractory symptoms are well-known, and long disease duration before diagnosis remains one of the most important poor prognostic indicators.[11] Good motivation to be engaged in treatment and reasonable expectations for treatment are the key features for a better outcome.

SUMMARY

FMD is often persistent and associated with significant disability and health care resource consumption. Neurologists often report finding interactions with such patients challenging, and specific services that can help with treatment are poorly developed, commonly falling between neurology and psychiatry services. An early diagnosis, with subsequent treatment involving rehabilitative and/or psychological treatments, can promote recovery. However, there are no consensus diagnostic and multidisciplinary treatment guidelines. Most of the diagnostic tests have been studied in small samples without proper validation.[9,19,21] Similarly, support from evidence-based medicine regarding FMD-specific treatments is still limited, and there is a lack of predictors of specific treatment outcomes and prognosis.[9] Medical professionals must still rely on expert recommendations and clinical experience. As research expands, subsequent adequate education of professionals across disciplines and the development of health care facilities are critical steps toward the improvement of the patients' outcomes through an early and correct diagnosis and disease-specific, evidence-based multidisciplinary management of FMD.

CLINICS CARE POINTS

- Functional movement disorder (FMD) is a genuine disorder. Symptoms are involuntary. Feigning is rare in clinical settings.

- Motor manifestations of FMD include abnormal movements (eg, tremor, dystonia, and myoclonus) or weakness that can be significantly altered by distraction, beliefs, and expectations.

- FMD is a rule-in clinical diagnosis based on the positive findings of internal inconsistency and incongruence/incompatibility with other neurologic conditions, which can be demonstrated using general maneuvers (demonstration of distractibility using a competitive motor or cognitive task) or phenotype-specific bed side tests (eg, Hoover's sign for weakness or entrainment test for tremor).

- Clinical tests for FMD diagnosis have a high specificity but may have low sensitivity, and multiple tests might be needed for a reliable demonstration of inconsistency and incongruence. In some cases, a battery of neurophysiological tests can corroborate the diagnosis (for tremor and myoclonus).

- People with FMD have a high prevalence of non-motor physical symptoms (eg, pain and fatigue) and psychological symptoms (eg, depression and anxiety).

- Unnecessary testing should be avoided to prevent iatrogenic harm because a better prognosis has been related to early diagnosis.

- It is beneficial to show the patients' positive signs of FMD, explain the effect of distraction during the clinical examination, and adequately communicate the diagnosis.

- Treatment should be individualized, multimodal, and started by the neurologist or neuropsychiatrist.

- Physiotherapy may be the initial treatment of choice for many patients with motor symptoms. Consensus recommendations for physiotherapy, occupational therapy, and speech and language therapy with phenotype-specific recommendations have been published.

- Psychological therapy for FND may also be helpful and is centered on exploring relationships between physical symptoms, thoughts, emotions, and behaviors, and identifying predisposing, precipitating, and perpetuating factors.

DISCLOSURE

T. Serranová: Grant by the Czech Ministry of Health Project AZV (NU20–04–0332) Charles University programme Cooperatio, the project National Institute for Neurologic Research (Programme EXCELES, ID Project No. LX22NPO5107)—Funded by the European Union—Next Generation EU.

SUPPLEMENTARY DATA

Supplementary data related to this article can be found online at https://doi.org/10.1016/j.ncl.2023.02.002.

REFERENCES

1. Stone J, Carson A, Duncan R, et al. Who is referred to neurology clinics?–the diagnoses made in 3781 new patients. Clin Neurol Neurosurg 2010;112(9):747–51.
2. Carson AS J, Sharpe M. Epidemiology and clinical impact of psychogenic movement disorders. In: Hallett M, Lang AE, Jankovic J, et al, editors. Psychogenic

Movement Disorders and Other Conversion Disorders. Cambridge: Cambridge University Press; 2011. p. 20–9.

3. Gargalas S, Weeks R, Khan-Bourne N, et al. Incidence and outcome of functional stroke mimics admitted to a hyperacute stroke unit. J Neurol Neurosurg Psychiatr 2017;88(1):2–6.

4. Gendre T, Carle G, Mesrati F, et al. Quality of life and psychiatric comorbidities comparisons in patients with functional (psychogenic) and organic movement disorders. Mov Disord 2018;33:S475.

5. Gupta A, Lang AE. Psychogenic movement disorders. Curr Opin Neurol 2009; 22(4):430–6.

6. Edwards MJ, Adams RA, Brown H, et al. A Bayesian account of 'hysteria'. Brain 2012;135(Pt 11):3495–512.

7. Erro R, Brigo F, Trinka E, et al. Psychogenic nonepileptic seizures and movement disorders: a comparative review. Neurol Clin Pract 2016;6(2):138–49.

8. Vechetova G, Slovak M, Kemlink D, et al. The impact of non-motor symptoms on the health-related quality of life in patients with functional movement disorders. J Psychosom Res 2018;115:32–7.

9. Aybek S, Perez DL. Diagnosis and management of functional neurological disorder. BMJ 2022;376:o64.

10. LaFaver K, Lang AE, Stone J, et al. Opinions and clinical practices related to diagnosing and managing functional (psychogenic) movement disorders: changes in the last decade. Eur J Neurol 2020;27(6):975–84.

11. Gelauff J, Stone J, Edwards M, et al. The prognosis of functional (psychogenic) motor symptoms: a systematic review. J Neurol Neurosurg Psychiatry 2014;85(2): 220–6.

12. American Psychiatric Association. Diagnostic and Statistical Manual of Mental Disorders. 5th Edition. Arlington, VA: American Psychiatric Association; 2013.

13. World Health Organization. International statistical classification of diseases and related health problems (11th Edition.), 2019. Available at: https://icd.who.int/.

14. Maggio J, Alluri PR, Paredes-Echeverri S, et al. Briquet syndrome revisited: implications for functional neurological disorder. Brain Communications 2020;2(2): fcaa156.

15. Lidstone SC, Costa-Parke M, Robinson EJ, et al. Functional movement disorder gender, age and phenotype study: a systematic review and individual patient meta-analysis of 4905 cases. J Neurol Neurosurg Psychiatry 2022;93(6):609–16.

16. Gasca-Salas C, Lang AE. Neurologic diagnostic criteria for functional neurologic disorders. Handb Clin Neurol 2016;139:193–212.

17. Fekete R, Baizabal-Carvallo JF, Ha AD, et al. Convergence spasm in conversion disorders: prevalence in psychogenic and other movement disorders compared with controls. J Neurol Neurosurg Psychiatry 2012;83(2):202–4.

18. Teodoro T, Cunha JM, Abreu LF, et al. Abnormal Eye and Cranial Movements Triggered by Examination in People with Functional Neurological Disorder. Neuro Ophthalmol 2019;43(4):240–3.

19. Daum C, Gheorghita F, Spatola M, et al. Interobserver agreement and validity of bedside 'positive signs' for functional weakness, sensory and gait disorders in conversion disorder: a pilot study. J Neurol Neurosurg Psychiatry 2015;86(4): 425–30.

20. van der Veen S, Klamer MR, Elting JWJ, et al. The diagnostic value of clinical neurophysiology in hyperkinetic movement disorders: A systematic review. Park Relat Disord 2021;89:176–85.

21. Daum C, Hubschmid M, Aybek S. The value of 'positive' clinical signs for weakness, sensory and gait disorders in conversion disorder: a systematic and narrative review. J Neurol Neurosurg Psychiatry 2014;85(2):180–90.
22. Fahn S, Williams DT. Psychogenic dystonia. Adv Neurol 1988;50:431–55.
23. Zutt R, Gelauff JM, Smit M, et al. The presence of depression and anxiety do not distinguish between functional jerks and cortical myoclonus. Park Relat Disord 2017;45:90–3.
24. Stone J, Reuber M, Carson A. Functional symptoms in neurology: mimics and chameleons. Practical Neurol 2013;13(2):104–13.
25. Parees I, Kojovic M, Pires C, et al. Physical precipitating factors in functional movement disorders. J Neurol Sci 2014;338(1–2):174–7.
26. Lagrand T, Tuitert I, Klamer M, et al. Functional or not functional; that's the question: can we predict the diagnosis functional movement disorder based on associated features? Eur J Neurol 2021;28(1):33–9.
27. Huys ACML, Beck B, Haggard P, et al. No increased suggestibility to placebo in functional neurological disorder. Eur J Neurol 2021;28(7):2367–71.
28. Stone J, Aybek S. Functional limb weakness and paralysis. Handb Clin Neurol 2016;139:213–28.
29. Stone J, Warlow C, Sharpe M. The symptom of functional weakness: a controlled study of 107 patients. Brain 2010;133(Pt 5):1537–51.
30. Schwingenschuh P, Espay AJ. Functional tremor. J Neurol Sci 2022;435:120208.
31. Deuschl G, Bain P, Brin M. Consensus statement of the Movement Disorder Society on Tremor. Ad Hoc Scientific Committee. Mov Disord 1998;13(Suppl 3):2–23.
32. Schrag A, Trimble M, Quinn N, et al. The syndrome of fixed dystonia: an evaluation of 103 patients. Brain 2004;127(Pt 10):2360–72.
33. Popkirov S, Hoeritzauer I, Colvin L, et al. Complex regional pain syndrome and functional neurological disorders: time for reconciliation. J Neurol Neurosurg Psychiatry 2019;90(5):608–14.
34. Frucht L, Perez DL, Callahan J, et al. Functional Dystonia: Differentiation From Primary Dystonia and Multidisciplinary Treatments. Front Neurol 2020;11:605262.
35. Ercoli T, Defazio G, Geroin C, et al. Sudden Onset, Fixed Dystonia and Acute Peripheral Trauma as Diagnostic Clues for Functional Dystonia. Mov Disord Clin Pract 2021;8(7):1107–11.
36. Hallett M. Functional (psychogenic) movement disorders - Clinical presentations. Park Relat Disord 2016;22(Suppl 1):S149–52.
37. Dreissen YEM, Cath DC, Tijssen MAJ. Functional jerks, tics, and paroxysmal movement disorders. Handb Clin Neurol 2016;139:247–58.
38. van der Salm SM, Erro R, Cordivari C, et al. Propriospinal myoclonus: clinical reappraisal and review of literature. Neurology 2014;83(20):1862–70.
39. Stamelou M, Saifee TA, Edwards MJ, et al. Psychogenic palatal tremor may be underrecognized: reappraisal of a large series of cases. Mov Disord 2012;27(9):1164–8.
40. Nonnekes J, Ruzicka E, Serranova T, et al. Functional gait disorders: A sign-based approach. Neurology 2020;94(24):1093–9.
41. Kaski D, Bronstein AM, Edwards MJ, et al. Cranial functional (psychogenic) movement disorders. Lancet Neurol 2015;14(12):1196–205.
42. Demartini B, Ricciardi L, Parees I, et al. A positive diagnosis of functional (psychogenic) tics. Eur J Neurol 2015;22(3):527–e536.
43. Ganos C, Martino D, Espay AJ, et al. Tics and functional tic-like movements: Can we tell them apart? Neurology 2019;93(17):750–8.

44. Martino D, Hedderly T, Murphy T, et al. The spectrum of functional tic-like behaviours: Data from an international registry. Eur J Neurol 2023;30:334–43.

45. Erro R, Bhatia KP. Unravelling of the paroxysmal dyskinesias. J Neurol Neurosurg Psychiatry 2019;90(2):227–34.

46. Feinstein A, Stergiopoulos V, Fine J, et al. Psychiatric outcome in patients with a psychogenic movement disorder: a prospective study. Neuropsychiatry Neuropsychol Behav Neurol 2001;14(3):169–76.

47. Perez DL, Aybek S, Popkirov S, et al. A Review and Expert Opinion on the Neuropsychiatric Assessment of Motor Functional Neurological Disorders. J Neuropsychiatry Clin Neurosci 2021;33(1):14–26.

48. Stone J, Carson A, Duncan R, et al. Which neurological diseases are most likely to be associated with "symptoms unexplained by organic disease". J Neurol 2012;259(1):33–8.

49. Walzl D, Solomon AJ, Stone J. Functional neurological disorder and multiple sclerosis: a systematic review of misdiagnosis and clinical overlap. J Neurol 2022; 269(2):654–63.

50. Onofrj M, Russo M, Carrarini C, et al. Functional neurological disorder and somatic symptom disorder in Parkinson's disease. J Neurol Sci 2022;433:120017.

51. Serranova T, Slovak M, Kemlink D, et al. Prevalence of restless legs syndrome in functional movement disorders: a case-control study from the Czech Republic. BMJ Open 2019;9(1):e024236.

52. Hallett M. Physiology of psychogenic movement disorders. J Clin Neurosci 2010; 17(8):959–65.

53. Schwingenschuh P, Saifee TA, Katschnig-Winter P, et al. Validation of "laboratory-supported" criteria for functional tremor. Mov Disord 2014;29:S423–4.

54. van der Stouwe AM, Elting JW, van der Hoeven JH, et al. How typical are 'typical' tremor characteristics? Sensitivity and specificity of five tremor phenomena. Park Relat Disord 2016;30:23–8.

55. Stone J. Functional neurological disorders: the neurological assessment as treatment. Practical Neurol 2016;16(1):7–17.

56. Gelauff JM, Rosmalen JGM, Carson A, et al. Internet-based self-help randomized trial for motor functional neurologic disorder (SHIFT). Neurology 2020;95(13): E1883–96.

57. Jordbru AA, Smedstad LM, Klungsoyr O, et al. Psychogenic gait disorder: A randomized controlled trial of physical rehabilitation with one-year follow-up. J Rehabil Med 2014;46:181–7.

58. Nielsen G, Buszewicz M, Stevenson F, et al. Randomised feasibility study of physiotherapy for patients with functional motor symptoms. J Neurol Neurosurg Psychiatry 2017;88(6):484–90.

59. Gandolfi M, Riello M, Bellamoli V, et al. Motor and non-motor outcomes after a rehabilitation program for patients with Functional Motor Disorders: A prospective, observational cohort study. NeuroRehabilitation 2021;48(3):305–14.

60. Gandolfi M, Sandri A, Geroin C, et al. Improvement in motor symptoms, physical fatigue, and self-rated change perception in functional motor disorders: a prospective cohort study of a 12-week telemedicine program. J Neurol 2022;269: 5940–53.

61. Nielsen G, Stone J, Matthews A, et al. Physiotherapy for functional motor disorders: a consensus recommendation. J Neurol Neurosurg Psychiatry 2015; 86(10):1113–9.

62. Nicholson C, Edwards MJ, Carson AJ, et al. Occupational therapy consensus recommendations for functional neurological disorder. J Neurol Neurosurg Psychiatry 2020;91(10):1037–45.

63. Baker J, Barnett C, Cavalli L, et al. Management of functional communication, swallowing, cough and related disorders: consensus recommendations for speech and language therapy. J Neurol Neurosur Psychiatr 2021;92(10):1112–25.

64. Gutkin M, McLean L, Brown R, et al. Systematic review of psychotherapy for adults with functional neurological disorder. J Neurol Neurosurg Psychiatry 2021;92:36–44.

65. Godena EJ, Perez DL, Crain LD, et al. Psychotherapy for Functional Neurological (Conversion) Disorder: A Case Bridging Mind, Brain, and Body. J Clin Psychiatry 2021;82(6):45–52.

66. Sharpe M, Walker J, Williams C, et al. Guided self-help for functional (psychogenic) symptoms: a randomized controlled efficacy trial. Neurology 2011;77(6):564–72.

67. Oriuwa C, Mollica A, Feinstein A, et al. Neuromodulation for the treatment of functional neurological disorder and somatic symptom disorder: a systematic review. J Neurol Neurosurg Psychiatry 2022;93(3):280–90.

68. Moene FC, Spinhoven P, Hoogduin KA, et al. A randomized controlled clinical trial of a hypnosis-based treatment for patients with conversion disorder, motor type. Int J Clin Exp Hypn 2003;51(1):29–50.

69. Garcin B, Mesrati F, Hubsch C, et al. Impact of Transcranial Magnetic Stimulation on Functional Movement Disorders: Cortical Modulation or a Behavioral Effect? Front Neurol 2017;8:338.

70. Lefaucheur JP, Aleman A, Baeken C, et al. Evidence-based guidelines on the therapeutic use of repetitive transcranial magnetic stimulation (rTMS): An update (2014-2018). Clin Neurophysiol 2020;131(2):474–528.

71. Dreissen YEM, Dijk JM, Gelauff JM, et al. Botulinum neurotoxin treatment in jerky and tremulous functional movement disorders: a double-blind, randomised placebo-controlled trial with an open-label extension. J Neurol Neurosurg Psychiatry 2019;90(11):1244–50.

72. Vizcarra JA, Lopez-Castellanos JR, Dwivedi AK, et al. OnabotulinumtoxinA and cognitive behavioral therapy in functional dystonia: A pilot randomized clinical trial. Park Relat Disord 2019;63:174–8.

73. Stone J, Hoeritzauer I, Brown K, et al. Therapeutic sedation for functional (psychogenic) neurological symptoms. J Psychosom Res 2014;76(2):165–8.

74. Bullock K, Won AS, Bailenson J, et al. Virtual Reality-Delivered Mirror Visual Feedback and Exposure Therapy for FND: A Midpoint Report of a Randomized Controlled Feasibility Study. J Neuropsychiatry Clin Neurosci 2020;32(1):90–4.

75. Saxena A, Godena E, Maggio J, et al. Towards an Outpatient Model of Care for Motor Functional Neurological Disorders: A Neuropsychiatric Perspective. Neuropsychiatr Dis Treat 2020;16:2119–34.

Using Verbally-Reported and Video-Observed Semiology to Identify Functional Seizures

Wesley T. Kerr, MD, PhD

KEYWORDS

- Ictal behavior • Psychogenic nonepileptic seizures (PNES) • Dissociative seizures
- Interview • Eye closure • Asynchronous movements

KEY POINTS

- A high-quality description of seizure semiology is critical to an accurate diagnosis but patients and nonclinical witnesses are untrained observers.
- High-quality videos of the entire body for the entire seizure are extremely valuable. When viewed by seizure specialists, diagnostic accuracy can be high but videos can contribute to falsely high confidence in less expert providers.
- No individual ictal behavior is perfectly diagnostic of epileptic or functional seizures and clinicians should look for the presence of multiple features that support a functional seizure diagnosis. The most reliable positive signs indicating functional seizures include ictal eye closure, ictal weeping, asynchronous limb movements, and hip thrusting. Epileptic seizures tend to be shorter and can include pathognomonic features such as head version, dystonic posturing, and automatisms.

INTRODUCTION

Functional seizures, also known as dissociative or psychogenic nonepileptic seizures (PNES) are involuntary, transient episodes of abnormal behavior, movement, awareness, or sensation that most likely represent brain network dysfunction driven by a range of predisposing and precipitating biopsychosocial factors.[1–3] Through neuroimaging studies, the field is beginning to understand functional seizures as a disorder of functional connectivity, where neuroanatomic circuits are altered to increase a patient's involuntary propensity to experience motor responses or other physical sensations related to changes in emotional cognition, emotional processing, or limbic reactivity, as well as reduced conscious awareness of these emotions and physical sensations.[4] However, this stress-diathesis model is just one of the multiple hypothesized mechanisms for an extremely heterogeneous condition. In contrast, epileptic

Department of Neurology, University of Michigan, 1500 East Medical Center Drive, Ann Arbor, MI 48109, USA
E-mail address: KerrWe@med.UMich.edu

Neurol Clin 41 (2023) 605–617
https://doi.org/10.1016/j.ncl.2023.02.003
0733-8619/23/© 2023 Elsevier Inc. All rights reserved.
neurologic.theclinics.com

seizures are the direct physical manifestation of hypersynchronous and hyperexcitable electrical activity in the brain caused by abnormal brain structure or function of ion channels.[5]

Due to the similarity in patient experience between epileptic and functional seizures, this article uses the noun, "seizure," as the descriptor for both events, whereas others prefer to use the terms spell, event, episode, or attack.[1,2,6] Although colloquial understanding of the word "seizure" implies an epileptic seizure, the official definition of seizure is "being taken by a condition."[6] This official definition is broad and can include seizures provoked by biological stressors (eg, severe head injury, alcohol withdrawal), epilepsy, cerebral hypoperfusion (eg, convulsive syncope), and biopsychosocial stressors (eg, functional seizures). This broad definition reflects the breadth of the differential diagnosis of paroxysmal events that should be considered when a patient has a seizure-like event.

Although the mechanisms causing seizures differ, it remains challenging to accurately differentiate between functional and epileptic seizures. Initially, almost all patients are presumed to have epileptic seizures and more than 80% of patients with functional seizures were prescribed antiseizure medication.[7] The average time to diagnosis of functional seizures was 9 years (median 3 years), during which time patients often have high health-care utilization and disability from uncontrolled seizures.[8–10] In a trial for convulsive status epilepticus, 10% of patients had prolonged functional seizures.[11] These diagnostic inaccuracies reflect that differentiating between epileptic and functional seizures is challenging.

For patients with functional seizures, an early and accurate diagnosis can be life changing. Early diagnosis was associated with improved long-term seizure control and quality of life.[12] Accurate diagnosis can cause immediate reductions in health-care utilization, including reduced emergency visits and reduced medication costs from antiseizure medications.[10] However, accurate diagnosis, education, and treatment does not necessarily lead to seizure freedom. With appropriate treatment, 80% of patients had at least a 50% reduction in seizure frequency but only 15% were seizure-free.[13]

With the goal of decreasing the interval between symptom onset and accurate diagnosis, this review focuses on how descriptions of ictal behavior can be used to accomplish this difficult and important task of identifying functional seizures. Although this article focuses on direct observation of ictal behavior by a nonclinical, clinical, or expert observer, it is important to note that other information can provide critical information to the diagnosis. A limitation of the International League Against Epilepsy criteria for diagnostic certainty of functional seizures is that there is no agreed upon definition of what constitutes a history "suggestive" of functional seizures.[14] In addition to clinical history, epileptiform abnormalities on electroencephalography (EEG) and epilepsy-associated abnormalities on neuroimaging can substantially increase the likelihood of epileptic seizures. However, 15% to 25% of patients with functional seizures had these epilepsy-associated abnormalities without also having comorbid epilepsy.[15,16] Conversely, patients with functional seizures frequently have been exposed to significant biopsychosocial stressors and commonly have numerous other medical problems.[7,17] Although not experienced by all patients, the most prominent biopsychosocial stressor in the literature is childhood sexual trauma. Other stressors include, but are not limited to, physical abuse, medical trauma, family discord, childhood maltreatment, and mild traumatic brain injuries.[17] Although the seizures themselves typically are the focus of a health-care encounter, these other data can be reported more consistently than ictal behavior.[18–20] However, ictal video-EEG monitoring remains the only method to definitively diagnose functional seizures. Due to limited availability and capacity for ictal video-EEG monitoring, clinicians should use all available information to build a clinical impression including conversation analysis, nonclinical witness descriptions, video-recordings, interictal EEG, and MRI.

The focus of a clinical encounter can be to differentiate between functional and epileptic seizures but we also must remember that patients may not fit cleanly into these dualistic categories. Around 10% of patients with functional seizures also have epileptic seizures, which may be difficult to differentiate even within the same patient.[21] Therefore, even in the presence of clear positive signs or symptoms suggesting functional seizures, best practice is to conduct standard neurodiagnostic testing to confirm the diagnosis and rule out concomitant structural dysfunction (eg, EEG and MRI for seizures).

BETWEEN THE WORDS: CONVERSATION ANALYSIS

When asking about the story of a typical seizure, pay attention to the context around the specific descriptions of ictal behavior in addition to the content.[22] This analysis of speech patterns in addition to speech content is called conversation analysis. By the health-care provider asking open-ended questions, the patient is allowed to set the priorities for what should be addressed in the visit. In epilepsy, and likely in functional seizures, addressing comorbidities can have a bigger impact on quality of life than focusing solely on seizure counts.[23] These open-ended questions do not take longer than closed (yes or no) questions and can provide critical information that may differentiate between functional and epileptic seizures.

In response to open-ended questions including "How can I help you today?," patients with functional seizures were less likely to bring up the seizures themselves and were more likely to describe the impact of seizures on the patient, or the environment in which seizures tend to occur.[22] In contrast, patients with epilepsy described seizures as an external force that took control of their bodies. Even if the patient loses awareness during seizures, patients with epilepsy often can recount a detailed description of the course of events. Patients with epileptic seizures also may use more speech that reflects "formulation effort" where pauses, "um," and other nonword expressions are used to reflect the difficulty of the description.[22]

Although most studies of conversation analysis focused on detailed analysis from linguists, one study demonstrated that neurology residents could be trained in detecting these concepts quickly.[24] Jenkins and colleagues developed a checklist to clearly define each of the linguistic features that helped differentiate functional seizures from epilepsy (**Table 1**).[24] Although these differences were statistically significant, these factors had insufficient reliability to be diagnostic without considering other data (area under the receiver operating curve of 84% calculated with 33 patients).

PATIENT AND NONCLINICAL WITNESS DESCRIPTIONS OF SEMIOLOGY

A fundamental aspect of a clinical encounter for seizures is obtaining a description of the seizures themselves from the patient and available witnesses. This section will detail important caveats about verbal or written history, followed by highlighting key descriptions of ictal behavior that can differentiate between functional seizures and other seizure causes.

Often patients are amnestic to the actual seizure; therefore, an accurate description requires a witness. Patients and witnesses are untrained observers and frequently have only been exposed to "seizure" through media and entertainment.[20] Seizures can be frightening, disabling, events where the patient is in crisis. Therefore, witnesses appropriately focus on patient safety as compared with being an objective observer.

Table 1
Conversational features to differentiate functional seizures from epilepsy

Conversational Feature	More Commonly Present in:
Patient volunteers descriptions of seizure semiology	Epilepsy
In response to inquiries, the patient readily provides more detailed descriptions	Epilepsy
The patient provides detailed descriptions of semiology	Epilepsy
Patient focuses more on symptoms of seizures than consequences of seizures or the situations in which they occurred	Epilepsy
Seizure descriptions are characterized by formulation effort	Epilepsy
The interview was challenging for me	Functional Seizures

Adapted from Jenkins, L., et al., Neurologists can identify diagnostic linguistic features during routine seizure clinic interactions: results of a 1-day teaching intervention. Epilepsy Behav, 2016. 64(Pt A): p. 257-261; with permission.

Consequentially, patient and caregiver reports of seizure semiology can be quite unreliable when compared with seizure semiology observed through video-EEG monitoring. These observers can reliably report some broad aspects of seizure but some of the more detailed diagnostic features may be missing or inaccurate. Therefore, although it is valuable to extract important details about ictal behavior verbally, it is inappropriate and unhelpful to forcibly interrogate patients and witnesses about minutiae or implicitly shame them if they are unable to provide definitive or consistent answers. For example, when describing versive movements, observers can be confused between the patient's left and the observer's left. To illustrate the limitations in the accuracy of seizure semiology, a computer-aided diagnostic tool to differentiate functional from epileptic seizures based on ictal behavior alone was not statistically superior to the naïve assumption that all patients had epilepsy.[19,20] In comparison, the Functional Seizures Likelihood Score that combined ictal behavior with other clinical information was able to correctly identify 77% of patients.[18]

Because of these limitations, the most reliable diagnostic features of ictal behavior focus on things that patients and witnesses can readily observe and describe well. Although there are more than 150 potential positive features indicative of functional seizures that have been described in peer-reviewed literature, key features that have been replicated in the largest, high-quality studies and meta-analyses are highlighted below and in **Table 2**.[18,25–27] However, none of these ictal behaviors were diagnostic in isolation.

Ictal eye closure: When eyes were closed during seizures, the seizures were 40-fold more likely to be functional as compared with epileptic.[18,27] However, eye closure was reported in 15% to 20% of patients.[18,20,27] These datasets included both forced eye closure, where increased effort was indicated by contraction of the periorbital facial muscles, as well as more passive eye closure. Other eye movements including eye opening, repetitive blinking, and eye fluttering were less reliable indicators.[19,27] Therefore, when eye closure is a feature of the seizure, the likelihood of functional seizures increases but when eye opening is noted, the likelihood was relatively unchanged.

Ictal weeping: Ictal weeping includes generation of tears or other similar emotional expressions either during or immediately after the seizure. This is differentiated from an "ictal cry," which describes an involuntary primal vocalization during an epileptic seizure.[20] When ictal weeping was reported, the likelihood of functional seizures increased 8-fold but this was only reported in 15% of patients with functional

Table 2 Most reliably verbally reported features of ictal behavior	
Ictal Behavior	**More Commonly Present in:**
Ictal eye closure	Functional seizures
Ictal weeping	Functional seizures
Hip thrusting	Functional seizures
Asynchronous limb movements	Functional seizures
Head version	Epilepsy
Automatisms	Epilepsy
Tonic-clonic movements	Epilepsy
Short seizures (<30 s)	Epilepsy
Long seizures (>5 min)	Functional Seizures

Data from Refs.[18,25–27]

seizures.[27] In comparison, the "ictal cry" only increased the likelihood of epilepsy 1.7-fold even though it was reported in 60% of patients with epilepsy.

Hip thrusting: Pelvic thrusting is sustained extension of the lower back and, more rarely, can include rhythmic upward thrusting driven primarily by the hips, as compared with the extremities. When pelvic thrusting is described, this increased the likelihood of functional seizures by 2.6-fold.[18,27,28] However, pelvic thrusting was only reported in 5% to 15% of patients with functional seizures.[18,27] Due to similarities in neuroanatomic localization, some experts generalize the specific sign of pelvic thrusting to include rhythmic or sustained extension of the upper chest and thoracic spine, or the head. These related signs have not been as diagnostic in other patient samples.[29] Hip thrusting can be a feature of frontal lobe epilepsy.[28]

Asynchronous limb movements: Asynchronous limb movements were defined by multiple movements in multiple limbs that did not seem synchronous or coordinated between these limbs. In bilateral or generalized epileptic seizures, the evolving epileptic seizure leads to abnormal hypersynchrony across both hemispheres that, most often, impairs awareness. When multiple limbs are involved without this widespread hypersynchronicity, the seizure semiology is incompatible with our knowledge of neuroanatomic localization of neurologic symptoms. This asynchronicity of limb movements was reported in 70% of patients with functional seizures across 3 studies and increased the likelihood of functional seizures 10-fold.[27] When absent, as it was in 98% of patients with epilepsy, it increased the likelihood of epilepsy 2.6-fold. Although mimics of asynchronous movements were not described in those studies, it is important to know that frontal lobe epilepsies can include repetitive, coordinated, and overlearned bilateral movements including but not limited to bicycling of legs and arms, clicking heels, and rocking of the hips. In comparison to asynchronous movements, these behaviorally similar movements did not accurately differentiate functional from epileptic seizures.

Head version: Forced deviation of the head when an epileptic seizure transitions from one side of the body to include bilateral tonic-clonic movements is a valuable sign to lateralize epileptic seizures to the contralateral hemisphere. This sign occurs due to hyperactivation of the ipsilateral frontal attention network, leading to a strong drive to attend to the contralateral side of the body. In clear versive movements, there is an overwhelming shift in attention with the eyes, head, and whole body causing sustained rotation.[30] When forced head version was reported, the likelihood of epileptic seizures increased by 5-fold.[27] This strong head version was only reported in 45% (25/56) of patients with epilepsy across 2 studies, as compared with 8% (1/12) patients with functional seizures. However, when this sign was originally being studied in patients with epilepsy, it became clear that less strong, nonspecific movements of the head in one direction did not provide lateralizing value. In comparison, nonspecific head movements in any direction or any type were reported in 20% to 40% of 1500 patients with either epileptic or functional seizures.[18]

Limb automatisms and tonic-clonic movements: There is mixed evidence regarding seizures including limb automatisms and tonic-clonic movements, especially when nonneurologists use those specific words. Limb automatisms are defined by repetitive, purposeless activities (eg, picking at clothing). Tonic-clonic movements alternate between a tonic, or stiff, phase of movement and a clonic, or jerking, phase of movement. In some large patient cohorts, these features meaningfully increased the likelihood of epileptic seizures but other large series did not replicate these findings.[18,27]

Seizure duration: Functional seizures tend to be longer than epileptic seizures.[20] From studies of status epilepticus, the average convulsive epileptic seizure in adults was between 90 and 120 seconds long, with 95% of seizures stopping before 3 minutes and 30 seconds without intervention.[11] This excludes the duration of the postictal period, which often can be hours. Therefore, seizures longer than 5 minutes should have a higher suspicion for functional seizures.[18,20] Alternatively, the patient could be experiencing recurrent status epilepticus, which is uncommon in adults without established epilepsy syndromes like Lennox-Gastaut syndrome. Due to status epilepticus being a neurologic emergency, it is generally advisable to avoid using a variation of the term "status" to describe prolonged functional seizures.

Conversely, a substantial minority of epileptic seizures can last less than 30 seconds.[20] These very short seizures are very uncommon in functional seizures; therefore, extremely brief seizures should raise the suspicion for epilepsy.

Syncope: Recurrent syncope is an important cause of *physiologic* nonepileptic seizures that typically is easier to differentiate from both functional and epileptic seizures due to presyncopal symptoms. The Calgary Syncope versus Seizure score identified key historical descriptions indicating syncope: preevent diaphoresis, ever having light-headedness spells, and association with prolonged sitting or standing.[31] The Paroxysmal Event and Observer Profiles also confirmed that syncope was associated with prolonged sitting or standing, palpitations, a pale appearance of the lips or skin, and limpness of the legs and arms.[25,26] Although symptoms of a panic attack without the emotion of panic can be a feature of functional seizures,[32] patients with syncope rarely reported the positive movements or sensations that were reported in epilepsy or functional seizures. When present, the convulsive phase of convulsive syncope typically lasts for less than 30 seconds and includes arrhythmic, asynchronous limb movements. These movements can sustain for longer periods when patients were unable to quickly improve cerebral hypoperfusion by laying down, which can occur when patients are restrained.

In addition to these most useful features of ictal behavior, health-care providers should be aware of features that did not meet this high level of evidence that are pervasive in discussion. Ictal incontinence has been discussed as a perfect sign of epileptic seizures but multiple studies have demonstrated that when asked uniformly to patients with functional seizures, this was inaccurate.[18,20] Similarly, lateral as compared with anterior ictal oral trauma to the tongue or cheek has been suggestive of epilepsy as compared with functional seizures but this has not been replicated in other larger datasets.[20] Additionally, side-to-side head shaking, body rocking, bicycling, vocalization, fluctuating course, stereotypy, postictal amnesia, and other postictal symptoms did not have a high diagnostic reliability across multiple studies.[27]

There also is insufficient data regarding the unique ictal behaviors of functional seizures in patients with comorbid intellectual disability or patients with mixed functional and epileptic seizures.[14,21] As compared with other patients, patients with intellectual disability and the elderly are more likely to have physiologic nonepileptic seizure-like events such as convulsive syncope and episodes of rage or confusion.[33] Therefore, more studies are needed to reliably describe these less common clinical scenarios.

Although these individual features of ictal behavior were helpful for identifying patients with possible or probable functional seizures, combinations of multiple suggestive features can indicate "possible" functional seizures.[14] However, observation of a seizure by a clinician, seizure-specialist, or ictal video-EEG is needed to improve the certainty of diagnosis.

VIDEO-OBSERVED AND EXPERT-OBSERVED SEMIOLOGY

Other than simultaneous video plus EEG, high-quality videos of seizures can be the most valuable piece of the diagnostic evaluation of functional seizures.[34] However, clinicians should avoid being overly confident in a video-based diagnosis without concomitant EEG in the absence of positive signs of functional seizures and when the quality of the video is poor.[35,36]

Video Quality, Availability, and Other Considerations

Despite the pervasive availability of smart phones and surveillance cameras, high-quality seizure videos were rarely available in adults.[36,37] This low rate may be because seizures are rare, unpredictable, and brief events; seizure observers prioritize patient safety over recording; many caregivers are not trained in what constitutes a quality video; lack of interacting with the patient during video; and viewing a seizure can be distressing.[38]

A quality video includes an unobstructed view of the entire patient before, during, and after the seizure.[39] This includes both a quality view of the face as well as all limbs, so that experts can look for, for example, dystonic posturing contralateral to hypermotor automatisms or eye closure. In the surgical evaluation of epilepsy, the earliest semiological signs help localize the early symptomatogenic zone, defined as the region of cortex involved in generating the symptoms associated with an epileptic seizure.[40] As the seizure spreads within and between cerebral hemispheres, more regions of brain are recruited and produce more symptoms that can overlap and contradict each other. Contradictory semiological features may seem functional. For example, in a focal to bilateral tonic-clonic epileptic seizure, ictal version of the head, eyes, and body localize the seizure onset to the contralateral side but late head version once the epileptic seizure has already bilateralized had low lateralizing value.[30,41] Additionally, a devolving bilateral tonic-clonic epileptic seizure may seem to have asynchronous limb movements.

Capturing the context preceding the seizure can raise concern for alternative seizure causes. For example, symptoms that only occur after an orthostatic challenge can raise concern for orthostatic tremor or convulsive vasovagal syncope. Additionally, dystonic posturing provoked by movement can raise concern for paroxysmal kinesigenic dyskinesia (PKD), which is associated with mutations in the Proline Rich Transmembrane Protein 2 (PRRT2) gene.[42] In addition to ruling out nonfunctional conditions, awareness of acute external and internal factors that lead up to functional seizures can be a key component of cognitive behavioral informed treatment. Training patients with functional seizures to improve their perception of internal stimuli can serve as a method to identify and address their preseizure state.[43]

After a seizure ends, a postseizure video can reveal a focal neurologic deficit indicating Todd paralysis, where a region involved in an epileptic seizure has postictal diminished function.[44] Although Todd paralysis typically is associated with limb weakness, it can apply to any region of cortex involved in seizure including a postictal facial droop or postictal Broca aphasia. When observed, a focused evaluation of the Todd paralysis on the video can reveal positive diagnostic signs of either epilepsy or Functional Neurological Disorder (FND) that are better described in articles about functional motor disorders.[45]

Additionally, functional seizures can have a waxing and waning character to the severity of seizure that must be distinguished from a cluster of epileptic seizures or status epilepticus.[29] By recording after (or between) seizures, there may be a greater chance to observe the very valuable start of subsequent seizures that can reveal if the seizure semiology progresses in a stereotyped fashion suggestive of epilepsy, as compared with the variability of functional seizures.

Diagnosis Based on Video-Observed Semiology

Although there are numerous large series that evaluate the diagnostic performance of features of reported ictal behavior, there are relatively few studies that describe the features that epileptologists used in those seizure videos to differentiate between functional seizures and epileptic seizures.[36–39,46] In the absence of these detailed descriptions, we return to the fundamental principles of behavioral localization based on neuroanatomy. The task of the expert is to create a map from each ictal behavior to a brain network. Functional seizures should not be based simply on ruling out epilepsy but, for clarity, it helps to describe the neuroanatomic correlates of epileptic seizures before describing how functional seizures do not respect these neuroanatomic boundaries.

In focal-onset epileptic seizures, the seizure starts in the seizure-onset zone then spreads to include the symptomatogenic zone, defined above.[40] As epileptic seizures evolve, the symptomatogenic zone can increase based on highly connected neuroanatomic pathways. Epileptic seizures also are caused by evolving rhythmic or periodic electrical activity; therefore, within each symptomatogenic zone, the ictal behavior often has a characteristic rhythm.

When a seizure localizes to a well-established neuroanatomic pathway, then the diagnosis can be determined with high confidence and accuracy even in absence of EEG data. For example, a limbic-onset seizure can begin with a lapse in awareness, followed by oral automatisms, then dystonic posturing of one limb and contralateral limb automatisms, followed by a "Figure 4" sign, then head and eye version before evolving into a bilateral tonic-clonic seizure. This series of events corresponds to symptomatogenic zones starting in the limbic system, then spreading to supplementary motor and other frontal areas, before asymmetric activation of the frontal eye field, and subsequent spread to the contralateral frontal lobe. When this exact series of events is observed, the likelihood of epileptic seizures is high. In general, if a patient exhibits extremely stereotyped ictal behavior that is pathognomonic for a particular localization of epilepsy, those seizures are likely to be epileptic (eg, Fencer's posture, self-stimulation in Sunflower syndrome, hyperventilation-induced absence seizures).

However, when more atypical ictal behavior is observed, the seizure expert must draw on their knowledge of other focal-onset or generalized-onset epilepsy syndromes to see if symptoms map onto those known conditions. One commonly reported positive sign of functional seizures was preserved awareness and memory throughout a bilateral motor seizure, which would require the involvement of bilateral motor networks and sparing of networks involved in awareness and memory.[27] Just as functional seizures are not a diagnosis of exclusion, not all seizures with atypical semiology are functional.

A key differential diagnosis for functional seizures is frontal lobe epilepsy.[3] Because of the complex functional neuroanatomical organization of the frontal lobe, seizures that originate there often have no warning and have explosive hypermotor symptoms, with a quick return to baseline. Although these features are similar to functional seizures, frontal lobe seizures are almost identical from seizure to seizure, whereas functional seizures will have qualitatively more variability. Additionally, as suggested by Autosomal Dominant Nocturnal Frontal Lobe Epilepsy associated with mutations in *CHRNA4*,[42] frontal lobe seizures often occur during sleep whereas functional seizures only occur during wakefulness. However, misdiagnoses can be made when the patient awakes from sleep but does not yet move and thereby seems to be sleeping and subsequently has a functional seizure.[47]

Although functional seizures are most commonly mistaken for epileptic seizures, there are other nonseizure conditions that can be appreciated on video. In addition to PKD, discussed above, clinicians should consider paroxysmal nonkinesigenic dyskinesia (PNKD) and focal dystonias. PNKD was associated with mutations in the *PNKD* gene and, most frequently, has onset in childhood. Focal dystonias tend to be more sustained than seizures and can have a "sensory trick" where symptoms abate with a specific sensory stimulus that often is atypical (eg, a finger on an ear).[45] Alternatively, an association with startling or emotional stimuli can raise suspicion for cataplexy in narcolepsy.[48] In the rare cases of malingering or factitious syndromes, the video potentially can capture objective evidence for voluntary generation of symptoms. However, outside medicolegal contexts, malingering and factitious disorders are exceptionally rare when compared with the prevalence of functional seizures and the suggestion of malingering or factitious symptoms substantially contributes to stigma in functional seizures.[49–51]

Although videos can give extremely valuable diagnostic information, it is important to remain humble about the level of diagnostic confidence that a video can lend. In studies of video-based diagnosis, epileptologists had 90% accuracy in differentiating functional seizures from epilepsy, which is distinctly less than the 1% rate of diagnostic revision rate after video-EEG monitoring.[36,46,52] In comparison, general neurologists and neurology residents had 75% accuracy but the residents' confidence in their diagnoses was higher than the epileptologists.[36] This reflects that video may give a less-expert observer a false sense of diagnostic certainty. To further emphasize the role of experience, the accuracy of nonneurologists was between 45% and 60%, including internal medicine physicians, emergency medicine physicians, and emergency medicine nurses.[52] These low-accuracy rates for nonneurology health-care providers highlight the need for increased education and management strategies to avoid, for example, intubation and high doses of antiseizure medications for prolonged functional seizures that were misdiagnosed as convulsive status epilepticus.[11]

SUMMARY

Functional seizures are a disabling condition that is defined by the presence of episodic, involuntary neurologic symptoms. A high-quality description of the seizures is fundamental to an accurate diagnosis. There are key semiological features that can support a positive diagnosis of possible functional seizures including ictal eye closure, ictal weeping, asynchronous movements, hip thrusting, and long seizures.

High-quality videos of seizures are extremely valuable but also are rarely available and difficult to obtain. When direct observation of multiple typical seizures by a seizure specialist is not possible, health care should recognize the inherent challenges faced by nonspecialists who attempt to describe distressing events. Therefore, ictal behavior should be one important component of a comprehensive evaluation to determine the cause of seizure and, thereby, identify the next steps in diagnosis and treatment.

CLINICS CARE POINTS

- A verbal history from untrained observers should focus on key features that these observers are readily able to understand and describe. These key features include ictal eye closure, ictal weeping, asynchronous movements, hip thrusting, and seizure duration greater than 5 minutes.

- Video documentation of seizures can be critical in the identification of functional seizures. Quality video captures the whole patient for the whole seizure and can include interaction with the patient.

- Reliable diagnosis based on semiology is expertise-dependent, with epileptologists being the most accurate, followed by neurologists and EEG technicians. The diagnostic accuracy of nonexperts can be around 50%.

DECLARATION OF INTERESTS

Dr W.T. Kerr has received honoraria from Medlink for review articles on this topic. Dr W.T. Kerr has consulting agreements for unrelated topics with SK Lifesciences, Radius Health, Janssen, and Biohaven Pharmaceuticals.

ACKNOWLEDGMENTS

This study was supported by grants from the National Institutes of Health, United States (NIH R25 NS089450 and NIH U24 NS107158).

REFERENCES

1. Asadi-Pooya AA, Brigo F, Mildon B, et al. Terminology for psychogenic nonepileptic seizures: making the case for "functional seizures". Epilepsy Behav 2020; 104(Pt A):106895.
2. Kerr WT, Stern JM. We need a functioning name for PNES: consider dissociative seizures. Epilepsy Behav 2020;105:107002.
3. Dickinson P, Looper KJ. Psychogenic nonepileptic seizures: a current overview. Review. Epilepsia 2012;53(10):1679–89.
4. Pick S, Goldstein LH, Perez DL, et al. Emotional processing in functional neurological disorder: a review, biopsychosocial model and research agenda. J Neurol Neurosurg Psychiatry 2019;90(6):704–11.
5. Fisher RS, Cross JH, French JA, et al. Operational classification of seizure types by the International League Against Epilepsy: position paper of the ILAE Commission for Classification and Terminology. Epilepsia 2017;58(4):522–30.
6. LaFrance WC Jr. Psychogenic nonepileptic "seizures" or "attacks"? It's not just semantics: seizures. Neurology 2010;75(1):87–8.
7. Kerr WT, Janio EA, Braesch CT, et al. Identifying psychogenic seizures through comorbidities and medication history. Epilepsia 2017;58(11):1852–60.

8. Walczak TS, Papacostas S, Williams DT, et al. Outcome after diagnosis of psychogenic nonepileptic seizures. Epilepsia 1995;36(11):1131–7.

9. Kerr WT, Zhang X, Hill CE, et al. Factors associated with delay to video-EEG in dissociative seizures. Seizure 2021;86:155–60.

10. Libbon R, Gadbaw J, Watson M, et al. The feasibility of a multidisciplinary group therapy clinic for the treatment of nonepileptic seizures. Epilepsy Behav 2019; 98(Pt A):117–23.

11. Kapur J, Elm J, Chamberlain JM, et al. Randomized trial of three anticonvulsant medications for status epilepticus. N Engl J Med 2019;381(22):2103–13.

12. Goldstein LH, Robinson EJ, Chalder T, et al. Moderators of cognitive behavioural therapy treatment effects and predictors of outcome in the CODES randomised controlled trial for adults with dissociative seizures. J Psychosom Res 2022; 158:110921.

13. Goldstein LH, Robinson EJ, Mellers JDC, et al. Cognitive behavioural therapy for adults with dissociative seizures (CODES): a pragmatic, multicentre, randomised controlled trial. Lancet Psychiatry 2020;7(6):491–505.

14. LaFrance WC Jr, Baker GA, Duncan R, et al. Minimum requirements for the diagnosis of psychogenic nonepileptic seizures: a staged approach: a report from the International League Against Epilepsy Nonepileptic Seizures Task Force. Review. Epilepsia 2013;54(11):2005–18.

15. Kerr WT, Lee JK, Karimi AH, et al. A minority of patients with functional seizures have abnormalities on neuroimaging. J Neurol Sci 2021;427:117548.

16. Adenan MH, Khalil M, Loh KS, et al. A retrospective study of the correlation between duration of monitoring in the epilepsy monitoring unit and diagnostic yield. Epilepsy Behav 2022;136:108919.

17. Kerr WT, Janio EA, Braesch CT, et al. An objective score to identify psychogenic seizures based on age of onset and history. Epilepsy Behav 2018;80:75–83.

18. Kerr WT, Janio EA, Chau AM, et al. Objective score from initial interview identifies patients with probable dissociative seizures. Epilepsy Behav 2020;2020(113): 107525.

19. Kerr WT, Zhang X, Janio EA, et al. Reliability of additional reported seizure manifestations to identify dissociative seizures. Epilepsy Behav 2021;115:107696.

20. Kerr WT, Chau AM, Janio EA, et al. Reliability of reported peri-ictal behavior to identify psychogenic nonepileptic seizures. Seizure 2019;67:45–51.

21. Baroni G, Piccinini V, Martins WA, et al. Variables associated with co-existing epileptic and psychogenic nonepileptic seizures: a systematic review. Seizure 2016;37:35–40.

22. Cornaggia CM, Gugliotta SC, Magaudda A, et al. Conversation analysis in the differential diagnosis of Italian patients with epileptic or psychogenic non-epileptic seizures: a blind prospective study. Epilepsy Behav 2012;25(4):598–604.

23. Boylan LS, Flint LA, Labovitz DL, et al. Depression but not seizure frequency predicts quality of life in treatment-resistant epilepsy. Research Support, Non-U.S. Gov't. Neurology 2004;62(2):258–61.

24. Jenkins L, Cosgrove J, Chappell P, et al. Neurologists can identify diagnostic linguistic features during routine seizure clinic interactions: results of a one-day teaching intervention. Epilepsy Behav 2016;64(Pt A):257–61.

25. Wardrope A, Jamnadas-Khoda J, Broadhurst M, et al. Machine learning as a diagnostic decision aid for patients with transient loss of consciousness. Neurol Clin Pract 2020;10(2):96–105.

26. Wardrope A, Newberry E, Reuber M. Diagnostic criteria to aid the differential diagnosis of patients presenting with transient loss of consciousness: A systematic review. Seizure 2018;61:139–48.

27. Muthusamy S, Seneviratne U, Ding C, et al. Using semiology to classify epileptic seizures vs psychogenic nonepileptic seizures: a meta-analysis. Neurol Clin Pract 2022;12(3):234–47.

28. Geyer JD, Payne TA, Drury I. The value of pelvic thrusting in the diagnosis of seizures and pseudoseizures. Neurology 2000;54(1):227–9.

29. Duncan AJ, Peric I, Boston R, et al. Predictive semiology of psychogenic non-epileptic seizures in an epilepsy monitoring unit. J Neurol 2022;269(4):2172–8.

30. Fotedar N, Gajera P, Pyatka N, et al. A descriptive study of eye and head movements in versive seizures. Seizure 2022;98:44–50.

31. Sheldon R, Rose S, Ritchie D, et al. Historical criteria that distinguish syncope from seizures. J Am Coll Cardiol 2002;40(1):142–8.

32. Hendrickson R, Popescu A, Dixit R, et al. Panic attack symptoms differentiate patients with epilepsy from those with psychogenic nonepileptic spells (PNES). Epilepsy Behav 2014;37:210–4.

33. Kerr WT, Sreenivasan SS, Allas CH, et al. Title: functional seizures across the adult lifespan: female sex, delay to diagnosis and disability. Seizure 2021;91: 476–83.

34. Beniczky SA, Fogarasi A, Neufeld M, et al. Seizure semiology inferred from clinical descriptions and from video recordings. How accurate are they? Epilepsy Behav 2012;24(2):213–5.

35. Samuel M, Duncan JS. Use of the hand held video camcorder in the evaluation of seizures. J Neurol Neurosurg Psychiatry 1994;57(11):1417–8.

36. Tatum WO, Hirsch LJ, Gelfand MA, et al. Assessment of the predictive value of outpatient smartphone videos for diagnosis of epileptic seizures. JAMA Neurol 2020;77(5):593–600.

37. Ramanujam B, Dash D, Tripathi M. Can home videos made on smartphones complement video-EEG in diagnosing psychogenic nonepileptic seizures? Seizure 2018;62:95–8.

38. Tatum WO, Hirsch LJ, Gelfand MA, et al. Video quality using outpatient smartphone videos in epilepsy: results from the OSmartViE study. Eur J Neurol 2021; 28(5):1453–62.

39. Ricci L, Boscarino M, Assenza G, et al. Clinical utility of home videos for diagnosing epileptic seizures: a systematic review and practical recommendations for optimal and safe recording. Neurol Sci 2021;42(4):1301–9.

40. Rosenow F, Luders H. Presurgical evaluation of epilepsy. Brain 2001;124(Pt 9): 1683–700.

41. Wyllie E, Luders H, Morris HH, et al. The lateralizing significance of versive head and eye movements during epileptic seizures. Neurology 1986;36(5):606–11.

42. de Gusmao CM, Garcia L, Mikati MA, et al. Paroxysmal genetic movement disorders and epilepsy. Front Neurol 2021;12:648031.

43. Reiter JM, Andrews D, Reiter C, et al. Taking control of your seizures. Treatments that work. Oxford University Press; 2015.

44. Xu SY, Li ZX, Wu XW, et al. Frequency and Pathophysiology of post-seizure Todd's paralysis. Med Sci Monit 2020;26:e920751.

45. Espay AJ, Aybek S, Carson A, et al. Current concepts in diagnosis and treatment of functional neurological disorders. JAMA Neurol 2018;75(9):1132–41.

46. Birca V, Keezer MR, Chamelian L, et al. Recognition of psychogenic versus epileptic seizures based on videos. Can J Neurol Sci 2021;21:1–9.

47. Duncan R, Oto M, Russell AJ, et al. Pseudosleep events in patients with psychogenic non-epileptic seizures: prevalence and associations. J Neurol Neurosurg Psychiatry 2004;75(7):1009–12.
48. Perez-Carbonell L, Mignot E, Leschziner G, et al. Understanding and approaching excessive daytime sleepiness. Lancet 2022;400(10357):1033–46.
49. Robson C, Lian OS. "Blaming, shaming, humiliation": Stigmatising medical interactions among people with non-epileptic seizures. Wellcome Open Res 2017; 2:55.
50. Rommelfanger KS, Factor SA, LaRoche S, et al. Disentangling stigma from functional neurological disorders: conference report and roadmap for the future. Front Neurol 2017;8:106.
51. Rawlings GH, Brown I, Stone B, et al. Written accounts of living with psychogenic nonepileptic seizures: a thematic analysis. Seizure 2017;50:83–91.
52. Wasserman D, Herskovitz M. Epileptic vs psychogenic nonepileptic seizures: a video-based survey. Epilepsy Behav 2017;73:42–5.

Functional Cognitive Disorder

Diagnosis, Treatment, and Differentiation from Secondary Causes of Cognitive Difficulties

Verónica Cabreira, MD, Laura McWhirter, PhD*, Alan Carson, MD

KEYWORDS

- Functional neurological disorder • Cognitive disorders
- Subjective cognitive impairment • Metacognition • Dementia
- Functional cognitive disorder

KEY POINTS

- A significant proportion of patients attending memory clinics have cognitive symptoms that despite being disabling do not progress to dementia, for whom a diagnosis of functional cognitive disorder (FCD) may be appropriate.
- Pathophysiological mechanisms of FCD encompass global metacognitive bias, heightened attentional focus, impaired emotional processing, and negative illness perceptions.
- Diagnosis of FCD is based on positive features of internal inconsistency gathered from the clinical history, patterns of communication, and behavior and adjunctive cognitive testing.
- Complementary investigations, including neuroimaging, are required if comorbidities or contributing pathologies are considered, but the possibility of incidental findings should always be discussed.
- There is an urgent need for effective treatments for FCD and promising therapies include metacognitive retraining, acceptance and commitment therapy, and cognitive-behavioral therapy modalities.

INTRODUCTION

A growing awareness of dementia as a public health problem in an aging population has led to increasing numbers of people seeking help for memory problems and a higher demand for clinical assessments. Clinicians increasingly encounter patients with memory complaints not due to neurodegenerative conditions[1] and that will not progress to dementia. In some cases, memory problems are secondary to primary

Centre for Clinical Brain Sciences, University of Edinburgh, Edinburgh, UK
* Corresponding author. Department of Clinical Neurosciences, Edinburgh Royal Infirmary, Little France, Edinburgh.
E-mail address: Laura.mcwhirter@ed.ac.uk

Neurol Clin 41 (2023) 619–633
https://doi.org/10.1016/j.ncl.2023.02.004
0733-8619/23/© 2023 Elsevier Inc. All rights reserved.
neurologic.theclinics.com

medical or psychiatric diagnoses, either alone or in combination, such as untreated sleep apnea, polypharmacy, or a major depressive episode. In others, the presence of internal inconsistency in the symptoms indicates a functional cognitive disorder (FCD) —a diagnostic category operationalized in 2020.[2]

A growing body of evidence supports positive diagnosis of FCD, based on specific clinical features (*not* exclusion of disease), and improved understanding of metacognitive profiles, interaction patterns, and other biopsychosocial-informed characteristics.[3,4] Functional cognitive symptoms are characterized by internal inconsistency and are not better explained by another neurologic, psychiatric, or systemic disorder (**Box 1** for diagnostic criteria).[2,5] FCD may comprise up to a quarter of the new referrals to tertiary memory clinics and is a common source of disability.[2,5–8] Improving awareness of FCD is a first step toward facilitating research into the diagnosis, prognosis, and treatment of this often neglected cause of cognitive difficulty.

FCD is understood under the functional neurological disorder (FND) umbrella. Although cognitive symptoms may occur in isolation for FCD patients, they are often part of a wider constellation of neurologic symptoms (**Fig. 1**).[9–11]

With hope of disease-modifying therapeutics on the horizon, the focus in neurodegenerative disease research has shifted to an earlier diagnosis and better diagnostic specificity. Improved specificity of non-neurodegenerative disease diagnoses, including FCD, should be an important part of this.

Terminology

The development of terminology acceptable to both clinicians and patients, and simultaneously reflecting the current *state of the art* was behind efforts to develop diagnostic criteria for FCD.[2] Recognition of and research into FCD have historically been undermined by various and overlapping terminologies. Some terms try to normalize the symptoms (eg, "worried well") whereas others try to explain the cause (eg,

---

Box 1
Diagnostic criteria for functional cognitive disorder

All of the following.

1. One or more *symptoms of impaired cognitive function* (suggesting a deficit in attention, concentration, and memory domains, usually in the form of amnestic blocks for overlearned information that they are able to later recall).[a]

2. Clinical *evidence of internal inconsistency* between self-reported symptoms and conversational abilities/everyday functioning/cognitive testing, as well as discrepancy between the level of concern demonstrated by the patient and their relatives.[2,3,5]

3. Symptoms or deficits that are not better explained by another medical or psychiatric disorder (a comorbid medical, psychiatric, or neurodegenerative disorder may co-occur with a functional diagnosis).

4. Symptoms or deficits that cause clinically significant distress or impairment in social, occupational, or other important areas of functioning (assessment for premorbid function including in workplace, preferably through a collateral informant, is often required).

[a] Although in many patients, the symptoms tend to remain stable without progression (or fluctuation) over time, a subset of patients revert to normal or slowly progress over time. We suggest that an early diagnosis based on positive features provides an opportunity for better prognostic communication and treatment referral, and reduces the risk of misdiagnosis and treatment harm.

For a review, refer to [2,11].

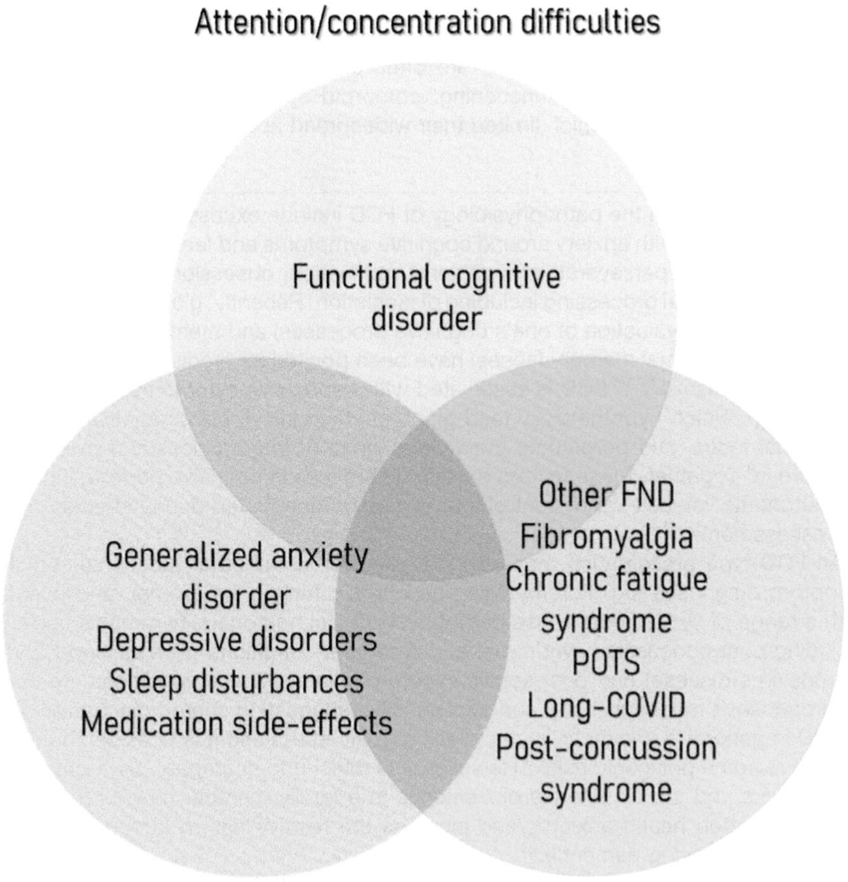

Fig. 1. Venn diagram demonstrating overlap between inattentive cognitive symptoms in several conditions, ranging from mental health diagnoses such as depression and generalized anxiety disorder to somatic symptoms and other functional disorders. The distinction lies in part in the presence and degree of internal inconsistency, in part in the severity of other symptoms, and in part in the direction and aims of treatment. FCD, Functional cognitive disorder; FND, Functional neurological disorder; POTS, Postural orthostatic tachycardia syndrome.

depressive pseudodementia). Often, when patients have subjective complaints without or with evidence of cognitive impairment on neuropsychometric tests, these are labeled as subjective cognitive impairment and mild cognitive impairment (MCI), respectively. As MCI can have a broad and multifactorial etiology, not all patients with MCI will progress to dementia. In fact, over the years, several consensus definitions have been established for MCI, essentially referring to a deterioration in cognitive function greater than expected with normal aging.[12,13] Yet, it continues to be used inconsistently, as illustrated by surveys across European countries and the United States.[14–16] In our experience, population-based identification of MCI cases may over-recruit people with FCD, especially in younger age strata. This puts patients with cognitive complaints at risk of misdiagnosis and iatrogenic harm through inappropriate treatments and predictions of decline. Historically, 'worried well' was reserved for patients who performed normally on routine cognitive assessments, and were generally reassured by explanations that their memory lapses fall under the range of a normal experience. Other terms such as 'benign senescent forgetfulness,' 'cogniform disorder,' and 'cogniform condition,' are often dismissive (or interpreted as such), highly dependent on overall functioning, comorbid symptoms, employment level, and other social factors, which limited their widespread application and adoption.

Pathophysiology

Factors implicated in the pathophysiology of FCD include excessive self-monitoring, attentional bias, health anxiety around cognitive symptoms and fear avoidance, negative illness beliefs, perseverative cognitions (rumination, obsession, and worry), and abnormal emotional processing including dissociation. Recently, global metacognitive error (inaccurate evaluation of one's cognitive processes) and memory perfectionism (intolerance of normal memory lapses) have been posited as predisposing or perpetuating mechanisms.[17,18] FCD is associated with depressive symptoms, anxiety, and neuroticism, which hypothetically feed global metacognitive bias, negatively impact attentional focus, and perpetuate the vicious circle of forgetfulness and perception of failure.[4,9] Together, these factors explain differences in cognitive performance under automatic versus explicit control that can be demonstrated during standard clinical assessments.[19]

An FCD-type presentation may also be seen across all other functional somatic symptom diagnoses (eg, fibromyalgia and chronic fatigue syndrome), and overlap with a range of syndromes whose pathophysiological homogeneity remains unclear, including post-concussion syndrome, and emergent conditions such as long-COVID (coronavirus disease) and post-sepsis syndromes (albeit these conditions are likely heterogeneous mechanistically and etiologically), suggesting shared mechanisms.[9]

FND in general is known to have a weak genetic effect and it is possible that FCD may have some polygenic risk.[20] However, it is difficult to segregate that from experiential risks and the experience of dementia in a family member may be important (with associated health anxiety), and increase the relative risk to attend a memory clinic, without having dementia.[21]

Of course, FCD is not the only cause of non-degenerative cognitive difficulties. The difference in clinical practice between, for example, depression with cognitive symptoms and an FCD lies in part in the presence and degree of internal inconsistency, in part in the severity of other (eg, affective) symptoms, and in part in the direction and aims of treatment. Not all patients with inconsistently present inattentive cognitive symptoms should receive a new diagnosis of FCD (see **Fig. 1**). However, even in cases where there are multiple contributors to cognitive difficulty or an alternative primary diagnosis (such as generalized anxiety disorder or major depression), understanding and identifying contributory FCD mechanisms can open additional treatment targets and can aid recovery.

Evaluation: Historical Features, Demographics, and Comorbidities

Clinical history and examination, and in some cases longitudinal follow-up, are key to making the diagnosis of FCD.[2,3,22–24] In the search for positive clinical features of FCD, close examination of communication profiles has been promising.[6,24] Overall, FCD patients report a higher number of memory complaints, can frequently date the onset of their memory failures with precision, and characteristically provide extensive and detailed descriptions of their memory difficulties, often with specific examples and additional unsolicited details,[3,6] whereas patients with cognitive impairment due to other causes tend to provide shorter, concrete answers.[22] Additionally, the ability to handle and recall all parts of compound questions[6,24] is often a sign of preserved working memory. Equally, although patients complain of episodic memory failures usually in the form of amnestic blocks (usually for overlearned information such as PINs, names of familiar places/people, and dates of birth), they are able to recall these episodes with great detail, and content repetitions in the clinic are rarely observed, in contrast with patients with dementia.[5,7,25] The nature of the complaints in FCD typically relates to impaired concentration: misplacing things, losing track during conversations, or forgetting the purpose of a task while doing it.[7] To further co-substantiate their complaints, FCD patients might mention others' observations of their memory using direct reported speech to establish comparisons with their previous memory.[6] There is often a discrepancy between the level of worry demonstrated by the patients and their relatives (in the opposite direction to that seen in neurodegenerative disease), with the patients being more concerned by their problems than others.[5,6,24] Indeed, frequently the patients are self-referred and attend the clinic alone, evidencing independent function.[26] Patients with neurodegenerative cognitive disorders often look to the support person accompanying them for help and answers,[6,24] a very specific behavior known as the head-turning sign.[27] Likewise, if the history suggests a slow onset, gradual progression, and loss of insight, a neurodegenerative disease is more likely.[24] Whereas people with FCD may report memory loss for both recent and remote events, a temporal gradient with relative preservation of remote events is more likely in Alzheimer's disease.

Pre-test probability is important in interpreting the clinical examination. Advancing age is the single strongest predictor of neurodegenerative disease, and FCD affects a comparatively younger fraction of the population, often affecting individuals in their early sixties, but it can also occur in the elderly population, making age unreliable as a sole diagnostic marker.[7,19,28] Education level and premorbid functional status (including any difficulties in the workplace and/or with other instrumental activities of daily living) are important hints to consider.[5] Anecdotally, patients with FCD may have higher levels of education: although this is a protective factor against neurodegenerative disease, it may also be associated with cognitively demanding occupations in which minor deficits are quickly noticed and/or perfectionistic traits/obsessive-compulsive personality.[29] Family history of neurodegenerative disease should not drive clinicians away from the possibility of FCD; as discussed above, having a close relative with dementia might increase vulnerability to FCD.[28]

Psychiatric comorbidities are commonly encountered in FCD, often in excess when compared with healthy controls and patients with neurodegenerative disorders, but significant overlap may occur in prodromal stages of neurodegeneration, predominantly in cases of the frontotemporal dementias spectrum. Patients with dysthymia, generalized anxiety disorder, obsessive-compulsive personality disorder, and depression might present with concentration difficulties that may or may not fulfill the criteria for FCD(5). However, it is worth noticing that approximately 50% of FCD patients are not depressed.[23,30] Several studies also found that sleep disturbances are commonly reported by patients with FCD.[5,28] Whether this reflects the effects of poor sleep on cognition, an increased self-monitoring of sleep, or comorbid conditions such as mood disorders, sleep-disordered breathing, or restless legs syndrome is less certain. FCD may be associated with multimorbidity and certainly with greater reporting of somatic symptoms.[22,31]

A key feature is the failure to relentlessly progress over time and toward dependence and death, the cardinal trajectory of neurodegenerative dementias. In contrast, FCD symptoms may persist without progression or may fluctuate over time. Some patients can revert to normal cognition, others remain stable, and a subset may slowly and incompletely progress over time.[2] Whereas some earlier studies suggested a

6 month to 1 year window before establishing a secure diagnosis of FCD, we support an early positive diagnosis, when possible, to prevent over- or misdiagnosis and further diagnostic delay. This is not to supplant the need for close follow-up, especially when symptoms present at an older age.

Differential Diagnosis

Several factors can contribute to experience of memory failures: mood and anxiety disorders, substance use/medication effects, pain, and sleep disturbances. Functional cognitive symptoms can occur in isolation or be part of a cascade of symptoms carrying an attentional burden; a 'side effect' of other things going on in the brain and the body (**Table 1**). Accordingly, FCD-type inattentive cognitive symptoms are in our

Table 1
Red flags that should prompt investigation for an alternative diagnosis

Red Flag	Alternative Diagnosis
Accompanying person being more concerned than the patient. Evidence of focal atrophy/metabolic changes on structural and functional (nuclear medicine) neuroimaging. Cognitive assessment suggesting impairment in a single domain such as single word comprehension or language production. Praxis, prosopagnosia, or visuospatial deficits. Greater difficulty to recall recent vs older events (temporal gradient).	Consider an alternative neurodegenerative disorder.
Prominent anhedonia, psychomotor retardation, apathy, and low mood.	Depression or frontal lobe lesions.
Gait impairment, cerebellar or movement disorder features (eg, chorea, extrapyramidal features).	Normal pressure hydrocephalus Other hereditary or sporadic conditions presenting with cognitive impairment including Huntington's disease, Lewy body dementia, or atypical parkinsonism
Preservation of implicit memory with episodic memory impairment.	Korsakoff's syndrome
Amnestic gap for a certain period with anterograde memory impairment	Transient global amnesia
Absence of decline or fluctuation over time.	Some patients with neurodegeneration and a high premorbid function may still have a cognitive performance under the normative range and have normal imaging for a certain period. Equally, patients with medical conditions, delirium/encephalopathy, or Lewy body dementia may present with cognitive symptoms with day-to-day variation.
Sudden onset of symptoms, often along with other neurologic symptoms, and especially in a patient with vascular risk factors.	Consider the possibility of a vascular etiology (eg, stroke).
Systemic symptoms (fatigue, daytime somnolence, weight, sweating, or skin abnormalities).	Consider investigation for other medical conditions (eg, metabolic, sleep, or cardiology disorders).

experience a near-universal complaint of those with other FND symptoms. Similarly, although there is limited evidence to support this apart from clinical experience and analogy to what occurs in Parkinson's disease and multiple sclerosis, FCD can be an anxiety-related prodrome of early neurodegeneration in a minority of patients.

In patients with a previous history of head trauma, it is important to accurately characterize the severity of the index injury (including loss of consciousness, history of bleeding, surgical interventions, retro- or anterograde amnesia) as a risk factor for poor cognition, as well as to inquire about common concomitant symptoms such as fatigue, headache, dizziness, or anxiety, all of which can increase worry and anxiety around cognitive symptoms.

The biopsychosocial-informed interview should include an inquiry about psychiatric symptoms and mental status examination. Symptoms of depression and anxiety, or post-traumatic symptoms (including dissociation), may be comorbid or contributory. In more severe cases, features of absolute anhedonia, loss of drive, early-morning wakening, and psychomotor retardation may indicate a severe depressive episode — a presentation in which cognitive decline has been described as 'depressive pseudodementia', requiring a different approach. Such a presentation will be best managed under psychiatry and might be considered an overlapping but distinct presentation from FCD.

If the patient has a history of vascular risk factors, cerebrovascular disease should be considered. The clinician must always consider other systemic and metabolic conditions such as decompensated heart failure, poorly controlled diabetes mellitus, or chronic obstructive pulmonary disease as contributors to the cognitive impairment; there may be opportunities to optimize management, and therefore, improve cognitive function.

As discussed, while patients' complaints in FCD suggest a deficit in attention, concentration, and sometimes memory domains, patients with dementia due to Alzheimer's disease are more likely to initially present with episodic memory impairment, orientation, or visuospatial deficits. Lewy body dementia may also initially present with attention and concentration deficits which fluctuate over time, although usually these are accompanied by visuospatial difficulties and parkinsonism on the neurologic examination. If the person or family members report behavioral changes, dietary changes, rigid habits, apathy, lack of insight, as well as attention and concentration impairment, frontotemporal lobar degeneration (behavioral variant) may be considered.

INVESTIGATIONS

FCD patients may not feel relieved by negative investigation results, and negative results per se are not a requirement of the diagnosis, which as discussed should be made based on the identification of positive clinical features of FCD.

Nevertheless, there are many situations where the clinical history and examination suggest possibilities of non-neurodegenerative causes of cognitive symptoms, comorbidities, or contributing pathologies for which additional investigations are useful. Baseline blood tests are often a pre-requisite for referral to tertiary memory services. Structural brain imaging (computerized tomography [CT] or MRI) can be helpful and, in some patients, reassuring; but the possibility of incidental findings is substantial, particularly with MRI.

Emerging Non-Imaging Biomarkers

Over the last two decades, CSF biomarkers reflecting Alzheimer's brain pathology have been developed for research purposes (clinical trial recruitment for population homogeneity). The last years have also seen the development of the first blood-based Alzheimer's disease biomarkers that can differentiate Alzheimer's disease from non-Alzheimer's disease dementias with excellent accuracy (eg, plasma pTau217, pTau181, and Aβ1–42).[32,33] Importantly, though, currently available Alzheimer's disease biomarkers lack sensitivity and specificity when applied broadly across a range of older patient populations. After a certain age amyloid is naturally deposited in the brain, and on a population basis, many people with positive Alzheimer's disease biomarker profiles will die of other causes without ever developing a clinical Alzheimer's dementia syndrome. In addition, other conditions, including FCD, can cause cognitive symptoms in patients with positive biomarkers for Alzheimer's disease[34]; in this group, the biomarker tests have the unhelpful effect of preventing access to treatment that might improve symptoms. Disease biomarker profiles are best used to augment data obtained in routine diagnostic evaluation.[32] Currently our concern is that patients with FCD, who are anxious and concerned about developing dementia, are at particular risk of incorrect interpretation of biomarker profiles.[35] Use of biomarker tests requires clear communication to make sure that patients understand the limited predictive value of positive tests in the absence of a clear clinical dementia syndrome.

Recognizing that only a proportion of patients with MCI will proceed to dementia, the American Academy of Neurology has recently issued a guideline on Recommendations for Assessing MCI that can be extrapolated for patients with FCD. These recommendations outline that a thorough investigation of MCI is important to assess for reversible causes of cognitive impairment and also address that, to date, there are no biomarkers to predict progression in patients with MCI, outside of the research field.[33]

There is considerable debate regarding the cost utility of testing for the APOE-ε4 allele. Although this is known to increase the risk of Alzheimer's disease, the information regarding the risk of disease progression portrayed by this allele is very limited. Plus, it was not found to be exceedingly prevalent in patients with subjective memory symptoms.[5] In those patients where FCD manifests as a prodromal stage of neurodegenerative dementia, being positive for APOE-ε4 would be unsurprising, but current evidence does not support widespread testing.

Structural and Functional Imaging

Structural imaging is useful to exclude alternative pathologies (eg, tumors) and is currently also employed to provide positive evidence for neurodegeneration or cerebrovascular disease. Care should be taken to not over-emphasize age-related changes such as mild generalized atrophy and T2/FLAIR white-matter hyperintensities, which often reflect underlying vascular risk factors. Although focal cerebral atrophy (specifically medial temporal lobe atrophy) may be a marker of Alzheimer's disease, a few studies found no association between global atrophy and objective cognitive performance or symptom severity in patients complaining of memory loss.[5,36] Longitudinal studies identified patterns of atrophy thought to be specific to Alzheimer's disease in individuals who in fact had non-progressive memory impairment.[37] Similarly, depressive symptoms in memory-clinic attenders were associated with variable superior temporal gyrus atrophy.[5,38] Conversely, absence of atrophy can be observed in earlier stages of neurodegeneration; nonetheless, a high negative predictive value can be attributed to the absence of atrophy in a patient with longstanding memory problems present for several years. Our practice is to clearly explain the possibility of incidental findings with the patient during a collaborative discussion about whether or not to scan.

Over the last decade, several modalities of functional (nuclear medicine-based) imaging, including fluorodeoxyglucose (FDG)-positron emission tomography (PET), single photon emission computed tomography (SPECT) scan, and Amyloid PET, were developed, and their utility explored for the diagnosis and management of patients with cognitive complaints. A change to regional blood flow identified on SPECT scans (or certain regional hypometabolism patterns on FDG-PET) would be another red flag for underlying brain pathology such as Alzheimer's disease or frontotemporal dementia. Young patients with unexplained MCI and long or atypical progression are the ones who can largely benefit from these advanced investigations if a molecular diagnosis becomes a limiting factor to access any novel disease-modifying therapies that may become available in the future. So far, concerns regarding therapeutic changes as a result of these investigations, safety, and available infrastructure are still ongoing issues. Functional MRI changes are a promising research area in other FND subtypes, and have helped unravel the pathophysiological mechanisms, but data for an FCD subtype of FND still lag.[5]

Neuropsychological testing

Although cognitive screening tests still form the core of many dementia diagnoses, the categorization of patients into clusters based on normative ranges has limitations. For some patients, apparent underperformance may reflect baseline function, whereas others with a higher cognitive reserve maybe later drop in performance, and therefore, reach a diagnosis. Thus, if used as a standalone 'dementia test', these screening tests will increase the number of false positive dementia diagnoses, including in those with FCD.[39]

Some patients with FCD score highly—or at least within healthy expected ranges—across neuropsychological tests. One view of FCD is of a disorder in which cognitive test performance is normal. However, studies in which people with FCD tend to perform reasonably well, similar to, or worse than healthy controls, but better than groups with MCI or dementia,[3,31] are significantly biased by use of criteria for a 'subjective' or functional diagnosis based on *normal* cognitive performances. In contrast, patients with FCD can find cognitive testing distressing; resulting in disrupted self-monitoring, expectation, and high levels of anxiety can significantly interfere with cognitive performance. Several FCD case series demonstrate underperformance, cognitive inconsistencies—mainly due to poor selective and divided attention[5,9,28,30]—and poor correlation between subjective symptom severity and objective cognitive performance.[5]

Detailed neuropsychological cognitive testing may be helpful in selected cases to identify domain-specific deficits or for tracking progression and response to treatment.

A few examples of positive clinical features of FCD during cognitive screening or neuropsychological testing include overt anxiety during simple tasks but not during more complex ones (eg, struggling with immediate recall and registration tasks but then performing well on delayed recall of the same items)[30]; a tendency to give 'approximate answers'; and an excessive concern about errors or an undue pessimism about their performance (in contrast with neurodegenerative patients who are not particularly worried about their performance or might not recognize their failures).[7] Another indicator is poor performance on easy parts of the test (eg, orientation, repetition of address) incongruent with reasonable day-to-day function.[7] Wakefield and colleagues were unable to find statistically significant differences between FCD and healthy controls on cognitive performance,[19] and argued that the cognitive deficits in FCD are usually context-dependent, and possibly not evident in calmer test environments.

Another area of controversy and debate is the use and interpretation of performance validity tests in patients with FCD. Patients with FND often do well on these tests; but patients with dementia may fail, even allowing for use of dementia or severe impairment profiles.[9,40] Careful interpretation and detailed explanation of what is being analyzed with these tests (qualitative vs quantitative performance) are needed alongside a clinical assessment of the patient's psychological state and motivation during testing.

Symptom trajectory and prognosis

A major concern for clinicians dealing with patients with memory concerns is the risk of misdiagnosis. Of 46 patients with a functional memory disorder who attended a memory clinic for follow-up examination 20 months after the diagnosis, the symptoms only resolved in 13% of the patients and only one patient had been diagnosed with dementia in that interval.[41] Given that the incidence of dementia during follow-up was exceedingly low, the risk of misdiagnosis of FCD where there is an underlying dementia appears low. On the other hand, this study provides solid evidence against FCD being a benign (spontaneously resolving) disorder. On the contrary, this is a disorder associated with significant morbidity and is in need of evidence-based treatments.

Few studies have examined patient trajectories in those defined as having FCD—the majority focusing on MCI populations. Population-based analysis over a period of 7 years found that 53% of individuals with MCI did not progress, and 35% actually reverted to normal cognition.[42] Taking more prescription medications was associated with being in the stable MCI and reverter groups, whereas having an APOE-ε4 genotype or a history of stroke was associated with progressive MCI.[42] Similarly, although some studies report on conversion rates of MCI to dementia at 1 year follow-up in the range of 15% to 30%, long-term follow-up studies find that many individuals do not convert to dementia even at a 10 year follow-up.[43] Given that, as demonstrated, FCD symptoms can persist over time,[41] it can be assumed that FCD patients accounted for some of these patients who maintained or reverted symptoms in the MCI population studies.[33]

Therapeutic options

Providing patients with FCD with a positive diagnosis allows us to break a cycle of diagnostic uncertainty. In every patient with FCD, the first step in treatment is a clear explanation of how attention is required to commit information to memory. A diagnostic framework using the biopsychosocial model (similar to other FND subtypes) may be adapted to the individual patient. The clinician might share data about the frequency of memory lapses in healthy adults[44] and may want to explore the concept of metacognition. The diagnosis should not be framed as one of exclusion, with an emphasis on negative investigations, and it is important to transparently discuss the internal inconsistencies that confirm the diagnosis.[45] It is particularly relevant to discuss factors that can contribute to cognitive symptoms, including occupational and social demands, cognitive perceptions and expectations, other symptoms such as pain or fatigue, and certain medications.

Currently, there are no approved medications for FCD. The role of psychopharmacology is reserved for the treatment of comorbid psychiatric disorders, such as depression, anxiety, obsessive-compulsive disorder, or attention deficit hyperactivity disorder (ADHD) with a clear developmental history.[46] Clinicians should try to reduce or wean patients from medications that can contribute to cognitive impairment (eg, opioids for pain, benzodiazepines, anticholinergic, and antihistamine drugs). Other medical problems, such as sleep disturbances earlier discussed, should be screened for and managed, alongside personal risk reduction plans (eg, exercise and vascular risk factor control). Patients with significant psychiatric comorbidities may need a referral to or collaborative management with a psychiatrist or neuropsychiatrist. We find neuropsychology intervention useful from both a diagnostic and therapeutic point of view.[5,11,14,46]

There is an urgent need for effective treatments for FCD. A survey conducted in the United Kingdom in 2015 found that 73% of memory service psychiatrists discharged these patients to primary care. Overall, there was no agreement on which treatment is the most appropriate, and treatments included doing nothing, reassurance, psychology assessment, community mental health team referral, or commencement of selective serotonin reuptake inhibitors.[14]

Suggested psychotherapeutic modalities include metacognitive retraining, acceptance and commitment therapy (ACT), and cognitive-behavioral therapy (CBT).[4] CBT and more specifically ACT are promising therapies to tackle the rigid thoughts and feelings toward memory lapses and to promote behavioral steps to optimize attention.[46] Metternich and colleagues conducted a randomized controlled trial to evaluate a novel group therapy consisting of psychoeducation, cognitive restructuring, stress management, relaxation, and mindfulness techniques in 40 patients with functional memory and attention disorder. The intervention provided significant improvement in a measure of memory self-efficacy at 6 months.[47] Similar results were obtained in a randomized trial focused on metamemory memory training over 10 sessions applied to patients with subjective memory complaints.[48] FCD-informed computerized cognitive training and rehabilitation is another promising avenue, with the advantage of overcoming limited resource availability and simultaneously accessing patients in their real-life environments.[49] Recently, Carpenter and colleagues explored the effectiveness of a novel computer-based training to improve the metacognitive ability in healthy adults over eight training sessions. The experimental group showed significant improvement in metacognitive ability compared with the control group and, interestingly, the poorer metacognitive ability was at baseline, the greater the benefits of the training.[50,51] A systematic review looking at interventions in patients with subjective cognitive decline confirmed a lack of high-quality research in this field and the need for more evidence-based treatment strategies.[52]

Future directions

Ongoing research should focus on a better understanding of FCD trajectories including predictors of progression and evidence-based interventions. Further validation of the different positive clinical features is needed, as well as further characterizing features that distinguish FCD from other non-neurodegenerative, neuropsychiatric conditions with prominent cognitive symptoms (eg, dissociative disorders). Exploring the neural substrates of metacognition in FCD using functional imaging techniques is another potential therapeutic avenue.[4,17]

CLINICS CARE POINTS

- FCD may comprise up to around a quarter of the new referrals to tertiary memory clinics.
- Even in cases where there are multiple contributors to cognitive difficulty or an alternative primary diagnosis (such as generalized anxiety disorder or major depression), understanding and identifying contributory FCD mechanisms can open additional treatment targets.

- In FCD, investigations are typically normal, but minor neuroimaging changes such as non-focal atrophy and mild white-matter changes do not exclude this diagnosis.

- FCD is not a diagnosis of exclusion; instead, it should be diagnosed based on positive features of internal inconsistency (historical and clinical clues as well as patterns of performance) and longitudinal follow-up.

- FCD patients often overperform or present a normal cognitive performance, but they may exhibit underperformances or cognitive inconsistencies.

- FCD can remain stable over the years, progress or revert to normal, and is associated with substantial disability.

DISCLOSURES

L. McWhirter receives funding from the Scottish Government Chief Scientist Office. L. McWhirter provides independent medical testimony in court cases regarding patients with functional disorders, is secretary of the British Neuropsychiatry Association, and receives research funding from the Scottish Government Chief Scientist Office. V. Cabreira has received funding from the European Union's Horizon 2020 research and innovation programme under the Marie Skłodowska-Curie grant agreement No 956673. This artilce reflects only V. Cabreira's view, the Agency is not responsible for any use that may be made of the information it contains. A J. Carson is a director of a limited personal services company that provides independent medical testimony in court cases on a range of neuropsychiatric topics on a 50% pursuer 50% defender basis, a paid associate editor of the Journal of Neurology Neurosurgery and Psychiatry, and unpaid president-elect of the International Functional Neurological Disorder Society.

REFERENCES

1. Larner AJ. Impact of the National Dementia Strategy in a neurology-led memory clinic: 5-year data. Clin Med 2014;14(2):216.
2. Ball HA, McWhirter L, Ballard C, et al. Functional cognitive disorder: dementia's blind spot. Brain 2020;143(10):2895–903.
3. Bailey C, Poole N, Blackburn DJ. Identifying patterns of communication in patients attending memory clinics: a systematic review of observations and signs with potential diagnostic utility. Br J Gen Pract 2018;68(667):e123–38.
4. Larner AJ. Functional Cognitive Disorders (FCD): how is metacognition involved? Brain Sci 2021;11(8):1082.
5. McWhirter L, Ritchie C, Stone J, et al. Functional cognitive disorders: a systematic review. Lancet Psychiatr 2020;7(2):191–207.
6. Elsey C, Drew P, Jones D, et al. Towards diagnostic conversational profiles of patients presenting with dementia or functional memory disorders to memory clinics. Patient Educ Couns 2015;98(9):1071–7.
7. Pennington C, Newson M, Hayre A, et al. Functional cognitive disorder: what is it and what to do about it? Practical Neurol 2015;15(6):436–44.
8. Pennington C, Ball H, Swirski M. Functional cognitive disorder: diagnostic challenges and future directions. Diagnostics 2019;9(4):131.
9. Teodoro T, Edwards MJ, Isaacs JD. A unifying theory for cognitive abnormalities in functional neurological disorders, fibromyalgia and chronic fatigue syndrome: systematic review. J Neurol Neurosurg Psychiatry 2018;89(12):1308–19.

10. Stone J, Pal S, Blackburn D, et al. Functional (Psychogenic) cognitive disorders: a perspective from the neurology clinic. J Alzheimers Dis 2015;48(Suppl 1): S5–s17.
11. Hallett M, Aybek S, Dworetzky BA, et al. Functional neurological disorder: new subtypes and shared mechanisms. Lancet Neurol 2022;21(6):537–50.
12. Dunne RA, Aarsland D, O'Brien JT, et al. Mild cognitive impairment: the manchester consensus. Age Ageing 2020;50(1):72–80.
13. McKhann GM, Knopman DS, Chertkow H, et al. The diagnosis of dementia due to Alzheimer's disease: recommendations from the National Institute on Aging-Alzheimer's Association workgroups on diagnostic guidelines for Alzheimer's disease. Alzheimers Dement 2011;7(3):263–9.
14. Bailey C, Bell SM, Blackburn DM. How the UK describes functional memory symptoms. Psychogeriatrics 2017;17(5):336–7.
15. Bertens D, Vos S, Kehoe P, et al. Use of mild cognitive impairment and prodromal AD/MCI due to AD in clinical care: a European survey. Alzheimer's Res Ther 2019; 11(1):74 [Internet].
16. Roberts JS, Karlawish JH, Uhlmann WR, et al. Mild cognitive impairment in clinical care: a survey of American Academy of Neurology members. Neurology 2010;75(5):425–31.
17. Bhome R, McWilliams A, Price G, et al. Metacognition in functional cognitive disorder. Brain Communications 2022;4(2):fcac041.
18. Larner A. Metacognition in functional cognitive disorder: contradictory or convergent experimental results? Brain Communications 2022;4(3):fcac138.
19. Wakefield SJ, Blackburn DJ, Harkness K, et al. Distinctive neuropsychological profiles differentiate patients with functional memory disorder from patients with amnestic-mild cognitive impairment. Acta Neuropsychiatr 2018;30(2):90–6.
20. Frodl T. Do (epi)genetics impact the brain in functional neurologic disorders? Handb Clin Neurol 2016;139:157–65.
21. Larner AJ. Subjective memory complaints: is family history of dementia a risk factor? J Neurol Sci 2013;333:e295.
22. McWhirter L, Ritchie C, Stone J, et al. Identifying functional cognitive disorder: a proposed diagnostic risk model. CNS Spectr 2021;27(6):754–63.
23. Bhome R, Huntley JD, Price G, et al. Clinical presentation and neuropsychological profiles of functional cognitive disorder patients with and without co-morbid depression. Cogn Neuropsychiatry 2019;24(2):152–64.
24. Reuber M, Blackburn DJ, Elsey C, et al. An interactional profile to assist the differential diagnosis of neurodegenerative and functional memory disorders. Alzheimer Dis Assoc Disord 2018;32(3):197–206.
25. Mirheidari B, Blackburn D, Harkness K, et al. Toward the automation of diagnostic conversation analysis in patients with memory complaints. J Alzheimers Dis 2017; 58(2):373–87.
26. Haussmann R, Mayer-Pelinski R, Borchardt M, et al. Extrinsic and intrinsic help-seeking motivation in the assessment of cognitive decline. Am J Alzheimers Dis Other Demen 2018;33(4):215–20.
27. Larner AJ. Neurological signs of possible diagnostic value in the cognitive disorders clinic. Practical Neurol 2014;14(5):332–5.
28. Bharambe V, Larner AJ. Functional cognitive disorders: demographic and clinical features contribute to a positive diagnosis. Neurodegener Dis Manag 2018;8(6): 377–83.
29. Then FS, Luck T, Angermeyer MC, et al. Education as protector against dementia, but what exactly do we mean by education? Age Ageing 2016;45(4):523–8.

30. Ball HA, Swirski M, Newson M, et al. Differentiating functional cognitive disorder from early neurodegeneration: a clinic-based study. Brain Sci 2021;11(6):800.

31. Aarts S, van den Akker M, Hajema KJ, et al. Multimorbidity and its relation to subjective memory complaints in a large general population of older adults. Int Psychogeriatr 2011;23(4):616–24.

32. van Maurik IS, Vos SJ, Bos I, et al. Biomarker-based prognosis for people with mild cognitive impairment (ABIDE): a modelling study. Lancet Neurol 2019; 18(11):1034–44.

33. Petersen RC, Lopez O, Armstrong MJ, et al. Practice guideline update summary: mild cognitive impairment: report of the guideline development, dissemination, and implementation subcommittee of the american academy of neurology. Neurology 2018;90(3):126–35.

34. Pai M-C, Wu C-C, Hou Y-C, et al. Evidence of plasma biomarkers indicating high risk of dementia in cognitively normal subjects. Sci Rep 2022;12(1):1192.

35. Dubois B, Villain N, Frisoni GB, et al. Clinical diagnosis of Alzheimer's disease: recommendations of the International Working Group. Lancet Neurol 2021; 20(6):484–96.

36. Striepens N, Scheef L, Wind A, et al. Volume loss of the medial temporal lobe structures in subjective memory impairment. Dement Geriatr Cogn Disord 2010;29(1):75–81.

37. Ferreira D, Falahati F, Linden C, et al. A 'disease severity index' to identify individuals with subjective memory decline who will progress to mild cognitive impairment or dementia. Sci Rep 2017;7:44368.

38. van Tol M-J, van der Wee NJA, van den Heuvel OA, et al. Regional brain volume in depression and anxiety disorders. Arch Gen Psychiatr 2010;67(10):1002–11.

39. Jansen WJ, Handels RL, Visser PJ, et al. The diagnostic and prognostic value of neuropsychological assessment in memory clinic patients. J Alzheimers Dis 2017;55(2):679–89.

40. McWhirter L, Ritchie CW, Stone J, et al. Performance validity test failure in clinical populations-a systematic review. J Neurol Neurosurg Psychiatry 2020;91(9): 945–52.

41. Schmidtke K, Pohlmann S, Metternich B. The syndrome of functional memory disorder: definition, etiology, and natural course. Am J Geriatr Psychiatr 2008;16(12): 981–8.

42. Ganguli M, Jia Y, Hughes TF, et al. Mild cognitive impairment that does not progress to dementia: a population-based study. J Am Geriatr Soc 2019;67(2):232–8.

43. Canevelli M, Grande G, Lacorte E, et al. Spontaneous reversion of mild cognitive impairment to normal cognition: a systematic review of literature and meta-analysis. J Am Med Dir Assoc 2016;17(10):943–8.

44. Mcwhirter L, King L, McClure E, et al. The frequency and framing of cognitive lapses in healthy adults. CNS Spectr 2021;27:331–8.

45. Stone J, Edwards M. Trick or treat? Showing patients with functional (psychogenic) motor symptoms their physical signs. Neurology 2012;79(3):282–4.

46. Poole NA, Cope SR, Bailey C, et al. Functional cognitive disorders: identification and management. BJPsych Adv 2019;25(6):342–50.

47. Metternich B, Schmidtke K, Härter M, et al. [Development and evaluation of a group therapy for functional memory and attention disorder]. Psychother Psychosom Med Psychol 2010;60(6):202–10.

48. Youn JH, Lee JY, Kim S, et al. Multistrategic memory training with the metamemory concept in healthy older adults. Psychiatry Investig 2011;8(4):354–61.

49. Freeburn J. Speech therapy: being understood clearly. In: LaFaver K, Maurer CW, Nicholson TR, et al, editors. Functional Movement disorder: an Interdisciplinary case-based approach. Cham: Springer International Publishing; 2022. p. 341–52.
50. Carpenter J, Sherman MT, Kievit RA, et al. Domain-general enhancements of metacognitive ability through adaptive training. J Exp Psychol Gen 2019; 148(1):51–64.
51. Bhome R, McWilliams A, Huntley JD, et al. Metacognition in functional cognitive disorder- a potential mechanism and treatment target. Cogn Neuropsychiatry 2019;24(5):311–21.
52. Bhome R, Berry AJ, Huntley JD, et al. Interventions for subjective cognitive decline: systematic review and meta-analysis. BMJ Open 2018;8(7):e021610.

Functional Speech and Voice Disorders

Approaches to Diagnosis and Treatment

Jennifer L. Freeburn, MS, CCC-SLP[a],*, Janet Baker, LACST, MSc, PhD[b]

KEYWORDS

- Functional neurological disorder • Functional movement disorder
- Functional speech disorder • Functional voice disorder • Psychogenic voice
- Psychogenic stutter • Conversion disorder

KEY POINTS

- Functional speech and voice disorders (FSVD) are common, may co-occur with other functional neurological disorder (FND) subtypes, and promote substantial patient distress.
- Diagnosis of FSVD is made following a comprehensive assessment where one or more positive "rule-in" clinical signs may be observed or elicited suggesting an FND cause.
- Therapeutic interventions combining symptomatic and behavioral strategies alongside targeted counseling by the speech and language therapist have the potential to substantially improve patients' functional speech and voice symptoms.

INTRODUCTION

Verbal communication is a primary vehicle for the human expression of needs, thoughts, and feelings as well as a crucial element of social participation. The impact of impairments in communication is extensive, affecting a person's social interactions, relationships, vocation, and overall quality of life.[1]

Disruptions to aspects of motor speech, voice, and language often develop in the setting of neurobiological disorders with a multitude of structural underpinnings including injury and disease. However, it has been well established that biopsychosocial factors may also contribute to communication difficulties, particularly those affecting the neuromotor aspects of speech production.[2] Functional neurological disorder (FND) encompasses a range of neurologic disturbances including motor, sensory, and cognitive symptoms that develop from disruptions in neural networks that mediate both neurophysiologic and intrapsychic processes as opposed to a

[a] Department of Speech, Language, and Swallowing Disorders, Massachusetts General Hospital, Boston, MA, USA; [b] Flinders University, Adelaide, Unit 111/3 Young Street, Randwick, NSW 2031, Australia
* Corresponding author. Functional Neurological Disorder Unit, Department of Neurology, Massachusetts General Hospital, 275 Cambridge Street, POB-3, Boston, MA 02114.
E-mail address: jfreeburn@partners.org

Neurol Clin 41 (2023) 635–646
https://doi.org/10.1016/j.ncl.2023.02.005
0733-8619/23/© 2023 Elsevier Inc. All rights reserved.

physiologic cause alone.[3,4] Functional speech and voice disorders (FSVD) represent one aspect of FND motor symptoms and may occur in isolation or as part of a larger symptom complex.[5,6]

FSVD are common and treatable disorders of communication. Ensuring that providers across disciplines are prepared with essential tools to identify these disorders and connect patients with the most appropriate avenues for the treatment is crucial. Furthermore, increasing the speech and language therapist (SLT) clinical knowledge base and confidence in the treatment of FSVD enables patients to more readily access high-quality care.

HISTORY

FSVD have been documented by physicians for more than 100 years. Within the field of speech and language therapy, the diagnostic classification and naming of these disorders has varied throughout the literature, often with a lack of consistency or clear operational guidelines.[7] The terms "functional," "psychogenic" and/or "conversion" have been used somewhat interchangeably to describe speech and voice disruptions occurring without distinct structural underpinnings.[8] In more recent times, a reversion to the term "functional" has been adopted. This is consistent with current trends in neurology and psychiatry, where "conversion disorder" is now preferentially referred to as FND.[9] It has been argued that the term "functional" is more etiologically and mechanistically neutral because although psychological stressors are often present, their identification is no longer considered a requirement to establish an FND diagnosis.[8,10] We would argue, however, that in a number of patients there seems to be some disturbance to interactions between a patient's psychological processes and sensorimotor function in FSVD, even though the exact mechanism precipitating these symptoms is not yet fully understood.

Graduate and postgraduate education and discipline-specific research programs for SLT have historically offered very limited formal training opportunities in the area of FSVD. As a result, SLTs often report difficulty understanding and managing communication impairments in the setting of FND.[11,12] However, more recent attention to the treatment of FND has highlighted the importance of SLT as part of a multidisciplinary treatment team.[13] Furthermore, recent consensus guidelines for SLT assessment and treatment of functional disorders of communication, swallowing, and cough have now added to the field's knowledge base.[14]

PREVALENCE

FND is common, with patients presenting to primary care, neurology, neuropsychiatry, and rehabilitation specialists including physical, occupational, and speech and language therapies.[4,15,16] An estimated 25% to 50% of patients with FND present with speech and voice symptoms as part of the clinical presentation.[2] Further data detailing the prevalence of FSVD with or without other functional symptoms are not available, perhaps in part due to historic misidentification and underreporting.[5,11,17]

EPIDEMIOLOGY

Functional speech disorders present more frequently in women versus men in a ratio of at least 2:1.[18] In the voice literature covering more broadly termed "functional" dysphonia, patient subgroups clearly defined as having "psychogenic" disorders present in a ratio of approximately 8:1 women to men.[19] FSVD may affect children and adults across the life span, although the prevalence in young children is unknown.[20,21]

ASSESSMENT OF FUNCTIONAL SPEECH AND VOICE DISORDERS

Patients may present to the clinic with sudden onset of isolated unexplained speech changes affecting articulation, voice, prosody, or fluency, or in association with an established FND diagnosis in which speech changes are one of several other presenting symptoms (eg, functional movement disorder, functional seizure, and so forth). Regardless, a thorough assessment is essential both for a confident differential diagnosis and as a basis for future therapy targets. Key elements of the assessment are highlighted here and have been further detailed in additional resources provided.[2,14,22,23]

Medical History and Psychosocial Interview

The initial interview is a clinician's opportunity to collect essential elements of the patient's history as well as any relevant predisposing/precipitating biopsychosocial factors preceding the patient's speech and/or voice changes.[14,24,25] The clinical interviewer should seek to understand the details surrounding the onset of speech/voice changes (eg, the date, any connected medical or personal events, rapidity of onset), the course of these speech changes since that time (eg, stable, worsening, or variable), and the impact of these communication changes on the patient's activities of daily living. It is recommended that the interviewer use both direct and open-ended questions that seek to understand the patient's experience and perspective on the presenting communication disruptions.

Skillful exploration of close family or community/relationship factors that may be perpetuating the patient's current symptoms will contribute to a more in-depth assessment. Here, it may be helpful to draw on ethnographic and narrative therapy interviewing styles to encourage discussion of psychosocial variables that the patient has recognized may be aggravating their present symptoms.[26,27]

Speech Data Collection and Analysis

The core components of FSVD assessment do not differ greatly from established principles of SLT assessment of motor speech and voice disorders more broadly. These tasks are outlined extensively elsewhere.[18,28] As FND can affect any and multiple areas of speech production, the assessment should include a thorough investigation of speech and voice subsystem functioning across a variety of verbal tasks.[2,23] Additional tasks that include a component of the patient's interests (eg, discussing preferred topics), distraction (eg, completing a card sort or visual trails task while speaking), and/or nonspeech vocalization (eg, humming/singing) may also be valuable to observing patient presentation across contexts.

The clinician's observation and auditory-perceptual analysis of patient performance during individual tasks and comparatively between tasks is essential for differential diagnosis. Therefore, audio and/or video recordings may be helpful for reviewing both auditory-perceptual ratings as well as any incongruities, inconsistencies, or evidence of normal speech and voice across time and assessment task.

DIFFERENTIAL DIAGNOSIS

A full workup examining underlying structural or other medical causes for speech and vocal dysfunction is an important part of differential diagnosis. Specifically, contributions from neurology, otolaryngology, gastroenterology, and respiratory medicine may be integral to the multidisciplinary team approach to assessment.[14] The role of the SLT is pivotal to the process of differential diagnosis by facilitating and observing any positive clinical signs during specifically targeted assessment activities of speech and voice. This also requires careful consideration of aspects of the patient's psychosocial history taken by the SLT during the initial or subsequent sessions.

Positive clinical signs of functional speech/voice disorder on examination include.

- Incongruity between initiation of voluntary functions while automatic functions are usually preserved (eg, patient cannot initiate voice during speech but produces a clear natural voice while yawning or laughing)
- Inefficient/nonergonomic patterns of movement, including clearly excessive effort
- Inconsistency with known structural neurologic disease patterns (eg, give-way tongue or jaw weakness, unusually variable patterns of fatigue)
- Internal inconsistency across tasks (eg, observable change to fluency based on context and topic), and/or overtly distractible (eg, normal phonation during spontaneous gross bodily movements or reflexive tasks such as laughter)
- Reversibility of symptoms and/or suggestibility wherein symptoms worsen with focused attention from the patient or the clinician
- Rapid modifiability of speech abnormalities, such that there is substantial improvement and even resolution of speech or voice symptoms within the diagnostic session
- Atypical agrammatism in the absence of aphasia

Further information on gathering and describing the distinguishing assessment features of FSVD have been extensively detailed elsewhere.[8,14,29]

Although historical information alone cannot be considered "rule-in" for an FND diagnosis, some reported patterns of onset, course, and precipitating events have been observed in both FVSD and other FND subtypes.[30–33] These include symptom onset that occurs:

- suddenly, while not directly attributable to another structural/neurologic condition;
- in association with a physical injury or illness (eg, upper respiratory tract infection, surgical intervention in adjacent structures, benign blunt injury to the face, mouth, or neck); and/or
- within the context of stressful life events and longer term difficulties including situations characterized by conflict over speaking out, powerlessness in the system, and lower perceived sense of agency.

Several common clinical manifestations of FSVD have been identified and may also help to contribute to differential diagnosis. Please see **Table 1** for a detailed listing of these common presentations. The sudden emergence of one or more of these symptom patterns outside of a known developmental or neurologically mediated cause may suggest a FSVD.[2,14,22,34] However, a departure from these patterns does not rule out FSVD given the known extent of heterogeneity of patient presentations. Furthermore, many patients may present with symptoms that span or vary between 2 or more common phenotypes.

It is important to note that the presence of overtly structural findings (eg, vocal fold pathologic condition, notable findings on brain imaging) does not exclude FSVD from the diagnosis. In fact, atypical features suggestive of functional neurologic symptoms may co-occur with neurologic pathologic condition and/or structural changes (eg, functional/psychogenic aphonia superimposed on a successfully medialized vocal fold paresis).[35] This highlights the importance of a thorough assessment by the SLT in consultation with the patient's full medical team to differentiate elements of the presentation resulting from structural damage/disease from those that are consistent with a FSVD.

Table 1 Common clinical presentations of functional speech/voice disorder	
Speech Phenotypes	
Functional stutter	Unusual and anomalous patterns of disfluency (sound repetitions, prolongations, and/or hesitation) with patterns incongruous with developmental stuttering
Functional "foreign accent"	Prosodic variations sometimes accompanied by articulatory errors and/or agrammatism that perceptually mimic an accent other than the patient's own
Functional "infantile" speech	Variable pattern of articulatory errors and/or intonation patterns that perceptually mimic childlike speech; may be accompanied by immature/idiosyncratic language patterns
Voice Phenotypes	
Functional aphonia/dysphonia	Sudden or intermittent loss of volitional control over the initiation and maintenance of normal phonation despite normal structure and function as demonstrated during laryngoscopy and clinical examination
Functional mutism	Involuntary failure to produce speech sounds, even during a whisper, or words may be mouthed with accurate but inaudible articulatory movements (distinct from selective mutism, which is a conscious voluntary refusal to speak in specific social contexts)
Mutational falsetto (puberphonia)	Abnormally high-pitched falsetto phonation after puberty despite normal low-pitched voice appropriate to age and gender being possible
Odynophonia	Pain associated with voice use out of proportion to normal structure and function as demonstrated during laryngoscopy and clinical examination

TREATMENT PRINCIPLES

Treatment of FSVD should be highly tailored to the individual patient's speech presentation, learning needs, motivation, and tolerance for the physical and cognitive demands of therapy sessions.[36] For a subset of patients experiencing FSVD, symptomatic therapy alone may lead to rapid resolution of the communication impairment. However, the complex biopsychosocial underpinnings of FND often necessitate therapeutic approaches that combine direct symptomatic treatment alongside exploration of predisposing and perpetuating psychosocial factors.[14]

Importantly, much of this exploratory counseling can be done by the SLT without additional training, simply by holding a psychotherapeutic mindset and allowing ample time for discussion of relevant psychosocial factors.[14,25] More formalized counseling models may also add value, although these do require additional SLT training and expertise. These may include educational and supportive person-centered approaches, action-oriented models with a focus on problem solving, motivational interviewing, systems theory and family dynamics, and/or cognitive behavioral therapy approaches. See **Box 1** and **Box 2** for illustrative (anonymized) examples of treatment principles in FSVDs.

Treatment Hierarchy

Although acknowledging the importance of an individualized approach to FSVD treatment, a set of core treatment principles combining both symptomatic and psychosocial approaches may be applied. This hierarchy of SLT treatment tasks is outlined

> **Box 1**
> **Treatment Case—Facilitating Change through Combined Symptomatic Treatment and Counseling**
>
> Laura, a 47-year-old cisgender white female, monolingual in English, presented to the outpatient neurology clinic with a constellation of symptoms including gait disturbance, dense retrograde amnesia, and an altered speech pattern consistent with FND as determined by the attending neurologist. The sudden onset of symptoms occurred ~1 week following a car accident during which the patient sustained a mild uncomplicated traumatic brain injury without loss of consciousness. Further psychosocial history included childhood abuse and longstanding anxiety. Laura reported no memory of her life before the accident but her husband described her as extremely high functioning at baseline, noting that she had been caregiving for an ailing relative in addition to working full-time before the accident. The patient was referred to SLT for further assessment and treatment.
>
> **Assessment**
>
> Rule-in features of FSVD on examination included give-way tongue weakness bilaterally to resistance, excessively consistent disfluency with visible effort, speech with variable articulatory breakdowns characteristic of developmental errors (eg, substitution of/t/for velar/k/and/w/for/ r/and/l/), immature prosodic abnormalities (eg, exaggerated pitch variation), and atypical agrammatic language patterns (eg, "I does it"; "me likey that").
>
> **Treatment**
>
> Following extensive education, the patient verbalized a basic understanding of the FND diagnosis by often repeating "my brain wires are crossed." She expressed initial doubt that treatment would be effective since, as she stated, "I don't remember that person" (regarding her former self).
>
> Laura was immediately stimulable for improved articulatory accuracy simply given visual models of placement (eg, showing interdental tongue placement of/l/), although with excess effort in all cases. She showed some improvement with less extreme effort during tasks of mimicking phrases and prosodic variation of celebrity videos. However, neither strategy translated into any spontaneous speech regardless of cuing.
>
> The clinician then encountered a sample of Laura's speech from before the car accident and FSVD onset on the patient's voicemail greeting. After listening to this short speech sample within a session, Laura became emotional and tearful. She was guided to reflect aloud on the differences between her prior and present speech, including the relative ease of her speech in that message. With ongoing counseling, she was encouraged to reflect further on changes to her family roles and relationships with others in the setting of FND, as well as what she had learned from others about her prior functioning. After additional structured reflection led by the SLT, Laura began to identify emotions associated with, in her words, feeling "detached from" and "less than" her former self.
>
> During the following treatment sessions, Laura made substantial gains in the fluency and accuracy of her speech output. Most notably, the excess effort that had marked nearly every utterance had almost entirely subsided. She began to apply articulatory and prosodic strategies during sentence and conversational level tasks with frequent self-corrections. She continued to make slow, steady gains toward a more typical speech pattern and report increased perception of control of her speech.

below, drawing on several detailed resources that provide more specific guidance on therapeutic techniques.[2,14,18,24,36]

1. Explain and provide education regarding the FSVD diagnosis.
   a. Demonstrate the rationale for the diagnosis, including explanation of positive functional signs demonstrated on examination.

Box 2
Treatment Case—Generalizing Normal Voice Through Counseling

Ben, a 15-year-old adolescent, presented with a 4-year history of severe dysphonia, diagnosed as a functional puberphonia (inappropriately high-pitched falsetto phonation, after normal healthy pubertal changes). He had been seen by numerous specialists from otolaryngology, speech pathology, and clinical psychology, with minimal involvement of his family.

Assessment

Laryngoscopic assessments confirmed normal laryngeal and vocal fold structures. However, severe supraglottic constriction interfered with the view and function of the true vocal folds. Botox administered to facilitate relaxation of this extreme pattern of supraglottic constriction had not been successful.

Despite all other signs of normal maturation beginning at the age of 11 years, Ben's vocal pitch remained abnormally high, with vocal instability and uncontrollable pitch breaks from his habitual falsetto phonation to a rough diplophonic (2 tones perceived simultaneously) voice. Ben was inexorably shy and appeared highly anxious, avoiding any eye contact. He did not report any stressful life events or longer term difficulties either at the time of onset of his pubertal changes or since the onset of his severe dysphonia. He did comment on his embarrassment and sense of desperation about his dysphonia, which was setting him apart from his peers. His parents and teachers were most concerned about the effect that this was having on his school attendance and friendships. The SLT delicately explored issues related to his maturing sexuality but Ben reported no concerns.

Treatment

Traditional symptomatic and behavioral techniques proved ineffective, and it took many months until Ben was able to produce any normal voice. During the sessions focused on symptomatic resolution, the SLT offered educational, motivational, and supportive counseling for both Ben and his family, with assurance that resolution was possible and that she (the SLT) would persevere for as long as they did.

Quite serendipitously, it was discovered by a family member that Ben's normal deep voice could be heard when he laughed while watching television. This offered an opening. A strategy was devised to record his voice, with his permission, during a particular program that he enjoyed, and for the first time, in the form of free uninhibited emotional laughter, the SLT recorded his normal voice at a pitch and quality appropriate to his age and maturity.

After weeks of tentative and variable use of his normal deep voice in the clinical setting, further generalization was encouraged. He and the SLT developed a "hierarchy of threat" identifying those family members, peers, teachers, or others that were relatively "safe," and he gradually consolidated his new voice first to these safe spaces and then to other settings.

Ben was encouraged to decide when he thought it was a good time to leave therapy, knowing that he could always return in the face of any relapse or concerns.[46] Some 5 months later, although he had maintained his normal voicing since discharge from treatment, he rang and asked if he could return briefly "to discuss a sensitive dilemma." He said he now thought ready to address "an issue that had plagued him" since the age of 12 when his voice started to break. This was his fear and realization that he may be gay. It was something that he could barely articulate for himself at the time, let alone share with his parents or others. In reflecting on the earlier conversations with his SLT about feelings or attitudes regarding his sexual maturity, he now proposed a connection between this underlying emotional dilemma and his difficulties in accommodating his natural voice.

---

    b. Supplement education with video and audio recordings of the patient's speech productions whenever possible.
2. Identify symptomatic behaviors and how they differ from typical speech/voice production.

    a. Support patient awareness of breakdowns using playback of speech samples.

    b. Discuss normal anatomic function and relatively low volitional effort and attention typically required for speech movements.

3. Introduce strategies to facilitate natural movement and/or regain volitional control.

    a. Encourage effortless and natural speech production through a variety of tasks such as reflexive sounds, automatic speech, imitation of the clinician or another speaker, and relaxation strategies.

    b. Praise any change in the atypical pattern, even if initially imperfect.

4. Build toward lengthier and more meaningful speech/voice production.

    a. Increase speech task complexity (eg, from sounds to phrases to sentences) as well as cognitive demands (eg, addition of background noise, incorporation of additional communication partners).

5. Help patients notice and challenge unhelpful illness beliefs and address any changeable psychosocial barriers to change.

    a. Integrate psychotherapeutically informed counseling to support patients in coping with negative emotions in anticipation of perceived threat in family, social, or work communication settings.[25,37]

6. Incorporate and generalize improved speech and voice behaviors into relevant daily communication with particular attention to the patient's interpersonal relationships and wider social contexts.

7. Discuss self-cueing strategies for possible setbacks/relapse and support the patient in identifying the appropriate timing and options for outreach to seek clinical help again in the future.

The initial steps of this hierarchy are crucial to supporting the patient's understanding of the diagnosis and beginning to build toward their increased sense of control over symptoms. In contrast, the steps following facilitation of natural movements are less prescriptive in order. Although the timing and extent of counseling integrated into symptomatic work may vary from one patient to the next, it is often essential to the success of generalizing change and/or supporting carryover to everyday communication contexts.

Complications for Treatment

Although patients generally begin to demonstrate at least some potential to change within the first session, there may be some factors that hinder progress in treatment. These barriers may be obvious at the assessment or may emerge during the treatment process. Although the factors discussed here may influence a patient's potential to improve with SLT treatment, it is not recommended that any factor alone be considered a reason to deny treatment.

- Patient readiness for change: A patient's acceptance of the FSVD/FND diagnosis is considered one of the most important factors in predicting a positive prognosis.[38] Similarly, the willingness to change is particularly essential for success in the treatment of FSVD. Understanding a patient's readiness to engage in treatment may begin with motivational interviewing although ultimately requires clinical observation across an initial series of treatment sessions.

- Indifference to or denial of the speech disruption: patients may deny issues with communication or express indifference toward the change. This apparent lack of distress may reduce the patient's motivation for the treatment and thereby stand in the way of progress.

- Significant medical comorbidities: Interfering (perpetuating) factors, most prominently including pain and fatigue, may limit the patient's tolerance for travel to clinic visits and/or participation in the treatment sessions themselves. In some cases, treatment specifically addressing pain may be recommended as a precursor to participation in SLT.[36]

- Worker's compensation and/or litigation related to the symptoms: The complications of pending legal cases including required second medical opinions, revisiting potentially traumatic events repeatedly during trials, and the implications of recovery and returning to threatening work environment before cases are settled may affect the progress and final outcomes for some patients.[14]

Clinical Outcomes

At this time, outcome data for the treatment of FSVD are limited.[10] Several reasons for the scarcity of empirical evidence have been suggested, including underreporting of speech and voice symptoms in FND literature, a historical lack of clear "rule-in" diagnostic criteria for FSVD, and problematic variations in terminology.[8,10,17,]

The existing publications on treatment outcomes in FSVD have demonstrated positive treatment results but have been largely confined to case samples or a subset of clinical presentations.[39–43] That said, multiple case studies have demonstrated excellent potential for patient improvement through SLT interventions combining symptomatic therapy with targeted counseling as described throughout this article.[2,29,35,36] A recently published retrospective case series of 20 patients reported positive but variable treatment outcomes in FSVD, with 15 patients showing improvement yet only 3 patients discharging from therapy without any symptoms.[44] This is largely aligned with data for patients within a broader spectrum of functional movement disorder, which has shown the potential for improvement yet with overall mixed outcomes.[45]

Without a doubt, further evidence is needed to better understand and predict therapeutic outcomes for patients with FSVD and to provide guidance for optimizing the timing, intensity, and frequency of SLT interventions.

SUMMARY

Professionals across medical disciplines will inevitably encounter FSVD and therefore will benefit from understanding the core features of the presentation of these disorders. A referral for comprehensive evaluation by SLT is often helpful in further identifying rule-in signs of a FSVD and assessing the patient's potential to benefit from therapeutic intervention. For the SLT, an increased understanding of the mechanisms of speech and voice disorders in FND is crucial, alongside building increased confidence for applying symptomatic treatment and in-depth counseling to form holistic biopsychosocial intervention for patients.

CLINICS CARE POINTS

Assessment
- Collection of patient history should explore details regarding onset of speech/voice changes, present pattern of changes (consistent vs sporadic), influence that communication changes have had on patient's activities of daily living, and relevant biopsychosocial variables.
- Examination must document performance across a variety of speech tasks, ideally supplemented by video or audio recording to aid in perceptual analysis.
- Differential diagnostic factors suggestive of FND should be documented specifically and may include a presentation consistent with known functional speech/voice subtypes, significant variability across tasks, and internal inconsistency.

Treatment

- Diagnostic therapy, education, and appropriate levels of counseling by the SLT are foundational to therapeutic efficacy.
- Strategies for facilitating motor change are patient-specific and focused on achieving increased automaticity and resumption of voluntary control over speech and voice output.
- Exploring psychosocial themes and offering supportive counseling may be relevant throughout the treatment hierarchy.
- Treatment goals should include resolution of functional speech and voice symptoms with psychological support for the patient to generalize their normalized speech/voice across daily communication settings.

DECLARATION OF INTERESTS

The authors have no relevant financial disclosures.

REFERENCES

1. Neumann S, Quinting J, Rosenkranz A, et al. Quality of life in adults with neurogenic speech-language-communication difficulties: A systematic review of existing measures. J Commun Disord 2019;79:24–5.
2. Utianski RL, Duffy JR. Understanding, recognizing, and managing functional speech disorders: current thinking illustrated with a case series. Am J Speech Lang Pathol 2022;31(3):1205–20.
3. Voon V, Cavanna A, Coburn K, et al. Functional neuroanatomy and neurophysiology of functional neurological disorders (Conversion Disorder). J Neuropsychiatry Clin Neurosci 2016;28:168–90.
4. Stone J, Burton C, Carson A. Recognising and explaining functional neurological disorder. BMJ 2020;371:m3745.
5. Baizabal-Carvallo JF, Jankovic J. Speech and voice disorders in patients with psychogenic movement disorders. J Neurol 2015;262(11):2420–4.
6. Chung DS, Wettroth C, Hallett M, et al. Functional speech and voice disorders: case series and literature review. Mov Disord Clin Pract 2018;5(3):312–6.
7. Payten CL, Chiapello G, Weir KA, et al. Frameworks, terminology and definitions used for the classification of voice disorders: a scoping review. J Voice 2022. https://doi.org/10.1016/j.jvoice.2022.02.009.
8. Baker J. Functional voice disorders: clinical presentations and differential diagnosis. In: Hallett M, Stone J, Carson A, editors. Handbook of clinical neurology functional neurologic disorders. Amsterdam: Elsevier; 2016. p. 379–88.
9. American Psychiatric Association. Diagnostic and statistical manual of mental disorders. In: Text revision). 5th edition. American Psychiatric Association Publishing; 2022.
10. Barnett C, Armes J, Smith C. Speech, language and swallowing impairments in functional neurological disorder: a scoping review. Int J Lang Comm Dis 2018;1–12.
11. Barnett C, Mitchell C, Tyson S. The management of patients with functional stroke: speech and language therapists' views and experiences. Disabil Rehabil 2022;44(14):3547–58.
12. Gregory C. Stern-Pooley R. Power, E. et al. "Luckily I haven't had one for a while": Current management of clients with functional psychogenic voice disorder by speech pathologists in Australia. FNDS Conference Poster Presentation; 2022.
13. LaFaver K, Ricciardi L. Interdisciplinary rehabilitation approaches in functional movement disorder. In: LaFaver K, Maurer C, Nicholson T, et al, editors.

Functional movement disorder: an interdisciplinary case-based approach. Cham: Springer; 2022. p. 353–65.

14. Baker J, Barnett C, Cavalli L, et al. Management of functional communication, swallowing, cough, and related disorders: consensus recommendations for speech and language therapy. J Neurol Neurosurg Psychiatry 2021;1–14.

15. Stone J, Carson A, Duncan R, et al. Who is referred to neurology clinics? –The diagnoses made in 3781 new patients. Clin Neurol Neurosurg 2010;112(9): 747–51.

16. Aybek S, Perez DL. Diagnosis and management of functional neurological disorder. BMJ 2022;376:o64.

17. De Letter M, Van Borsel J, Penen K, et al. Non-organic language disorders: three case reports. Aphasiology 2012;26:867–79.

18. Duffy JR. Motor speech disorders: substrates, differential diagnosis, and management. 4th Edition. Elsevier; 2020.

19. Baker J. The role of psychogenic and psychosocial factors in the development of functional voice disorders. Int J Speech Lang Pathol 2008;10:210–30.

20. Sunde KE, Hilliker DR, Fischer PR. Understanding and managing adolescents with conversation and functional disorders. Pediatr Rev 2020;41(12):630–41.

21. Bennett K, Diamond C, Hoeritzauer I, et al. A practical review of functional neurological disorder (FND) for the general physician. Clin Med 2021;21(1):28–36.

22. Aronson A, Bless D. Clinical voice disorders. 4th Edition. New York: Thieme; 2009.

23. Maurer C, Duffy JR. Functional speech and voice disorders. In: LaFaver K, Maurer C, Nicholson T, et al, editors. *Functional movement disorder: an interdisciplinary case-based approach*. Cham: Springer; 2022. p. 157–68.

24. Butcher P, Elias A, Cavalli L. Understanding and treating psychogenic voice disorder: a cognitive behaviour framework. West Sussex: Wiley; 2007.

25. Baker J. Psychosocial perspectives on the management of voice disorders. Compton Publishing; 2017.

26. Westby CE, Burda AN, Mehta Z. Asking the right questions in the right ways: Strategies for ethnographic interviewing. The ASHA Leader 2003;8:4–17. https://leader.pubs.asha.org/doi/10.1044/leader.FTR3.08082003.4.

27. Di Lollo A, Neimeyer RA. Counselling in speech-language pathology and audiology. San Diego: Plural Publishing; 2014.

28. Dysarthria in adults. American speech-language-hearing association. 2022. Retrieved 08/2022 from. www.asha.org/Practice-Portal/Clinical-Topics/Dysarthria-in-Adults/.

29. Duffy JR. Functional speech disorders: clinical manifestations, diagnosis, and management. In: Hallett M, Stone J, Carson A, editors. *Handbook of clinical neurology functional neurologic disorders*. Amsterdam: Elsevier; 2016. p. 379–88.

30. Frazier P, Merians A, Misono S. Perceived control and voice handicap in patients with voice disorders. Health Psychol 2017;36(11):1105–8.

31. Ludwig L, Pasman JA, Nicholson T, et al. Stressful life events and maltreatment in conversion (functional neurological) disorder: systematic review and meta-analysis of case-control studies. Lancet Psychiatr 2018;5:307–20.

32. Espay AJ, Aybek S, Carson A, et al. Current concepts in diagnosis and treatment of functional neurological disorders. JAMA Neurol 2018;75:1132–41.

33. Perez DL, Aybek A, Popkirov S, et al. A review and expert opinion on the neuropsychiatric assessment of motor functional neurological disorders. J Neuropsychiatry Clin Neurosci 2021;33:14–26.

34. McWhirter L, Miller N, Campbell C, et al. Understanding foreign accent syndrome. J Neurol Neurosurg Psychiatry 2019;1–5.
35. Baker J. Psychogenic voice disorders and traumatic stress experience: a discussion paper with two case reports. J Voice 2003;17(3):308–18.
36. Freeburn J. Speech therapy: being understood clearly. In: LaFaver K, Maurer C, Nicholson T, et al, editors. *Functional movement disorder: an interdisciplinary case-based approach*. Cham: Springer; 2022. p. 341–52.
37. Miller T, Deary V, Patterson J. Improving access to psychological therapies in voice disorders: a cognitive behavioural therapy model. Curr Opin Otolaryngol Head Neck Surg 2014;22:201–5.
38. LaFaver K, Lang AE, Stone J, et al. Opinions and clinical practices related to diagnosing and managing functional (psychogenic) movement disorders: changes in the last decade. Eur J Neurol 2020;1–10.
39. Roth CR, Aronson AE, Davis LJ Jr. Clinical studies in psychogenic stuttering of adult onset. J Speech Hear Disord 1989;54(4):634–46.
40. Duffy JR, Baumgartner J. Psychogenic stuttering in adults with and without neurologic disease. J Med Speech Lang Pathol 1997;5(2):75–95.
41. Roy N, Dietrich M, Blomgren M, et al. Exploring the neural bases of primary muscle tension dysphonia: a case study using functional magnetic resonance imaging. J Voice 2017;33:183–94.
42. Carding P, Bos-Clark M, Fu S, et al. Evaluating the efficacy of voice therapy for functional organic and neurological voice disorders. Clin Otolaryngol 2017;42: 201–17.
43. Deary V, McColl E, Carding P, et al. A psychosocial intervention in the treatment of functional dysphonia: Complex intervention development and pilot randomized control trial. Pilot Feasibility Stud 2018;4. https://doi.org/10.1186/s40814-018-0240-5.
44. Goldstein AN, Paredes-Echeverri S, Finkelstein SA, et al. Speech and language therapy: a treatment case series of 20 patients with functional speech disorder. Neurorehab 2023 (in press).
45. Gelauff J, Stone J, Edwards M, et al. The prognosis of functional (psychogenic) motor symptoms: a systematic review. J Neurol Neurosurg Psychiatry 2014;84: 220–6.
46. Baker J. The therapeutic relationship once established, need never be broken. IJSLP 2010;12(4):309–12.

Persistent Postural-Perceptual Dizziness

Review and Update on Key Mechanisms of the Most Common Functional Neuro-otologic Disorder

Jeffrey P. Staab, MD, MS[a,b],*

KEYWORDS

- Functional dizziness • Functional neurological disorder • Locomotion
- Persistent postural-perceptual dizziness • Perception of motion • Postural control
- Spatial orientation

KEY POINTS

- Persistent postural-perceptual dizziness (PPPD) is the most common chronic neuro-otologic disorder in primary care settings, neurologic practices, and specialized dizziness clinics.
- PPPD is a functional neuro-otologic (vestibular) disorder, a recognized subtype of functional neurological disorder. Its primary pathophysiologic processes are alterations in functioning of neurologic systems that manage postural control, locomotion, and spatial orientation.
- PPPD is precipitated by various conditions that cause vestibular symptoms or disrupt balance and promoted by excessive body vigilance, aberrant illness–related beliefs, and overreliance on visual cues for spatial orientation.
- Emerging data suggest that PPPD is perpetuated by misperceptions of motion that shift top-down priorities from controlling fluid locomotion to maintaining postural stability.
- Treatment with individualized vestibular rehabilitation exercises, serotonin reuptake inhibitors, and cognitive behavioral therapy alone or in combination reduces the substantial handicap of PPPD for most patients.

[a] Department of Psychiatry and Psychology, Mayo Clinic, 200 1st Street Southwest, Rochester, MN 55905, USA; [b] Department of Otorhinolaryngology–Head and Neck Surgery, Mayo Clinic, 200 1st Street Southwest, Rochester, MN 55905, USA
* Department of Psychiatry and Psychology, Mayo Clinic, 200 1st Street Southwest, Rochester, MN 55905.
E-mail address: staab.jeffrey@mayo.edu

Neurol Clin 41 (2023) 647–664
https://doi.org/10.1016/j.ncl.2023.04.003
0733-8619/23/© 2023 Elsevier Inc. All rights reserved.
neurologic.theclinics.com

INTRODUCTION

Persistent postural-perceptual dizziness (PPPD) was defined as a chronic functional neuro-otologic (vestibular) disorder for the International Classification of Vestibular Disorders in 2017[1] and International Classification of Diseases, 11th edition in 2022.[2] Its core symptoms are nonvertiginous dizziness, unsteadiness, and swaying or rocking (nonspinning) vertigo that are present most hours of the day, most days of the week (**Box 1**, criterion A). Patients describe their dizziness as heavy-, light-, or foggy-headedness and unsteadiness as wobbling, swaying, or rocking, which may not be observable by others. Some patients report subtle illusions that fixed objects in the environment are not quite still. Once PPPD is established, symptoms are exacerbated by upright posture (sitting or standing), active and passive movement, and exposure to environments with complex or moving visual stimuli (see **Box 1**, criterion B). A recent study of patients examined within 90 days of new-onset vestibular symptoms found that 50% experienced difficulties with at least one of these exacerbating factors, but hypersensitivity to all 3 was strongly associated with development of PPPD.[3] PPPD may be precipitated by peripheral or central vestibular disorders, other medical conditions, and periods of psychological distress (see **Box 1**, criterion C) that can cause vestibular symptoms or disrupt balance. The proportions of these precipitants were examined in 2 cross-sectional investigations of patients with chronic subjective dizziness, a predecessor of PPPD,[4,5] and 2 retrospective studies of patients meeting criteria for PPPD.[6,7] Peripheral or central vestibular disorders (eg, benign paroxysmal positional vertigo, unilateral peripheral vestibulopathies, stroke)

Box 1
Diagnostic criteria for persistent postural-perceptual dizziness from the International Classification of Vestibular Disorders

A. One or more symptoms of dizziness, unsteadiness, or nonspinning vertigo are present on most days for 3 months or more.
  1. Symptoms last for prolonged (hours-long) periods of time but may wax and wane in severity.
  2. Symptoms need not be present continuously throughout the entire day.

B. Persistent symptoms occur without specific provocation but are exacerbated by 3 factors:
  1. Upright posture
  2. Active or passive motion without regard to direction or position
  3. Exposure to moving visual stimuli or complex visual patterns

C. The disorder is precipitated by conditions that cause vertigo, unsteadiness, dizziness, or problems with balance including acute, episodic, or chronic vestibular syndromes, other neurologic or medical illnesses, or psychological distress.
  1. When the precipitant is an acute or episodic condition, symptoms settle into the pattern of criterion A as the precipitant resolves, but they may occur intermittently at first, and then consolidate into a persistent course.
  2. When the precipitant is a chronic syndrome, symptoms may develop slowly at first and worsen gradually.

D. Symptoms cause significant distress or functional impairment.

E. Symptoms are not better accounted for by another disease or disorder.

Reprinted from Staab JP, Eckhardt-Henn A, Horii A, Jacob R, Strupp M, Brandt T, Bronstein A (2017) Diagnostic criteria for persistent postural-perceptual dizziness (PPPD): Consensus document of the committee for the Classification of Vestibular Disorders of the Barany Society. J Vestib Res 27(4):191-208 with permission of IOS Press and the authors.

triggered PPPD in 21% to 25% of patients. Neurologic illnesses also triggered about one-quarter of cases, although specific diagnoses varied among studies: vestibular migraine (11%–25% of patients), mild traumatic brain injury (3%–15%), and dysautonomias (1%–7%). Psychiatric disorders, particularly panic and generalized anxiety disorders, were identified in 20% to 25% of patients in 3 studies,[4–6] with a higher rate of 42% in the fourth report.[7] Medical conditions including paroxysmal cardiac dysrhythmias and metabolic illnesses precipitated 3% to 11% of cases. To warrant a diagnosis of PPPD, patients must have distressing or impairing symptoms (see **Box 1**, criterion D). The final criterion (see **Box 1**, criterion E) ensures proper consideration of patients' entire clinical presentations in making final diagnoses by ruling PPPD in (or out), either as a sole diagnosis or coexisting with other illnesses.[1,8,9] A diagnosis of PPPD, similar to diagnoses of other functional neurological disorder subtypes,[10] is made by positively identifying its key features. Criterion E does not mean that PPPD is a diagnosis of exclusion.[1,8,9]

EPIDEMIOLOGY

After PPPD was defined in 2017, 5 studies gave information about its prevalence in clinical settings.[11–15] Among adults in primary care, 14.4% of 229 patients presenting to a general internal medicine clinic with chief complaints of vestibular or balance symptoms were diagnosed with PPPD.[16] Among adults in neurology clinics, studies from 3 countries,[11–13] including 2 that were quite large (N = 9200, N = 21,267),[12,13] found a remarkably consistent point prevalence of 20% (range 19.0%–21.8%) in patients referred for vestibular complaints. Among adults in a dedicated multidisciplinary dizziness clinic, 53.4% of 292 patients with chronic dizziness had PPPD either as their sole diagnosis (9.2%) or more commonly coexisting with other illnesses (44.2%).[14] Among children and adolescents in a tertiary pediatric balance clinic, 7.3% of 1021 patients were diagnosed with PPPD.[15] In a nonclinical study,[17] situations that exacerbate symptoms of PPPD, such as self-motion and exposure to moving visual stimuli (see **Box 1**, criterion B), also bothered substantial portions (10%–50%) of people without neuro-otologic diagnoses (cohorts of research volunteers, students, paid on-line survey participants). To date, no systematic epidemiologic investigations of PPPD have been conducted in the general population.

In studies of adult patients with PPPD, average ages ranged from 53 to 59 years and women outnumbered men by 2:1,[11,13,14] which is consistent with data on patients with phobic postural vertigo[18] and chronic subjective dizziness.[4] In one study of children, adolescents, and young adults, the average age was 14.6 years (range 8–22 years) and women outnumbered men by 5:1.[15]

The incidence of PPPD following precipitating events is unknown but may be estimated from a systematic review of 13 prospective and retrospective investigations predating publication of the definition of PPPD. These studies examined chronic PPPD-like dizziness following acute vestibular syndromes, mostly vestibular neuritis and benign paroxysmal positional vertigo, in 780 patients.[18] The percentage of patients in whom dizziness persisted for at least 3 months after inciting illnesses ranges from 7.5% to 53% (weighted mean of 26.3%). A retrospective review of patients who presented to a tertiary neurotology center within 90 days of new-onset vestibular symptoms suggested that the incidence of PPPD could be at the lower end of that range.[3] In that study, only 8/155 (5.2%) patients developed PPPD over 18 months of follow-up. Seven of eight patients met criteria for PPPD at the time of their initial evaluations except for the 3-month duration of illness, suggesting that PPPD may consolidate within a short period of time after precipitating illnesses for most patients who develop the disorder. If this finding is verified in future investigations, then it would inform strategies for early identification of patients at risk for PPPD, potentially minimizing long-term disability and secondary psychiatric comorbidity.[19,20]

DIAGNOSTIC CONSIDERATIONS

The initial clinical course of PPPD depends on the nature of precipitating illnesses. When triggered by acute vestibular syndromes (eg, vestibular neuritis), symptoms of PPPD begin to consolidate as the acute illnesses resolve.[1,3] Patients do not have asymptomatic intervals. Instead, their symptoms evolve from acute vertigo of precipitating illnesses into chronic nonvertiginous symptoms and hypersensitivities of PPPD. When precipitants are episodic vestibular syndromes (eg, benign paroxysmal positional vertigo, vestibular migraine, panic disorder), symptoms of PPPD may begin in full after the first attack, such that patients have no symptom-free intervals between attacks, or they may occur transiently at first, and then gradually extend throughout interictal periods until they consolidate into the disorder.[1] The least common cases are precipitated by chronic conditions such as degenerative neurologic or otologic disorders or gradually worsening generalized anxiety disorder or postural orthostatic tachycardia syndrome that often begin insidiously. In such cases, onset of hypersensitivity to complex or moving visual stimuli when patients are stationary may presage PPPD because this clinical feature would not be expected in other chronic disorders that cause persistent vestibular or balance symptoms.[1,8,9] Some investigators have used the term "primary" PPPD to denote its onset in patients without identifiable structural neurologic or otologic precipitants.[6] This unfortunate designation overlooks "other medical illnesses or periods of psychological distress,"[1] especially the latter, as possible triggers. The experience of this investigator's multidisciplinary team composed of otologists, neurologists, audiologists, physical therapists, psychiatrists, and psychologists suggests that specific precipitants of PPPD can be found in more than 90% of cases, with exceptions typically representing patients with unclear early histories and insufficient medical records to identify precipitants with certainty.[5]

Incorporating 2 self-report questionnaires, the well-known Dizziness Handicap Inventory (DHI)[21] and the new Niigata PPPD Questionnaire (NPQ),[22] into initial evaluations of patients with vestibular and balance symptoms may help to identify those with PPPD. In a retrospective study of patients with chronic vestibular symptoms, DHI scores greater than 60 were highly specific (specificity = 0.88) for the presence of functional or psychiatric vestibular disorders, particularly PPPD, whereas scores less than or equal to 30 were highly specific (specificity = 0.98) for their absence.[23] A similarly high specificity for the presence of PPPD with DHI scores greater than 60 was found in data reported by Staibano and colleagues[14] The 12-item NPQ focuses on the 3 exacerbating factors of PPPD (criterion B). In a retrospective study of patients examined within 3 months of new-onset vestibular symptoms, NPQ scores greater than or equal to 27 were highly sensitive (sensitivity = 0.88) but not very specific (specificity = 0.52) for identifying individuals at risk for PPPD.[3] If these results are validated in future studies, then the NPQ could be used as a sensitive screening tool for detecting PPPD among patients with subacute vestibular symptoms, whereas the DHI could aid identification of PPPD with high specificity in patients with chronic vestibular complaints.

DIFFERENTIAL DIAGNOSIS

The defining manuscript for PPPD details its differential diagnosis.[1] Pitfalls include attributing chronic symptoms to previous acute or active episodic vestibular syndromes and overlooking coexisting PPPD when other chronic illnesses are present. When PPPD is triggered by acute vestibular syndromes, the diagnostic challenge is to determine if the acute syndrome has resolved completely or the patient has compensated fully for residual vestibular deficits. For episodic vestibular syndromes, the challenge is to recognize the pattern of recurrent attacks of vestibular symptoms lasting seconds (benign paroxysmal positional vertigo, vestibular paroxysmia), minutes (panic attacks), hours (Menière disease, vestibular migraine), or days (vestibular migraine) superimposed on PPPD. For chronic triggers, the challenge is to determine if coexisting PPPD has developed.[1,8,9] As noted earlier, the presence of visually induced dizziness when patients are stationary can be helpful.[9] The diagnostic criteria of PPPD do not include symptoms or signs of altered stance or gait, near falls, or falls, so the presence of any of these merits consideration of structural, metabolic, and functional gait disorders.[9]

INVESTIGATIONS OF PERSISTENT POSTURAL-PERCEPTUAL DIZZINESS

Pathophysiologic models of PPPD matured through 3 iterations. Evidence from physiologic, psychological, and neuroimaging investigations of predecessors of PPPD and PPPD itself has converged around 7 processes: (1) possible predisposition by an anxiety diathesis; (2) promotion by anxiety-related responses to precipitating events; (3) altered control of posture, gait, and gaze; (4) visual dependence; (5) poor spatial cognition; (6) altered activity and connectivity in vestibular and visual cortices, hippocampus, and frontal lobes; and most recently, (7) misperception of motion.

Trait and state anxiety—obsessive compulsive personality traits were part of the definition of phobic postural vertigo.[24] Two cross-sectional studies of patients with chronic subjective dizziness[25,26] and one of patients with PPPD[27] found elevated levels of neurotic personality traits compared with patients with other vestibular disorders,[25,26] healthy volunteers,[26] and population norms.[27] In a complementary prospective study,[28] patients with personality traits opposite of neuroticism, namely higher resilience and sense of coherence, were less likely to develop chronic dizziness following acute or episodic vestibular disorders than those without these protective characteristics. However, unpublished data from a large cohort of patients with PPPD did not find any personality traits outside of population norms (Korean Balance Society Multicenter Working Group 2020. The characteristics of persistent postural perceptual dizziness in Korea. XXXI Bárány Society Congress, Madrid, Spain, May 2022, poster FP1225).

Some investigations predating PPPD found that patients with preexisting personal or family histories of anxiety disorders were at increased risk of developing chronic dizziness after acute vestibular syndromes[29–31] but others did not.[32,33] One observational study suggested that patients with preexisting anxiety disorders had increased risk of prolonged anxiety after experiencing acute vestibular syndromes.[31]

Body vigilance and negative illness perceptions—in studies predating PPPD[30,32,34] and one pilot study of patients with PPPD,[35] heightened body vigilance (ie, conscious attention to sensations of dizziness and unsteadiness) and negative illness perceptions (eg, worrisome thoughts about causes, consequences, and controllability of vestibular symptoms) were the psychological factors most strongly associated with persistence of dizziness following acute or episodic vestibular syndromes. Another study found that these factors were associated with severity of dizziness-related handicap.[36]

Altered control of stance, gait, and gaze—a consistent picture emerged about changes in postural control and gait from studies of patients with PPPD and its predecessors. Patients with phobic postural vertigo[37] and chronic subjective dizziness[38] stiffened their stance by cocontracting lower leg muscles. Patients with phobic postural vertigo had lower thresholds than normal individuals for engaging closed-loop feedback to control posture.[39] Stiffening the lower body increased sway in the upper body in a portion of patients with chronic subjective dizziness during static posturography[38] and in nearly all patients with PPPD on conditions 5 and 6 of the Sensory Organization Test.[40] Compared with normal individuals, patients with phobic postural vertigo had slower mean gait speed, shorter mean stride length, a wider base of support, and fractional increase in duration of 2-footed support while walking.[41] Their gaze shifts were 25% slower than normal, with end-gaze oscillations indicative of overcontrolled movement.[42]

Visual dependence—visual dependence is the tendency to rely more strongly on visual than vestibular or somatosensory inputs to determine spatial orientation. In a prospective study,[32] the combination of visual dependence and high body vigilance recorded within 48 hours of onset of acute vestibular neuritis predicted persistent PPPD-like chronic dizziness rather than recovery at 6 month. In a cross-sectional study,[43] patients with PPPD performed poorer than healthy controls on a measure of visual dependence.

Cognition—patients with PPPD performed quite poorly on the virtual Morris Water Maze test, which assesses spatial navigation and memory.[44] Their ability to use visual cues to navigate was worse than patients with unilateral vestibular deficits and healthy control volunteers. Patients with PPPD scored worse than patients with vestibular migraine, Menière disease, and benign paroxysmal positional vertigo and poorer than population norms on the Cognitive Failure Questionnaire, a self-report of momentary cognitive slips, absent-mindedness, and inattentiveness,[45] suggesting that patients with PPPD divert cognitive resources from spatial orientation and other valued activities to heightened vigilance about dizziness and conscious control of posture.

Neuroimaging—a recent review summarized results from 13 neuroimaging studies on patients with PPPD and its predecessors.[46] They included 4 resting state and 6 task-related (sound-evoked or caloric vestibular stimulation, virtual reality visual stimulation) functional brain imaging studies. All but one compared patients with healthy controls; the other compared women with PPPD with women who had recovered from acute illnesses that caused dizziness. Three studies investigated brain structure in patients versus healthy controls using surface-based or voxel-based morphometry. Despite differing patient populations and neuroimaging methods, a common pattern of decreased activity and functional connectivity in patients versus controls was found in areas associated with the multimodal vestibular cortex (eg, right posterior insula, parietal operculum, and surrounding regions), with reduced cortical folding and grey-matter volumes in these areas. Hippocampal connectivity to frontal, parietal, and cerebellar regions also was decreased. In contrast, connectivity between the prefrontal cortex and primary visual and motor regions was increased in patients versus controls, modulated by state anxiety and neuroticism. In a task-related functional MRI (fMRI) study comparing women with PPPD to an age-matched cohort that recovered from acute dizziness, standardized pictures designed to evoke negative versus neutral emotions activated brain regions associated with visuospatial processing (parahippocampal gyrus, intraparietal sulcus) rather that emotion processing (amygdala, orbitofrontal cortex) in patients with PPPD. The comparison group showed the expected activation of the amygdala.[47]

Altered perception of motion—patients with PPPD had lower thresholds than normal individuals for perceiving rotation[48] and misperceived (overestimated) both head tilt[49] and postural sway amplitude, the latter to a greater extent than patients with bilateral vestibulopathy and normal individuals standing on foam.[50]

PATHOPHYSIOLOGIC MODELS

The first pathophysiologic model of PPPD was derived from hypotheses about mechanisms underlying its predecessors.[5,8] It focused on high trait and state anxiety as triggers for a shift to high-risk postural control (stiffened posture and visual dependence). However, PPPD may occur in patients without identifiable anxiety, and the fMRI study using emotional pictures indicated that patients with PPPD may respond more to spatial than emotional aspects of visual stimuli.[47]

Work undertaken after the definition of PPPD was published found that patients had a reduced threshold for detecting motion and misperceived their own motion.[48–50] In addition, physiologic studies identified the importance of interhemispheric processing to resolve spatial and temporal ambiguities in data from peripheral vestibular organs, leading to a second-generation model.[51] It included Bayesian processing, alterations in self-agency, and top-down control of reflexive and overlearned behaviors, which also appeared in models of other functional neurological disorder subtypes.[52] This model brought attentional bias and misperception of motion to the forefront, which was consistent with patients' experiences and research data but left unexplained the curious observation of poor spatial orientation on the virtual Morris Water Maze test[44] and corresponding neuroimaging data showing reduced connectivity in the hippocampus.[46]

A third-generation model (**Fig. 1**) added an element that incorporated findings about spatial orientation. Hierarchical, adaptive systems, such as those supporting spatial orientation and locomotion, require master controllers. In optimal control theory, master controllers contain cost functions that enumerate constraints and prioritize key parameters to optimize performance of specific tasks.[53] **Table 1** compares cost functions for postural stability and fluid locomotion. These cost functions differ substantially, meaning that standing and walking are driven by different sets of top-down commands. Maintaining stance in low- versus high-risk situations also differs in ways that were investigated in healthy volunteers standing at ground level versus on elevated platforms.[54,55] In the optimal control model of **Fig. 1**, misperception of motion breaks the time constraint of using high-risk postural control transiently (ie, only when needed, **Table 1**), thereby limiting normal flexibility in shifting sets. The cost function for high-risk postural control restricts the focus of spatial orientation to immediate surroundings of the support surface because stabilizing stance does not require operations outside this narrow envelope. Patients stuck in high-risk postural control have little need to engage brain networks supporting orientation in a broader environment. Indeed, patients with phobic postural vertigo restricted their gaze to nearby objects when walking,[49,56] indicating that they applied elements of high-risk postural control to locomotion. Persistent application of the cost function for high-risk postural control maintains priorities on postural stability over fluid locomotion. **Table 2** shows how this third-generation model of PPPD aligns symptoms commonly reported by patients with research findings from physiologic, psychological, and neuroimaging investigations.

TREATMENT

Treatment strategies for PPPD were carried over from phobic postural vertigo and chronic subjective dizziness including vestibular rehabilitation, serotonin reuptake inhibitors, and cognitive behavioral therapy, either alone or in combination (see Refs.[5,8,9]

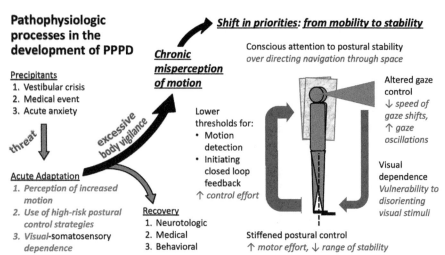

Fig. 1. Model of the pathophysiologic processes presumed to precipitate, provoke, and perpetuate PPPD. Following the arrows from the top left, PPPD may be triggered by any condition that causes vestibular symptoms or disrupts balance. The threat to postural stability inherent in these conditions prompts physiologic shifts that include heightened sensitivity to motion, engagement of high-risk postural control strategies, and preference for visual cues to determine spatial orientation and guide locomotion. Under normal circumstances, these return to normal as the inciting event resolves or remits. In the setting of excessive body vigilance, however, altered sensitivities to self- and object motion become chronic, as patients instinctively shift their priority from fluid locomotion to stabilization of perceived excessive postural sway. With that, as shown around the silhouette, attention to the dynamics of postural stability predominates over a natural focus on spatial orientation and locomotion through the wider world with resultant overcontrol of posture and gaze and continued overreliance on visual inputs.

for detailed reviews). No fully powered, randomized controlled trials have been completed to date, but since 2002 more than 1000 patients have been included in studies of these 3 treatments for PPPD and its predecessors. Studies in patients diagnosed with PPPD are summarized next.

Vestibular rehabilitation—in a retrospective review and telephone follow-up of 26 patients with PPPD, nearly all participants valued the educational component of a single in-person clinic visit and 14 (56%) reported clinically significant benefits from subsequent at-home exercises.[57] Patients improved their tolerance for self-motion more than visual stimuli. A randomized pilot study found no difference between outcomes of 15 patients treated with home-based vestibular exercises versus 15 treated in-clinic.[58] Mean improvements at 12 weeks were just at the minimal clinically important difference (MCID) of 18 points on the DHI. In a prospective study of 6 weeks of therapist-directed vestibular rehabilitation, 60 patients achieved a mean reduction of DHI scores from 55 (high-moderate handicap) to 36 (low-moderate handicap), exceeding the MCID. Twenty-seven patients (45%) achieved final DHI scores less than 30 (mild handicap).[59] In a randomized pilot trial, investigators tested the feasibility of psychologically informed vestibular rehabilitation, which combined cognitive behavior therapy techniques (eg, psychoeducation, relaxation training, reframing of excessive attention to posture and movement), with vestibular exercises targeting maladaptive postural control strategies and motion sensitivity (N = 20) versus standard vestibular

Table 1
Comparison of cost functions for postural stability versus fluid locomotion

Variable	Standing (Low Risk)	Standing (High Risk)	Walking Smoothly
Constraints (on movement)	• Sway path constrained at limits of stability. • Specific path not relevant.	• Sway path constrained within narrower (safer) limits. • Specific path not relevant.	Path optimized: • To reach target or • Maintain desired trajectory and • Avoid obstacles
Set point or target (spatial orientation)	• Gravity (static)	• Gravity (static)	• Trajectory (dynamic)
Data streams and weighting (sensory inputs)	• Internal data are adequate (vestibular, proprioceptive)	• Internal data are adequate (vestibular, proprioceptive) • External data are desired (primarily visual—overweighted)	• External data are required (primarily visual)
Operating envelope (environment)	• Support surface (narrow)	• Support surface (narrow)	• Path and destination (wide)
Tolerance for error (trigger for input from controller)	• High	• Low	• Variable
Duration	• Not constrained	• Transient (typically momentary)	• Not constrained
Energy expenditure	• Minimized	• Not constrained	• Minimized, adjusted to demand • Constrained by physical fitness

Reprinted from J Vestib Res 27(4), Staab JP, Eckhardt-Henn A, Horii A, Jacob R, Strupp M, Brandt T, Bronstein A, Diagnostic criteria for persistent postural-perceptual dizziness (PPPD): Consensus document of the committee for the Classification of Vestibular Disorders of the Barany Society, 191-208, Copyright (2017), with permission from IOS Press. The publication is available at IOS Press through http://dx.doi.org/10.3233/VES-170622.

Table 2
Effects of shifting control priorities from fluid locomotion to postural stability

Shifts in Functioning	Clinical Symptoms[a]	Physiologic and Psychological Data	Neuroimaging Data[46]
Increased attention to motion	• **Symptoms of dizziness, unsteadiness, and swaying/rocking vertigo** • Mental fatigue—distracting effects of attention to motion	• Increased body vigilance[32,35] • Poor scores on Cognitive Failure Questionnaire[45]	• Reduced *activity* and *connectivity* in regions of the multimodal vestibular cortex[b] in resting state and during vestibular and visual stimulation • Reduced *activity* in precuneus and cuneus during resting state
Misperception of motion	• **Symptoms exacerbated by active motion** • **Symptoms exacerbated by passive motion**	• Lower threshold for detection of motion of self[48] • Overestimation of head roll[49] • Overestimation of postural sway[50]	
Stiffened posture	• **Symptoms exacerbated by upright posture** • Reduced balance confidence	• Smaller static sway area[38] • Reduced limits of dynamic stability[40]	—
Increased postural control effort	• Physical fatigue – increased effort of standing	• Lower threshold for engaging closed loop feedback control[39]	—
Altered gait "walking on ice"	• Physical fatigue—increased effort of walking	• Shorter stride length[41] • Wider base of support[41] • Increased fraction of stride with 2-footed support[41]	—
Visual dependence	• **Symptoms exacerbated by exposure to moving visual stimuli or complex visual patterns**	• Impaired performance on functional head impulse test[43] • Increased deviation of subjective visual vertical[32]	• Increased *activity* in the primary visual cortex (V1, V2, V3) in proportion to symptom severity during visual motion stimulation • Increased *connectivity* between frontal regulatory regions[c] and visual association (V3, V4) cortices modulated by anxiety and neuroticism • Increased *connectivity* between sensorimotor network[d] and occipital visual network[e]

| Altered gaze control | • Inertial illusions with gaze shifts
• Sensations of stationary objects oscillating slightly in space | • Reduced speed of gaze shifts with end-gaze oscillations[42]
• Narrowed gaze range during ambulation[56] | — |
| Impaired spatial navigation | • Uneasiness in challenging environments | • Impaired performance on virtual Morris Water Maze test[44] | • Decreased activity and connectivity of hippocampi (L > R) to multiple brain regions |

[a] Symptoms in *bold* are included in the diagnostic criteria of PPPD. Others are commonly reported by patients with PPPD.
[b] The multimodal vestibular cortical network includes the right middle and posterior insula, parietal operculum, and posterior perisylvian regions of the temporal and parietal lobes.
[c] Frontal regulatory regions include the inferior frontal gyrus, anterior cingulate gyrus, and anterior insula.
[d] The sensorimotor network includes sensorimotor cortex, supplementary motor area, and secondary somatosensory cortex.
[e] The occipital visual network includes primarily the occipital poles.
Please see the text for additional information on these references.[32,35,38–46,48–50,56]

rehabilitation (N = 20).[60] Acceptability of the enhanced approach was good. Treatment outcomes favored it on cognitive and behavioral variables, although not strongly on vestibular symptoms.

Medication—a retrospective review[61] of 197 patients with PPPD treated with selective serotonin reuptake inhibitors (SSRIs), mostly escitalopram, with or without adjunctive benzodiazepines, mostly clonazepam, found that outcomes mirrored results of older studies,[5,8,9] with 65% of all patients being much improved or very much improved on medication. An 8-week prospective, 2-arm comparison trial of sertraline alone (N = 45) versus sertraline plus cognitive behavioral therapy (CBT) (N = 46) (no inactive control) showed that sertraline alone decreased mean DHI scores from 54 (moderate) to 26 (mild), similar to older studies, whereas sertraline plus CBT decreased mean DHI scores from 54 (moderate) to 15 (mild), a significant improvement over sertraline alone, despite using lower doses of medication.[62] **Table 3** lists dosing strategies for 2 commonly used SSRIs, sertraline and escitalopram, and one commonly used serotonin norepinephrine reuptake inhibitor (SNRI), venlafaxine.

Psychotherapy—Waterston and colleagues[7] conducted a retrospective review of 150 patients with PPPD treated with CBT over a 5-year period, finding a reduction in mean DHI scores from 50 (moderate) to 24 (mild). In a prospective study of 6 weeks of acceptance and commitment therapy (which stems from CBT) plus vestibular rehabilitation, 27 patients with PPPD had a reduction in mean DHI scores from 49 (moderate) to 26 (mild) at 6-month follow-up.[63] **Table 4** lists key principals for vestibular rehabilitation and psychotherapy.

These investigations of patients with PPPD produced results consistent with treatment studies of its predecessors[5,8,9] in finding that vestibular rehabilitation, pharmacotherapy with SSRIs/SNRIs, and psychotherapy with cognitive behavioral techniques reduced mean dizziness-related handicap from moderate (ie, interfering with daily activities) to mild (ie, nagging but not impairing) levels. These treatments may be combined based on clinical circumstances and patients' preferences. Axer and colleagues[64] reported that treatment using individualized combinations started during a week-long intensive outpatient program produced sustained benefits for 305 patients with PPPD at 6-month follow-up.

Emerging treatments (neuromodulation)—the first studies using neuromodulation therapies for PPPD were completed with mixed results. Eren and colleagues[65] treated 16 patients for 4 weeks with noninvasive vagal nerve stimulation scheduled twice daily and when needed for symptom flares. Participants experienced statistically significant improvements in quality of life and coexisting depressive symptoms (reduced from mild at baseline) but had limited improvement in PPPD symptoms (only 1 of 3 metrics

Table 3
Dosing strategies for selected serotonergic medications for persistent postural-perceptual dizziness

Medication	Initial Dose[a]	Titration Schedule	Maintenance Dose[b]
Sertraline	12.5–25 mg daily	25 mg every 2 wk	50–200 mg daily
Escitalopram	2.5–5 mg daily	5 mg every 2 wk	10–20 mg daily
Venlafaxine XR	37.5 mg daily	37.5 mg every 2 wk	75–225 mg daily

[a] Lower starting doses may be needed for patients who report sensitivity to medications.
[b] Continue maintenance medication for a minimum of 1 year (see text for details). Higher maintenance doses may be needed for patients with comorbid anxiety or depressive disorders.

Table 4 Targets for physical and psychological rehabilitation for persistent postural-perceptual dizziness	
Symptom	**Intervention**
Conscious attention to posture and motion (excessive body vigilance)	• Cognitive reframing • Mental relaxation (eg, imagery)
Stiffened postural control (usually present) Functional stance abnormalities (may coexist)	• Muscle relaxation or distraction (eg, simple mental tasks) while standing • Normalize natural sway and weight distribution
Altered gait and gaze (when present)	• Muscle relaxation or distraction (eg, simple mental tasks) while walking • Normalize natural gait with and without head and eye movements, to include balance confidence exercises when needed
Visually induced dizziness	• Habituation exercises—exposure to increasingly complex or moving visual stimuli (in vivo and virtual reality options) and performance of tasks requiring precise visual focus (reading printed materials, use of devices with electronic screens)
Reduced involvement in activities (usually present)	• Exposure schedule—gradually restore engagement in necessary and valued activities

reached statistical significance), although 1 of 2 measures of postural sway improved significantly. Im and colleagues[66] treated 12 patients with PPPD using transcranial direct current stimulation (tDCS) applied to the left dorsolateral prefrontal cortex (lDLPFC) for 20 minutes, 5 times per week, for 3 weeks. When compared with 12 patients randomized to the same course of sham treatments, active tDCS produced no differences in dizziness handicap, balance confidence, anxiety, or depressive symptoms posttreatment or at 1- or 3-month follow-ups. As of this writing, one small trial of repetitive transcranial magnetic stimulation of the lDLPFC was completed with results forthcoming.

The pathophysiologic model of **Fig. 1** offers insights for advancing treatment of PPPD. It suggests that patients may need specific interventions (physiotherapy or psychotherapy) to counter misperceptions of motion. San Pedro Murillo and colleagues[50] reported anecdotal benefits from showing patients video feedback of their perceived versus observed sway. The model also offers a framework for hypothesizing about bottom-up and top-down sites of action of SSRIs/SNRIs, given studies finding that serotonin modulated gains of second-order neurons in the vestibular nuclei,[67] serotonin 2A receptors are present in pathways linking vestibular inputs to the amygdala via the parabrachial nuclei,[68] and that administration of SSRIs may influence spatial working memory,[69] sustained attention,[70] and choices about gathering data versus taking action.[68,71]

SUMMARY

Formal diagnostic criteria for PPPD were included in the International Classification of Vestibular Disorders and the International Classification of Diseases, 11th edition.

Clinical epidemiologic studies found PPPD to be the most common cause of chronic dizziness in primary care (14% of all patients with chief complaints of vestibular symptoms), neurologic clinics (20% of all patients with chief complaints of vestibular symptoms), and specialized dizziness centers (>50% of all patients). Physiologic studies identified multiple alterations in functioning of postural control and spatial orientation systems, and neuroimaging investigations found changes in activity and connectivity in brain regions associated with these crucial components of locomotion. Conceptual models of PPPD continue to evolve in sophistication, now offering better insights into pathophysiologic mechanisms that may lead to refinements in physical therapy, psychotherapy, medication management, and neuromodulation.

CLINICS CARE POINTS

- PPPD is the most common cause of chronic vestibular symptoms in medical settings from primary care to subspecialty clinics. It should be at the top of the differential diagnosis for patients with persistent vestibular and balance complaints.

- PPPD must be ruled in using its diagnostic criteria. It is not a diagnosis of exclusion. Guidance for working through the differential diagnosis of potential precipitants and coexisting conditions may be found in the open access (free) manuscript that defined PPPD, available at https://content.iospress.com/articles/journal-of-vestibular-research/ves622.

- Treatment with individualized vestibular rehabilitation, a moderate dose of an SSRI or SNRI, and cognitive behavioral therapy, alone or in combination, reduces symptom severity by greater than 50% in most patients, although it may take 3 to 6 months to achieve that improvement.

DISCLOSURE

Dr J.P. Staab was supported by grant W81XWH1810760 from the US Army Medical Research and Materiel Command via the Congressionally Directed Medical Research Program. He had no commercial or financial conflicts of interest.

REFERENCES

1. Staab JP, Eckhardt-Henn A, Horii A, et al. Diagnostic criteria for persistent postural-perceptual dizziness (PPPD): Consensus document of the committee for the Classification of Vestibular Disorders of the Barany Society. J Vestib Res 2017;27(4):191-208. Available at https://content.iospress.com/articles/journal-of-vestibular-research/ves622 and can be downloaded free of charge. Accessed March 26, 2023.
2. World Health Organization. AB32.0 Persistent Postural-Perceptual Dizziness. In: ICD-11 for Mortality and Morbidity Statistics (Version: 01/2023). Available at: https://icd.who.int/browse11/l-m/en#/http://id.who.int/icd/entity/2005792829 Accessed March 26, 2023.
3. Kabaya K, Tamai H, Okajima A, et al. Presence of exacerbating factors of persistent perceptual-postural dizziness in patients with vestibular symptoms at initial presentation. Laryngoscope Investig Otolaryngol 2022;7(2):499–505.
4. Staab JP, Ruckenstein MJ. Expanding the differential diagnosis of dizziness. Arch Otolaryngol Head Neck Surg 2007;133:170–6.
5. Staab JP. Behavioural neuro-otology. In: Bronstein AM, editor. Oxford textbook of vertigo and imbalance. Oxford, UK: Oxford University Press; 2013. p. 333–46.

6. Habs M, Strobl R, Grill E, et al. Primary or secondary chronic functional dizziness: Does it make a difference? A DizzyReg study in 356 patients. J Neurol 2020;267: 212–22.

7. Waterston J, Chen L, Mahony K, et al. Persistent postural-perceptual dizziness: Precipitating conditions, co-morbidities and treatment with cognitive behavioral therapy. Front Neurol 2021;12:795516.

8. Dieterich M, Staab JP. Functional dizziness: from phobic postural vertigo and chronic subjective dizziness to persistent postural-perceptual dizziness. Curr Opin Neurol 2017;30(1):107–13.

9. Staab JP. Persistent postural-perceptual dizziness. Semin Neurol 2020;40(1): 130–7.

10. Hallett M, Aybek S, Dworetzky BA, et al. Functional neurological disorder: new subtypes and shared mechanisms. Lancet Neurol 2022;21(6):537–50.

11. Adamec I, Meaški SJ, Skorić MK, et al. Persistent postural-perceptual dizziness: Clinical and neurophysiological study. J Clin Neurosci 2020;72:26–30.

12. Xue H, Chong Y, Jiang ZD, et al. Etiological analysis on patients with vertigo or dizziness. Zhonghua Yixue Zazhi 2018;98(16):1227–30.

13. Kim HJ, Lee JO, Choi JY, et al. Etiologic distribution of dizziness and vertigo in a referral-based dizziness clinic in South Korea. J Neurol 2020;267:2252–9.

14. Staibano P, Lelli D, Tse D. A retrospective analysis of two tertiary care dizziness clinics: a multidisciplinary chronic dizziness clinic and an acute dizziness clinic. J Otolaryngol Head Neck Surg 2019;48:11.

15. Wang A, Fleischman KM, Kawai K, et al. Persistent postural-perceptual dizziness in children and adolescents. Otol Neurotol 2021;42(8):e1093–100.

16. Ishizuka K, Shikino K, Yamauchi Y, et al. The clinical key features of persistent postural perceptual dizziness in the general medicine outpatient setting: A case series study of 33 patients. Intern Med 2020;59(22):2857–62.

17. Powell G, Derry-Sumner H, Rajenderkumar D, et al. Persistent postural perceptual dizziness is on a spectrum in the general population. Neurology 2020; 94(18):e1929–38.

18. Trinidade A, Cabreira V, Goebel JA, et al. Predictors of persistent postural-perceptual dizziness (PPPD) and similar forms of chronic dizziness precipitated by peripheral vestibular disorders: a systematic review. J Neurol Neurosurg Psychiatry 2023. https://doi.org/10.1136/jnnp-2022-330196.

19. Huppert D, Strupp M, Rettinger N, et al. Phobic postural vertigo – a long-term follow-up (5 to 15 years) of 106 patients. J Neurol 2005;252:564–9.

20. Staab JP. Chronic subjective dizziness. Continuum: Lifelong Learning in Neurology (Minneap Minn) 2012;18:1118–41.

21. Jacobson GP, Newman CW. The development of the Dizziness Handicap Inventory. JAMA Otolaryngol Head Neck Surg 1990;116:424–7.

22. Yagi C, Morita Y, Kitazawa M, et al. A validated questionnaire to assess the severity of persistent postural-perceptual dizziness (PPPD): The Niigata PPPD Questionnaire (NPQ). Otol Neurotol 2019;40:e747–52.

23. Graham MK, Staab JP, Lohse CM, et al. A comparison of dizziness handicap inventory scores by categories of vestibular diagnoses. Otol Neurotol 2021;42(1): 129–36.

24. Brandt T, Dieterich M. Phobischer Attacken Schwankschwindel, ein neues Syndrom? Munch Med Wschr 1986;28:247–50.

25. Staab JP, Rohe DE, Eggers SD, et al. Anxious, introverted personality traits in patients with chronic subjective dizziness. J Psychosom Res 2014;76(1):80–3.

26. Chiarella G, Petrolo C, Riccelli R, et al. Chronic subjective dizziness: Analysis of underlying personality factors. J Vestib Res 2016;26(4):403–8.
27. Yan Z, Cui L, Yu T, et al. Analysis of the characteristics of persistent postural-perceptual dizziness: A clinical-based study in China. Int J Audiol 2016;56:1–5.
28. Tschan R, Best C, Beutel ME, et al. Patients' psychological well-being and resilient coping protect from secondary somatoform vertigo and dizziness (SVD) 1 year after vestibular disease. J Neurol 2011;258:104–12.
29. Best C, Tschan R, Eckhardt-Henn A, et al. Who is at risk for ongoing dizziness and psychological strain after a vestibular disorder? Neuroscience 2019;164:1579–87.
30. Heinrichs N, Edler C, Eskens S, et al. Predicting continued dizziness after an acute peripheral vestibular disorder. Psychosom Med 2017;69:700–7.
31. Staab JP, Ruckenstein MJ. Chronic dizziness and anxiety: Effect of course of illness on treatment outcome. Arch Otolaryngol Head Neck Surg 2005;131(8):675–9.
32. Cousins S, Kaski D, Cutfield N, et al. Predictors of clinical recovery from vestibular neuritis: A prospective study. Ann Clin Transl Neurol 2017;4:340–6.
33. Godemann F, Koffroth C, Neu P, et al. Why does vertigo become chronic after neuropathia vestibularis? Psychosom Med 2004;66(5):783–7.
34. Godemann F, Siefert K, Hantschke-Bruggemann M, et al. What accounts for vertigo one year after neuritis vestibularis—anxiety or a dysfunctional vestibular organ? J Psychiatr Res 2005;39:529–34.
35. Trinidade A, Harman P, Stone J, et al. Assessment of potential risk factors for the development of persistent postural-perceptual dizziness: A case-control pilot study. Front Neurol 2021;11:601883.
36. Wolf J, Sattel H, Limburg K, et al. From illness perceptions to illness reality? Perceived consequences and emotional representations relate to handicap in patients with vertigo and dizziness. J Psychosom Res 2020;130:109934.
37. Krafczyk S, Schlamp V, Dieterich M, et al. Increased body sway at 3.5–8 Hz in patients with phobic postural vertigo. Neurosci Lett 1999;259:149–52.
38. Ödman M, Maire R. Chronic subjective dizziness. Acta Otolaryngol 2018;128:1085–8.
39. Wuehr M, Pradhan C, Novozhilov S, et al. Inadequate interaction between open- and closed-loop postural control in phobic postural vertigo. J Neurol 2013;260(5):1314–23.
40. McCaslin DL, Shepard NT, Hollman JH, et al. Characterization of postural sway in patients with persistent postural-perceptual dizziness (PPPD) using wearable motion sensors. Otol Neurotol 2022;43(2):e243–51.
41. Schniepp R, Wuehr M, Huth S, et al. Gait characteristics of patients with phobic postural vertigo: Effects of fear of falling, attention, and visual input. J Neurol 2014;261:738–46.
42. Schröder L, von Werder D, Ramaioli C, et al. Unstable gaze in functional dizziness: A contribution to understanding the pathophysiology of functional disorders. Front Neurosci 2021;15:685590.
43. Teggi R, Gatti O, Cangiano J, et al. Functional head impulse test with and without optokinetic stimulation in subjects with persistent postural perceptual dizziness (PPPD): Preliminary report. Otol Neurotol 2020;41:e70–5.
44. Breinbauer HA, Contreras MD, Lira JP, et al. Spatial navigation is distinctively impaired in persistent postural perceptual dizziness. Frontiers Neurol 2020;10:1361.

45. Rizk HG, Sharon JD, Lee JA, et al. Cross-sectional analysis of cognitive dysfunction in patients with vestibular disorders. Ear Hear 2020;41:1020–7.

46. Indovina I, Passamonti L, Mucci V, et al. Brain correlates of persistent postural-perceptual dizziness: A review of neuroimaging studies. J Clin Med 2021; 10(18):4274.

47. von Sohsten Lins EMD, Bittar RSM, Bazan PR, et al. Cerebral responses to stationary emotional stimuli measured by fMRI in women with persistent postural-perceptual dizziness. Int Arch Otorhinolaryngol 2021;25(3):e355–64.

48. Wurthmann S, Holle D, Obermann M, et al. Reduced vestibular perception thresholds in persistent postural-perceptual dizziness - a cross-sectional study. BMC Neurol 2021;21:394.

49. Yagi C, Morita Y, Kitazawa M, et al. Head roll-tilt subjective visual vertical test in the diagnosis of persistent postural-perceptual dizziness. Otol Neurotol 2021; 42(10):e1618–24.

50. San Pedro Murillo E, Bancroft MJ, Koohi N, et al. Postural misperception: a biomarker for persistent postural-perceptual dizziness. J Neurol Neurosurg Psychiatry 2023;94(2):165–6.

51. Arshad Q, Saman Y, Sharif M, et al. Magnitude estimates orchestrate hierarchal construction of context-dependent representational maps for vestibular space and time: Theoretical implications for functional dizziness. Front Integr Neurosci 2022;15:806940.

52. Edwards MJ, Bhatia KP. Functional (psychogenic) movement disorders: merging mind and brain. Lancet Neurol 2012;11:250–60.

53. VanLandingham HF. Introduction to digital control systems. New York, NY: MacMillan Publishing Company; 1985. p. 347–91.

54. Cleworth TW, Adkin AL, Allum JHJ, et al. Postural threat modulates perceptions of balance-related movement during support surface rotations. Neuroscience 2019; 404:413–22.

55. Cleworth TW, Inglis JT, Carpenter MG. Postural threat influences the conscious perception of body position during voluntary leaning. Gait Posture 2018;66:21–5.

56. Penkava J, Bardins S, Brandt T, et al. Spontaneous visual exploration during locomotion in patients with phobic postural vertigo. J Neurol 2020;267(Suppl 1): 223–30.

57. Thompson KJ, Goetting JC, Staab JP, et al. Retrospective review and telephone follow-up to evaluate a physical therapy protocol for treating persistent postural-perceptual dizziness: A pilot study. J Vestib Res 2015;25(2):97–103.

58. Teh CS, Abdullah NA, Kamaruddin NR, et al. Home-based vestibular rehabilitation: A feasible and effective therapy for persistent postural perceptual dizziness (a pilot study). Ann Otol Rhinol Laryngol 2023;132(5):566–77.

59. Nada EH, Ibraheem OA, Hassaan MR. Vestibular rehabilitation therapy outcomes in patients with persistent postural-perceptual dizziness. Ann Otol Rhinol Laryngol 2019;128(4):323–9.

60. Herdman D, Norton S, Murdin L, et al. The INVEST trial: a randomised feasibility trial of psychologically informed vestibular rehabilitation versus current gold standard physiotherapy for people with persistent postural perceptual dizziness. J Neurol 2022;269(9):4753–63.

61. Min S, Kim JS, Park HY. Predictors of treatment response to pharmacotherapy in patients with persistent postural-perceptual dizziness. J Neurol 2021;268(7): 2523–32.

62. Yu Y-C, Xue H, Zhang Y-X, et al. Cognitive behavior therapy as augmentation for sertraline in treating patients with persistent postural-perceptual dizziness. Bio-Med Res Int 2018. Article ID 8518631.

63. Kuwabara J, Kondo M, Kabaya K, et al. Acceptance and commitment therapy combined with vestibular rehabilitation for persistent postural-perceptual dizziness: A pilot study. Am J Otolaryngol 2020;41(6):102609.

64. Axer H, Finn S, Wasserman A, et al. Multimodal treatment of persistent postural-perceptual dizziness. Brain Behav 2020;10(12):e01864.

65. Eren OE, Filippopulos F, Sönmez K, et al. Non-invasive vagus nerve stimulation significantly improves quality of life in patients with persistent postural-perceptual dizziness. J Neurol 2018;265(Suppl 1):63–9.

66. Im JJ, Na S, Kang S, et al. A randomized, double-blind, sham-controlled trial of transcranial direct current stimulation for the treatment of persistent postural-perceptual dizziness (PPPD). Front Neurol 2022;13:868976.

67. Licata F, Li Volsi G, Maugeri G, et al. Serotonin-evoked modifications of the neuronal firing rate in the superior vestibular nucleus: A microiontophoretic study in the rat. Neuroscience 1993;52:941–9.

68. Balaban CD. Neural substrates linking balance control and anxiety. Physiol Behav 2002;77:469–75.

69. Cano-Colino M, Almeida R, Compte A. Serotonergic modulation of spatial working memory: predictions from a computational network model. Front Integr Neurosci 2013;7:71.

70. Wingen M, Kuypers KP, van de Ven V, et al. Sustained attention and serotonin: a pharmaco-fMRI study. Hum Psychopharmacol 2008 Apr;23(3):221–30.

71. Livermore JJA, Holmes CL, Cutler J, et al. Selective effects of serotonin on choices to gather more information. J Psychopharmacol 2021;35(6):631–40.

Functional Neurological Disorder: Diagnostic Pitfalls and Differential Diagnostic Considerations

Sara A. Finkelstein, MD, MSc[a],*, Stoyan Popkirov, PD, MD[b],*

KEYWORDS

- Functional neurological disorder • Functional seizures • Nonepileptic seizures
- Functional movement disorder • Misdiagnosis

KEY POINTS

- There are numerous potential diagnostic pitfalls with respect to making a diagnosis of functional neurological disorder (FND).
- Diagnosis should be made based on specific rule-in examination signs or characteristic semiological features; diagnostic certainty increases with robustly positive signs and multiple signs being present.
- Some typical characteristics of FND can occasionally be seen in epileptic seizures, movement disorders, and primary psychiatric disorders, underscoring caution when diagnosis is based solely on these nonspecific features.
- Differential diagnosis should include both neurologic and psychiatric considerations.

INTRODUCTION

Functional neurological disorder (FND) is characterized by symptoms generated primarily through maladaptive changes in neural computation, rather than a discrete structural nervous system pathologic condition. Presentations include paroxysmal events resembling seizures or syncope, as well as persistent dysfunctions in the domains of movement, sensation, and cognition. FND subtypes are generally grouped according to chief neurologic complaint (eg, functional tremor, functional seizures, persistent dizziness)[1] but presentations usually include a variety of additional

---

Both authors contributed equally to the article.
[a] Department of Neurology, Functional Neurological Disorder Unit, Massachusetts General Hospital, Harvard Medical School, 55 Fruit Street, Boston, MA 20114, USA; [b] Department of Neurology, University Hospital Knappschaftskrankenhaus Bochum, In der Schornau 23-25, Bochum 44892, Germany
* Corresponding authors.
E-mail addresses: safinkelstein@mgh.harvard.edu (S.A.F.); popkirov@gmail.com (S.P.)

Neurol Clin 41 (2023) 665–679
https://doi.org/10.1016/j.ncl.2023.04.001
0733-8619/23/© 2023 Elsevier Inc. All rights reserved.

symptoms,[2] and cluster analyses have failed to delineate clear-cut phenotypical categories.[3,4] Current models for FND highlight several mechanisms that may contribute to symptoms, including errors in predictive processing shaped by internally generated symptom representations based on innate defensive mechanisms (eg, freezing reaction), acquired beliefs (eg, from past or concurrent illness), and impaired self-agency (the sense of being in control of one's movement).[5,6] Symptoms can be modulated by various forms of affect dysregulation such as hyperarousal, fatigue, and dissociative tendencies, as well as dysregulation of the attention system.

In neurologic practice, FND is one of the more commonly encountered conditions. Although FND has long been neglected and even disregarded, the last 2 decades have seen a steep increase in research and clinical attention to FND as a common, characteristic, and treatable condition at the intersection of neurology and psychiatry. Recognition, communication, and management of FND hinges on a reliable diagnostic process, which has been reshaped by a plethora of studies from "diagnosis by exclusion" into modern phenotype-based diagnosis.[1,7]

The diagnostic process consists of recognizing characteristic examination or semiological (in the case of functional seizures) features. For example, observing that a patient has their eyes shut tightly during a convulsive episode and actively resists passive eye opening is typical of functional seizures and simultaneously incompatible with a generalized epileptic seizure, in which large-scale neural synchronization disables this type of reflexive behavior. The neurologic exam can further support an FND diagnosis by demonstrating variability of function that depends on attention or expectation. For example, in the case of a positive Hoover's sign, leg weakness resolves once attention is shifted and muscle contraction becomes automatic. Finally, some clinical features, such as "tremor entrainment," can demonstrate involvement of voluntary motor function, even when the patient lacks a subjective sense of agency. Clinical characteristics and signs that can help establish an FND diagnosis have been reviewed extensively in recent years and should be actively explored and tested in any neurologic assessment.[1,7,8]

Despite efforts to streamline workup in suspected FND, a range of potential pitfalls need to be acknowledged. Some brain disorders can produce impairments in affect and attention regulation that can both predispose to and mimic FND. FND coexists with other neurologic pathologic conditions at a rate of 10% to 20%.[9,10] Changes in attention, arousal, and expectation during clinical assessment can modulate and amplify symptoms of other neurologic disease (so-called functional overlay) and potentially misdirect the diagnostic process. Problems with mobility and cognition can be secondary to musculoskeletal or psychiatric conditions that are left unexplored by neurologists (eg, protective limping or cognitive difficulties in the setting of decompensated mental health concerns). Finally, the predictive accuracy of clinical signs strongly depends on the relative incidence of FND in that particular setting and population (pretest probability).

As with any phenotype-based diagnosis, one needs to be cautious to avoid misdiagnosis. A common clinical reflex is to minimize this risk by a long list of technical examinations or to refrain from making a firm FND diagnosis. This approach is common across neurology and can be ascribed to a preference to "err on the side of caution." However, a look at the rate of misdiagnosis of FND and the invasiveness of wrong treatment should promote clinicians to further evaluate which of these two scenarios is truly "cautious."[11,12]

This review will take a phenotype-based approach and highlight relevant diagnostic pitfalls in the assessment of suspected functional stroke mimics, functional seizures, and functional movement disorders (FMDs), as well as psychiatric disorders that can mimic FND.

GENERAL PITFALLS

As the method for diagnosis of FND has shifted from a "rule out" to a "rule in" disorder—that is, relying on signs on examination or semiological features (in the case of functional seizures)—there has been an increasing push to highlight unreliable diagnostic markers that should *not* be used to make a diagnosis of FND. Many of these diagnostic pitfalls focus on an overreliance on patient demographics or historical features, in line with many other conditions (eg, one would not diagnose Parkinson disease based on male sex and older age). These general pitfalls that cut across FND subtypes have been reviewed in detail elsewhere[13,14] and are summarized in **Table 1** below.

Functional Stroke Mimics

FND accounts for up to 8% of acute stroke admissions.[15,16] In addition to the general principles and challenges of recognizing and establishing an FND diagnosis,[7] the assessment for suspected stroke has to be completed under intense time pressure in order to salvage the maximum therapeutic potential of intravenous thrombolysis and mechanical thrombectomy. However, even within this short timeframe and without the universal availability of immediate MRI, FND can often be diagnosed with a sufficient degree of confidence to withhold unnecessary treatment. The diagnostic principles and clinical signs relevant to this specific situation have been reviewed recently in *Stroke*.[17]

Most acute FND presentations that go through stroke workup include limb weakness, for which several clinical signs and examination techniques have been shown

Table 1
General diagnostic pitfalls for functional neurological disorder

Pitfall	Notes
A history of anxiety, depression, or other psychiatric disorder	Although the percentage of patients with psychiatric comorbidity is higher in the FND population than the general population, this is also true of many other neurologic disorders (eg, epilepsy) and should not be used to confirm or refute a diagnosis
Antecedent stressor	The need for a stressor immediately preceding onset of FND symptoms was removed from the revised diagnostic criteria in the Diagnostic and Statistical Manual of Mental Disorders (DSM-5) and is not reflective of all patient experiences
Diagnostic signs are only weakly positive on examination	Diagnostic signs when seen in isolation (ie, only one positive sign) or when only marginally positive should be interpreted with caution
Positive signs are present on examination but seem contingent on significant pain	Pain-contingent immobilization or compensatory movements are usually experienced as somewhat willful, although FND symptoms are not
The patient is "too normal" and therefore cannot have FND	FND should not be ruled in or out based on personality factors

to confidently predict FND. These include give-way weakness, drift without pronation for arm weakness, and Hoover sign for leg weakness. Although studies have shown positive predictive values of such clinical signs of up to nearly 100%, in clinical practice, one needs to be aware of certain pitfalls.

For example, Hoover sign, which demonstrates restored leg function with diverted attention, can be falsely positive in patients with isolated ischemia in the supplementary motor area.[18,19] More generally, reduced motor function that is counterintuitively made worse by attentional focus and improved with distraction can be found in parietal lobe lesions or degeneration.[20,21] The "drift without pronation" sign has shown near perfect accuracy identifying FND[22] but small thalamic infarctions can sometimes cause irregular drift, even combined with give-way weakness on isometric strength testing.[23,24] Inconsistency of motor function, which is a hallmark of FND, can be found in the rare case of isolated "astasia" due to small infarcts. This inability to stand in the absence of limb ataxia or weakness on isometric muscle testing is classically described with thalamic lesions[25,26] but has also been reported with other small infarcts.[27]

An important pitfall regarding functional (hemi-)sensory symptoms is that well-known diagnostic signs such as midline splitting or splitting of vibration sense have shown critically low discriminatory power in several studies and should thus only support an FND diagnosis if more reliable (motor) signs are also present.[28–30] "Nonanatomical" distributions of sensory disturbance such as glove-like patterns can be found in small cortical strokes.[31] Many other signs to identify functional sensory symptoms have not been sufficiently tested to be useful for firm decision-making during stroke workup.[17]

In addition to rare false-positive signs of FND, a major potential pitfall lies in making the diagnosis based on "circumstantial evidence." For example, panic at symptom onset can be associated with FND but is actually quite common in stroke.[32] Similarly, common FND precipitants such as migraine or peripheral injury can also be found at the onset of cerebrovascular stroke.[33,34] Demographic characteristics associated with FND, such as young age, female sex, or low socioeconomic status, can affect pretest probability of various tests but should never by themselves factor into the diagnostic decision-making.

In summary, the main pitfalls for making a misdiagnosis of stroke-like FND are (1) an overreliance on a single diagnostic sign, which can be a false positive (especially one that has not been validated empirically or if a given sign is only marginally present), (2) an oversight of minor concomitant symptoms that are not functional (eg, facial droop in supplementary motor area infarct with false-positive Hoover sign[18]), and (3) allowing demographic or psychological factors to unduly bias the diagnostic process.

Functional/Dissociative Seizures

Functional seizures, also known as dissociative or psychogenic nonepileptic seizures, are paroxysmal events that comprise a range of autonomic and dissociative symptoms, usually combined with stereotypical involuntary movements such as convulsions or falls.[6] They are thought to develop from affect dysregulation but can also be triggered by conditioned or autosuggestive cues.[6] Clinically, they can resemble epileptic seizures and syncope and are often misdiagnosed as such.[12]

Although there is ample evidence and research on the misdiagnosis of functional seizures as epilepsy,[35] the reverse problem has also been noted. An early study on misdiagnoses of seizure disorders showed that among 64 patients with suspected functional seizures and conclusive video-electroencephalography (EEG)-assessment, 14 (22%) were revealed to have a different underlying cause: convulsive syncope (1), paroxysmal dyskinesia (1), and focal epilepsy of mesial-frontal (5), mesial-parietal (1), and temporal lobe origin (6).[36] Since then, sources of possible misdiagnoses have been explored, although usually within highly selected populations referred to epilepsy-monitoring units. Although the focus of this article is on pitfalls as they relate to semiological features, there have also been many attempts to differentiate functional from epileptic seizures based on biomarkers, and potential pitfalls of common biomarkers are reviewed briefly in **Table 2**.

A possible pitfall for falsely diagnosing a functional seizure is emotional experiences as triggers. This has been reported in rare cases of focal and generalized (reflex-)epilepsy.[37,38] Although identifying precipitants is important for complete diagnostic formulations and for identifying points of therapeutic leverage in functional seizures, their diagnostic utility is likely very limited and should not bias semiology-based diagnosis.

A more common (although still rare) potential pitfall is the observation of marked emotional expression during seizures, especially ictal fear, which has been reported as a diagnostically misleading feature of parietal, frontal, and temporal lobe epilepsy.[39–41] Similarly, ictal dissociation in the form of derealization and depersonalization has also been described in focal epilepsy arising from frontal, temporal, and parietal areas.[42,43] When assessing an unknown seizure disorder with ictal emotional or dissociative experiences, the differential diagnosis of epilepsy becomes very likely when the seizures are very stereotypical and short-lasting (<2 minutes).[40,44,45] In epileptic seizures, longer duration is associated with an increased complexity of semiology,[46] which means that diagnostically unambiguous motor features are likely to appear.

Table 2
Biomarker data to diagnose functional versus epileptic seizures—potential pitfalls

Test	Potential Pitfall
EEG	False positive: Normal variants produced during drowsiness (eg, hypnagogic hypersynchrony), sleep (eg, wicket spikes), or hyperventilation can be mistaken for epileptiform abnormalities; nonspecific EEG changes common in patients with functional seizures[49] False negative: Deep seizure foci, for example, in the frontal lobe or insula, may not demonstrate ictal or interictal scalp EEG changes[50,51]
MRI	False positive: Nonspecific white matter abnormalities common in patients with functional seizures[49]
Prolactin	Levels highly depend on timing in relation to seizure (ideally drawn 10–20 min following seizure); studies have demonstrated potential for both false positives and false negatives; studies regarding ability of prolactin to discriminate between epileptic vs functional seizures show varied results; should only be used as adjunctive, not stand-alone, test[49,52]
Lactate	Ideal cutoff for differentiating between epileptic vs functional seizure has not been well established; not useful for events without major hyperkinetic component (eg, generalized convulsions); level depends on timing of sample (studies typically collecting sample within 2 h of event)[53,54]
Creatinine kinase (CK)	Nonspecific and may be elevated in a number of clinical situations outside of epileptic seizure[52]; not useful for events without major hyperkinetic component (eg, generalized convulsions)
White blood cell count	Nonspecific and may be elevated in a number of clinical situations outside of epileptic seizure[52]

Although thrashing movements, coactivation tremor, and other motor features observed during functional seizures are easily recognized as nonepileptic in most cases,[47] a further possible diagnostic pitfall has been reported in misattributing unusual patterns of movement and integrated behavior (interaction with environment) in hyperkinetic epileptic seizures. In this regard, again, highly invariable seizure semiology in an individual patient (stereotypy) as a sign of structurally determined motor sequences indicates epilepsy, regardless of how complex or interactional the observed behavior might be.[45,48] As with focal seizures in general, hyperkinetic epileptic seizures almost invariably last less than 2.5 minutes.[45] Anytime elementary motor signs such as clonic or tonic limb movements are recognized among more atypical, complex, or emotionally meaningful ictal patterns, the diagnostic decision should also tilt toward epileptic seizures.

In summary, although known diagnostic principles will likely help identify most convulsive functional seizures with a low rate of misdiagnosis, highly stereotypical attacks that last shorter than 2 minutes should be cause for in-depth evaluation, even if emotional behavior or dissociative experiences are prominent.

Movement Disorders

FMD can encompass both hypokinetic and hyperkinetic movement symptoms (for a full review of phenotypes, see article by Serranova and colleagues in this issue[55]). FMD and many other movement disorders lack reliable or readily accessible biomarkers. As such, a considerable importance is placed on having a high level of familiarity with the physical examination findings for FMD but also of other movement disorders, in order to make the diagnosis correctly and feel confident that another concurrent pathologic condition is not also present.

Available quantitative data regarding reliability of rule-in signs for FMD has indicated that degree of confidence in the diagnosis based on these signs may vary depending on the movement disorder in question. Functional tremor, the most common FMD, has rule-in features of distractibility and entrainment that have high sensitivity and specificity.[56] Functional gait disorder, however, can vary considerably in terms of presentation, with several patterns having a high specificity for a functional gait disorder (such as a dragging, monoplegic leg or knee buckling) but low sensitivity.[57,58] Although historical and demographic features cannot typically be used as the basis for the diagnosis of FMD, they may help to frame pretest probability during an assessment. For example, a new onset tic disorder in an adult (versus early childhood onset) increases suspicion for FND. Similarly, a focal dystonia that is fixed from onset is a strong indicator of functional neurological etiology (and in fact is a defining feature). People with FMD also often have other functional neurological symptoms present, and these should be screened for on history because they can help to paint a clearer picture of a broader FND syndrome.[59]

It is important to consider that there can sometimes be considerable overlap in examination signs of both FMD and movement disorders of other causes (summarized in **Table 3**). In the case of tremor, for example, variability in amplitude is common both with functional tremor and essential tremor. Similarly, while reversibility and distractibility are typically considered hallmarks of FND, dystonia due to other neurologic causes can have both of these features (eg, paroxysmal exercise-induced dyskinesia, improvement of a focal or segmental dystonia with running or walking backwards). Thus, neurologists and resident trainees should be aware that a "one size fits all" approach to rule-in signs for FMD cannot be readily applied—rather, a more nuanced understanding of which signs will differentiate functional neurological

Table 3
Overlap features in functional neurological disorder and other movement disorders

Phenomenology	Features Present in Both FND and Other Movement Disorders	Notes
Tremor[60]	Amplitude variability	Common in essential tremor, Parkinsonian tremor
	Worsening with stress and anxiety	Common to most tremor types, regardless of cause
	Irregularity in amplitude and frequency	Common in dystonic tremor, although irregularity is consistent in given patient
Gait[61]	Improvement with alternate motor pattern (eg, walking backwards)	May be seen in dystonic gait
	Inconsistency over time	May be seen in dystonic gait, frontal ataxia
Dystonia[56]	Change with alternative motor patterns (eg, voluntary action or exercise)	
	Abnormal posturing	
	Associated tremor	
Myoclonus/Jerky movements[62]	Triggered by stimulus	May be present with cortical myoclonus, brainstem myoclonus, startle syndromes (hyperekplexia)
Tics[63]	Warning/build-up beforehand (premotor urge)	
	Suggestibility/worsening with attention	
	Suppressibility	Uncommonly present with functional tics but has been noted in the literature
	Coprophenomena	
	Variability in tics over time	Less likely to be fully stereotyped movements in functional tics
Parkinsonism[64]	Rest tremor	In FND, will have other characteristics of functional tremor
	Rigidity	In FND, due to paratonia and should improve with motor distraction in contrast to Parkinson disease, where motor distraction can increase rigidity (Froment's maneuver)
	Gait: initiation difficulty, slowness, stiffness	
	Slowness of movement	In FND, typically effortful and distractible and may vary across tasks, absence of decrement during finger tapping
		(continued on next page)

Table 3 (continued)		
Phenomenology	**Features Present in Both FND and Other Movement Disorders**	**Notes**
	Positive pull test	In functional parkinsonism, may have bizarre response to pull test, test may be positive with tapping on shoulders only
Paroxysmal dyskinesia[62]	Intermittent motor symptoms with premonitory sensations	Can be seen in paroxysmal kinesigenic, nonkinesigenic, and exercise-induced dyskinesia—in these instances would typically have a consistent pattern and trigger

from other pathologic conditions reliably, based on specific movement disorder type, is needed.

One important diagnostic pitfall to recognize with regards to overdiagnosis of FMD is equating unusual movement patterns to a functional neurologic cause. Many other movement disorders can look bizarre, especially if the patient is using compensatory strategies to try and mask the movements or has a comorbid pathologic condition leading to multiple contributors to a complex physical examination picture. "Bizarre" presentations have been well-described in gait disorders including Parkinson disease,[65] higher level cortical dysfunction, as well as other rarer pathologic conditions such as genetic dystonias and stiff-person syndrome.[66,67] As such, diagnosis should not be based solely on an unfamiliar or strange-looking presentation. Instead, the clinician should return to a systematic examination to look for evidence that is known to be consistent with FMD versus another cause.

In a recent large cohort study, slightly more than 20% of patients with FMD were noted to have an additional neurologic disorder, and the possibility of comorbidity should be considered during the diagnostic process.[10] The case of functional parkinsonism deserves special mention here because this has been shown to coexist in some cases with Parkinson disease.[68] There has also been some evidence to indicate that a functional neurologic presentation may precede or coincide with diagnosis of Parkinson disease.[69]

Psychiatric Disorders

There is considerable comorbidity of FND with psychiatric disorders such as anxiety, depression, and posttraumatic stress disorder (PTSD).[59,70,71] Drawing a diagnostic line between manifestations of entities such as complex PTSD or panic attacks and FND can sometimes be difficult. For example, is a staring spell in which a person is awake, but unaware and unresponsive, best categorized as a "nonconvulsive" functional seizure or as another form of dissociation (eg, do they have PTSD *with* dissociative symptoms or PTSD *and* comorbid functional seizures)? Neurologists receive variable amounts of exposure to psychiatry throughout the course of their training, but in many instances this remains a particular blind spot for them. Thus, for the neurologist, there are a couple points of consideration when it comes to diagnostic pitfalls for FND as they relate to psychiatric disease manifestation. First, neurologists should strive for a neuropsychiatric, biopsychosocial-informed formulation that includes active psychiatric concerns (ie, not falling into the pitfall of an *incomplete* diagnosis). By extension, they need to consider the possibility that a psychiatric diagnosis might be a better descriptor for symptoms, with consideration given to what label may be the most therapeutically meaningful for the patient. Second, neurologists need to be aware of that in some cases a primary psychiatric disorder can mimic FND (ie, not falling into the pitfall of the *wrong* diagnosis). To avoid both of these issues, neurologists diagnosing FND will need a reasonable amount of familiarity with psychiatric disease manifestations (as well as the opportunity to collaborate/consult with mental health colleagues who can potentially assist in refining the differential diagnosis for neuropsychiatrically complex cases).

Anxiety and panic attacks

Anxiety can have either broad (as in the case of generalized anxiety disorder) or situation-specific (as in the cases of social anxiety, phobias, and so forth) manifestations, and a proportion of patients with an anxiety disorder may exclusively or concurrently suffer from panic disorder with panic attacks.[72] Anxiety disorders (typically with all types, always with panic disorder) are characterized by psychological and/or physical manifestations of a fight or flight response.[73] As such, there can be considerable overlap between symptoms of anxiety/panic and FND with regards to autonomic arousal. For example, many patients with functional seizures experience these types of symptoms as warning signs before their seizures.[74] Autonomic arousal can also cause neurologic symptoms such as paresthesias or dizziness, or "staring spells" due to dissociation. As discussed above, consideration should be given to a complete neuropsychiatric formulation and what diagnostic label may be the most useful, based in part on what type of treatment is being recommended. In someone presenting with a history of anxiety and panic attacks, with hypermotor events of full-body shaking with autonomic arousal and without electrographic (EEG) correlate, a diagnostic label of FND would likely be appropriate. By contrast, in someone with a similar anxiety history presenting with prolonged (nonepileptic) staring spells without hypermotor features but with numbness and tingling, a subjective feeling of weakness, tremulousness, and dissociation, this could be framed as FND or as a panic attack with prominent bodily symptoms and dissociation (and which formulation is presented may depend on a number of factors); either formulation should consider both the neurologic and psychiatric symptom manifestations and their interplay.

Two particular diagnoses to highlight are illness anxiety disorder (formerly hypochondriasis) and somatic symptom disorder. Overlapping features of these disorders and FND include having a high level of bodily focused attention and monitoring, avoidance behaviors, or hypervigilance. Both can be differentiated from FND by a lack of clear rule-in neurologic signs or semiological features typical of FND. For a review of these conditions, please see article by Sauer and colleagues in this issue.[75]

Posttraumatic stress disorder

PTSD has a high rate of comorbidity with FND, with one study showing that up to 60% of patients with FND indicate PTSD symptoms on self-report surveys, including manifestations of hyperarousal of the autonomic nervous system.[71] A recent study also proposed a trauma subtype of FND, with patients with probable PTSD showing increased FND symptom severity.[76] This high degree of overlap exemplifies the difficulty in categorizing neuropsychiatric conditions with overlapping cause and biology into discrete nosologic categories. Neuroimaging studies on FND and PTSD have revealed some shared biological underpinnings such as cingulo-insular structural alterations, which may represent sites of stress-mediated neuroplasticity.[77] Persons with PTSD may experience strong dissociation, which can manifest as staring spells or periods of low responsiveness. Significant cognitive symptoms may be present, including problems with memory and attention. This brings up similar considerations as with anxiety regarding which diagnostic label is most appropriate based on individual patient and symptom factors and again highlights the need for a transdiagnostic biopsychosocial formulation. Additionally, care should be taken not to mistake core PTSD symptoms, such as periods of dissociative memory loss and poor attention, for stand-alone FND, such as functional cognitive disorder. In particular, more research is needed to understand the boundaries between the spectrum of dissociative disorders (including PTSD with prominent dissociation) and functional cognitive disorder.

Depression

Depressive disorders can present with a number of symptoms that overlap with FND, including fatigue, pain (eg, as in the case of premenstrual dysphoric disorder), problems with sleep, and cognitive struggles.[78] In particular, regarding the presence of cognitive symptoms, depressive "pseudodementia" remains a significant differential diagnostic consideration where a functional cognitive disorder is being queried. Although fatigue, pain, and sleep problems are often part of the overall FND symptom complex, they are only supportive diagnostic features. As such, in the absence of more FND-specific motor or sensory symptoms, alternative diagnostic considerations — of which there are several, with a depressive disorder only representing one possibility — should be considered. Additionally, non-specific symptoms such as pain and fatigue should generally be evaluated in their own right regardless of an FND diagnosis.

Psychotic spectrum disorders

Although schizophrenia, schizoaffective disorder, delusional disorder, and FND seem to have little comorbidity (likely <1%),[59] and florid psychosis is typically readily recognizable, prodromal symptoms of psychosis have a greater potential to be mistaken for FND. These symptoms can precede the onset of a clear psychosis by weeks or months (or in some cases years), and can include unusual body sensations or sensory abnormalities, somatic preoccupations, cognitive difficulties, problems with communication, and impaired stress tolerance.[79,80] Clues to a primary psychotic spectrum disorder (e.g., schizophrenia) being the underlying diagnosis, as opposed to FND, include isolation and withdrawal from social functioning (whereas with FND they may withdraw from social activities but often still have a close care provider or express a desire for such), impaired personal hygiene and grooming, lack of energy or initiative, and a blunted or inappropriate affect.

SUMMARY

Diagnosis of FND relies on the clinical examination, during which rule-in signs consistent with the diagnosis should be assessed for. Clinicians should consider their degree of certainty in the diagnosis based on the clinical picture, and consideration could be given to use of "probable" or "possible" FND categories if diagnosis is unclear due to the absence of robust rule-in signs or when only one sign is present, for example. Although not discussed at length in this article, the possibility of concurrent neurologic or psychiatric disorders should be considered as a routine part of the assessment. There are several commonly encountered diagnostic pitfalls regarding an FND diagnosis, which vary based on FND phenotype. Neurologists and neurologic trainees should be aware of these pitfalls, in order to bring a high level of clinical acumen and diagnostic certainty to the assessment of this population.

CLINICS CARE POINTS

- In the setting of stroke-like symptoms, avoid an overreliance on a single diagnostic sign, oversight of minor concomitant symptoms that are not functional, or being biased by demographic or psychological factors.

- Highly stereotyped seizure-like episodes of less than 2 minutes in duration should be cause for in-depth evaluation, even if emotionally charged behavior or dissociative experiences are prominent.

- FMD subtypes will have varying signs of overlap with other movement disorders. Diagnosis of FMD should not be made based on the presence of "bizarre" movements.

- Anxiety, depression, PTSD, and prodromal psychosis all have features that can potentially overlap with or mimic FND, such as increased autonomic arousal, cognitive symptoms, somatic preoccupations, and periods of decreased responsiveness.

REFERENCES

1. Aybek S, Perez DL. Diagnosis and management of functional neurological disorder. BMJ 2022;376. https://doi.org/10.1136/BMJ.O64.
2. Butler M, Shipston-Sharman O, Seynaeve M, et al. International online survey of 1048 individuals with functional neurological disorder. Eur J Neurol 2021;28(11): 3591–602.
3. Forejtová Z, Serranová T, Sieger T, et al. The complex syndrome of functional neurological disorder. Psychol Med 2022. https://doi.org/10.1017/S0033291721005225. Published online.
4. Duwicquet C, de Toffol B, Corcia P, et al. Are the clinical classifications for psychogenic nonepileptic seizures reliable? Epilepsy Behav 2017;77:53–7.
5. Hallett M, Aybek S, Dworetzky BA, et al. Functional neurological disorder: new subtypes and shared mechanisms. Lancet Neurol 2022;21(6):537–50.
6. Popkirov S, Asadi-pooya AA, Duncan R, et al. The aetiology of psychogenic non-epileptic seizures : risk factors and comorbidities. Epileptic Disord 2019;21(6): 529–47.
7. Perez DL, Aybek S, Popkirov S, et al. A Review and Expert Opinion on the Neuropsychiatric Assessment of Motor Functional Neurological Disorders. J Neuropsychiatry Clin Neurosci 2021;33(1):14–26.
8. Espay AJ, Aybek S, Carson A, et al. Current concepts in diagnosis and treatment of functional neurological disorders. JAMA Neurol 2018;75(9):1132–41.
9. Kutlubaev MA, Xu Y, Hackett ML, et al. Dual diagnosis of epilepsy and psychogenic nonepileptic seizures: Systematic review and meta-analysis of frequency, correlates, and outcomes. Epilepsy Behav 2018;89:70–8.
10. Tinazzi M, Geroin C, Erro R, et al. Functional motor disorders associated with other neurological diseases: Beyond the boundaries of "organic" neurology. Eur J Neurol 2021;28(5):1752–8.
11. Langevin JP, Skoch J, Sherman S. Deep brain stimulation of a patient with psychogenic movement disorder. Surg Neurol Int 2016;7(Suppl 35):S824–6.

12. Jungilligens J, Michaelis R, Popkirov S. Misdiagnosis of prolonged psychogenic non-epileptic seizures as status epilepticus: epidemiology and associated risks. J Neurol Neurosurg Psychiatry 2021;92(12). https://doi.org/10.1136/JNNP-2021-326443.

13. Walzl D, Carson AJ, Stone J. The misdiagnosis of functional disorders as other neurological conditions. J Neurol 2019;266(8):2018–26.

14. Perez DL, Hunt A, Sharma N, et al. Cautionary notes on diagnosing functional neurologic disorder as a neurologist-in-training. Neurol Clin Pract 2020;10(6):484–7.

15. Gargalas S, Weeks R, Khan-Bourne N, et al. Incidence and outcome of functional stroke mimics admitted to a hyperacute stroke unit. J Neurol Neurosurg Psychiatry 2017;88(1):2–6.

16. Wilkins SS, Bourke P, Salam A, et al. Functional Stroke Mimics: Incidence and Characteristics at a Primary Stroke Center in the Middle East. Psychosom Med 2018;80(5):416–21.

17. Popkirov S, Stone J, Buchan AM. Functional neurological disorder: A common and treatable stroke mimic. Stroke 2020;51(5):1629–35.

18. Mohebi N, Arab M, Moghaddasi M, et al. Stroke in supplementary motor area mimicking functional disorder : a case report. J Neurol 2019;266(10):2584–6.

19. Mathew P, Batchala PP, Eluvathingal Muttikkal TJ. Supplementary Motor Area Stroke Mimicking Functional Disorder. Stroke 2018;49(2):e28–30.

20. Ghika J, Ghika-Schmid F, Bogousslasvky J. Parietal motor syndrome: A clinical description in 32 patients in the acute phase of pure parietal strokes studied prospectively. Clin Neurol Neurosurg 1998;100(4):271–82.

21. Ercoli T, Stone J. False Positive Hoover's Sign in Apraxia. Mov Disord Clin Pract 2020;7(5):567–8.

22. Daum C, Aybek S. Validity of the "Drift without pronation" sign in conversion disorder. BMC Neurol 2013;13:31.

23. Bogousslavsky EN, Regli F, Assal G. The Syndrome of Unilateral Tuberothalamic Artery Territory Infarction. Stroke 1986;17. Available at: http://ahajournals.org. Accessed 30 September, 2022.

24. Sacco RL, Bello JA, Traub R, Brust JCM. Selective Proprioceptive Loss From a Thalamic Lacunar Stroke. Available at: http://ahajournals.org. Accessed 30 September, 2022.

25. Lee PH, Lee JH, Joo US. Thalamic infarct presenting with thalamic astasia. Eur J Neurol 2005;12(4):317–9.

26. Masdeu JC, Gorelick PB. Thalamic astasia: inability to stand after unilateral thalamic lesions. Ann Neurol 1988;23(6):596–603.

27. Zhang J, Xing S, Li J, et al. Isolated astasia manifested by acute infarct of the anterior corpus callosum and cingulate gyrus. J Clin Neurosci 2015;22(4):763–4.

28. Rolak LA. Psychogenic sensory loss. J Nerv Ment Dis 1988;176(11):686–7.

29. Gould R, Miller BL, Goldberg MA, et al. The validity of hysterical signs and symptoms. J Nerv Ment Dis 1986;174(10):593–7.

30. Chabrol H, Peresson G, Clanet M. Lack of specificity of the traditional criteria of conversion disorders. Eur Psychiatr 1995;10:317–9.

31. Gass A, Szabo K, Behrens S, et al. A diffusion-weighted MRI study of acute ischemic distal arm paresis. Neurology 2001;57(9):1589–94.

32. Koksal EK, Gazioglu S, Boz C, et al. Factors associated with early hospital arrival in acute ischemic stroke patients. Neurol Sci 2014;35(10):1567–72.

33. Tentschert S, Wimmer R, Greisenegger S, et al. Headache at Stroke Onset in 2196 Patients With Ischemic Stroke or Transient Ischemic Attack. Stroke 2005; 36(2). https://doi.org/10.1161/01.STR.0000151360.03567.2B.

34. Yeboah K, Bodhit A, al Balushi A, et al. Acute ischemic stroke in a trauma cohort: Incidence and diagnostic challenges. Am J Emerg Med 2019;37(2):308–11.

35. Xu Y, Nguyen D, Mohamed A, et al. Frequency of a false positive diagnosis of epilepsy : A systematic review of observational studies. Seizure: European Journal of Epilepsy 2016;41:167–74.

36. Parra J, Iriarte J, Kanner AM. Are we overusing the diagnosis of psychogenic non-epileptic events? Seizure 1999;8(4):223–7.

37. Tamune H, Taniguchi G, Morita S, et al. Emotional stimuli-provoked seizures potentially misdiagnosed as psychogenic non-epileptic attacks: A case of temporal lobe epilepsy with amygdala enlargement. Epilepsy Behav Case Rep 2017;9:37–41.

38. Woods RJ, Gruenthal M. Cognition-induced epilepsy associated with specific emotional precipitants. Epilepsy Behav 2006;9(2):360–2.

39. Frazzini V, Cousyn L, Navarro V. Semiology, EEG, and neuroimaging findings in temporal lobe epilepsies. Handb Clin Neurol 2022;187:489–518.

40. LaFrance WC, Benbadis SR. Differentiating frontal lobe epilepsy from psychogenic nonepileptic seizures. Neurol Clin 2011;29(1):149–62.

41. McGonigal A, Bartolomei F. Parietal seizures mimicking psychogenic nonepileptic seizures. Epilepsia 2014;55(1):196–7.

42. Parvizi J, Braga RM, Kucyi A, et al. Altered sense of self during seizures in the posteromedial cortex. Proc Natl Acad Sci U S A 2021;118(29). https://doi.org/10.1073/pnas.2100522118/-/DCSupplemental. e2100522118.

43. Heydrich L, Marillier G, Evans N, et al. Depersonalization- and derealization-like phenomena of epileptic origin. Ann Clin Transl Neurol 2019;6(9):1739–47.

44. Seneviratne U, Minato E, Paul E. How reliable is ictal duration to differentiate psychogenic nonepileptic seizures from epileptic seizures? Epilepsy Behav 2017;66: 127–31.

45. Bonini F, McGonigal A, Trébuchon A, et al. Frontal lobe seizures: From clinical semiology to localization. Epilepsia 2014;55(2):264–77.

46. Jenssen S, Gracely EJ, Sperling MR. How long do most seizures last? A systematic comparison of seizures recorded in the epilepsy monitoring unit. Epilepsia 2006;47(9):1499–503.

47. Tatum WO, Hirsch LJ, Gelfand MA, et al. Assessment of the predictive value of outpatient smartphone videos for diagnosis of epileptic seizures. JAMA Neurol 2020;77(5):593–600.

48. Fayerstein J, McGonigal A, Pizzo F, et al. Quantitative analysis of hyperkinetic seizures and correlation with seizure onset zone. Epilepsia 2020;61(5):1019–26.

49. Baslet G, Bajestan SN, Aybek S, et al. Evidence-based practice for the clinical assessment of psychogenic nonepileptic seizures: A report from the american neuropsychiatric association committee on research. Journal of Neuropsychiatry and Clinical Neurosciences 2021;33(1):27–42.

50. Chowdhury FA, Silva R, Whatley B, et al. Localisation in focal epilepsy: a practical guide. Pract Neurol 2021;21(6):481–91.

51. Laoprasert P, Ojemann JG, Handler MH. Insular epilepsy surgery. Epilepsia 2017; 58(Suppl 1):35–45.

52. Sundararajan T, Tesar GE, Jimenez XF. Biomarkers in the diagnosis and study of psychogenic nonepileptic seizures: A systematic review. Seizure 2016;35:11–22.

53. Doğan EA, Ünal A, Ünal A, et al. Clinical utility of serum lactate levels for differential diagnosis of generalized tonic–clonic seizures from psychogenic nonepileptic seizures and syncope. Epilepsy Behav 2017;75:13–7.

54. Matz O, Zdebik C, Zechbauer S, et al. Lactate as a diagnostic marker in transient loss of consciousness. Seizure 2016;40:71–5.

55. Serranová T., DiVico I. and Tinazzi M., Functional movement disorder: assessment and treatment, Neurol Clin. Published online April 20, 2023. https://doi.org/10.1016/j.ncl.2023.02.002.

56. van der Stouwe AMM, Elting JW, van der Hoeven JH, et al. How typical are "typical" tremor characteristics? Sensitivity and specificity of five tremor phenomena. Parkinsonism Relat Disord 2016;30:23–8.

57. Daum C, Gheorghita F, Spatola M, et al. Interobserver agreement and validity of bedside "positive signs" for functional weakness, sensory and gait disorders in conversion disorder: A pilot study. J Neurol Neurosurg Psychiatry 2015;86(4):425–30.

58. Nonnekes J, Růžička E, Serranová T, et al. Functional gait disorders: A sign-based approach. Neurology 2020;94(24):1093.

59. Tinazzi M, Morgante F, Marcuzzo E, et al. Clinical Correlates of Functional Motor Disorders: An Italian Multicenter Study. Mov Disord Clin Pract 2020;7(8):920–9.

60. Hess CW, Hsu AW, Yu Q, et al. Increased variability in spiral drawing in patients with functional (psychogenic) tremor. Hum Mov Sci 2014;38:15–22.

61. Demartini B. Functional gait disorder. In: LaFaver K, Maurer CW, Nicholson TR, et al, editors. Functional movement disorder: an interdisciplinary case-based approach. Cham, Switzerland: Springer Nature; 2022. p. 135–46.

62. Dreissen YEM, Gelauff JM, Tijssen MAJ. Functional jerky movements. In: LaFaver K, Maurer CW, Nicholson TR, et al, editors. Functional movement disorder: an interdisciplinary case-based approach. Cham, Switzerland: Springer Nature; 2022. p. 103–14.

63. Mainka T, Ganos C. Functional tics. In: LaFaver K, Maurer CW, Nicholson TR, et al, editors. Functional movement disorder: an interdisciplinary case-based approach. Cham, Switzerland: Springer Nature; 2022. p. 147–56.

64. Akkaoui MA, Degos B, Garcin B. Functional parkinsonism. In: LaFaver K, Maurer CW, Nicholson TR, et al, editors. Functional movement disorder: an interdisciplinary case-based approach. Cham, Switzerland: Springer Nature; 2022. p. 93–102.

65. Růžička E, Zárubová K, Nutt JG, et al. Silly walks" in Parkinson's disease: unusual presentation of dopaminergic-induced dyskinesias. Mov Disord 2011;26(9):1783.

66. McKeon A, Robinson MT, McEvoy KM, et al. Stiff-man syndrome and variants: clinical course, treatments, and outcomes. Arch Neurol 2012;69(2):230–8.

67. Wilcox RA, Winkler S, Lohmann K, et al. Whispering dysphonia in an Australian family (DYT4): a clinical and genetic reappraisal. Mov Disord 2011;26(13):2404–8.

68. Akkaoui MA, Geoffroy PA, Roze E, et al. Functional motor symptoms in parkinson's disease and functional parkinsonism: A systematic review. Journal of Neuropsychiatry and Clinical Neurosciences 2020;32(1):4–13.

69. Wissel BD, Dwivedi AK, Merola A, et al. Functional neurological disorders in Parkinson disease. J Neurol Neurosurg Psychiatry 2018;89(6):566–71.

70. Garcin B, Villain N, Mesrati F, et al. Demographic and clinical characteristics of patients with functional motor disorders: the prospective Salpêtrière cohort. medRxiv 2021;2021. https://doi.org/10.1101/2021.02.04.21251123.

71. Gray C, Calderbank A, Adewusi J, et al. Symptoms of posttraumatic stress disorder in patients with functional neurological symptom disorder. J Psychosom Res 2020;129. https://doi.org/10.1016/J.JPSYCHORES.2019.109907.
72. American Pyschiatric Association. Diagnostic and statistical manual of mental disorders. 5th edition. Arlington, VA: American Psychiatric Association; 2013.
73. Gale C, Davidson O. Generalised anxiety disorder. BMJ 2007;334:579–81.
74. Indranada AM, Mullen SA, Wong MJ, et al. Preictal autonomic dynamics in psychogenic nonepileptic seizures. Epilepsy Behav 2019;92:206–12.
75. Sauer K.S., Witthöft M. and Rief W., Somatic Symptom Disorder and Health Anxiety: Assessment and Management, *Neurol Clin*. Published online April 20, 2023. https://doi.org/10.1016/j.ncl.2023.02.009.
76. Paredes-Echeverri S, Guthrie AJ, Perez DL. Toward a possible trauma subtype of functional neurological disorder: Impact on symptom severity and physical health. Front Psychiatry 2022;13:2583.
77. Perez DL, Matin N, Barsky A, et al. Cingulo-insular structural alterations associated with psychogenic symptoms, childhood abuse and PTSD in functional neurological disorders. J Neurol Neurosurg Psychiatry 2017;88(6):491–7.
78. Hamilton M. Frequency of Symptoms in Melancholia (Depressive Illness). Br J Psychiatr 1989;154(2):201–6.
79. George M, Maheshwari S, Chandran S, et al. Understanding the schizophrenia prodrome. Indian J Psychiatry 2017;59(4):505.
80. Larson MK, Walker EF, Compton MT. Early signs, diagnosis and therapeutics of the prodromal phase of schizophrenia and related psychotic disorders. Expert Rev Neurother 2010;10(8):1347–59.

Toward a Precision Medicine Approach to the Outpatient Assessment and Treatment of Functional Neurological Disorder

David L. Perez, MD, MMSc[a,b,]*, Sara Finkelstein, MD, MSc[a],
Caitlin Adams, MD[a,b], Aneeta Saxena, MD[a]

KEYWORDS

- Functional neurological disorder • Functional seizures
- Functional movement disorder • Functional cognitive disorder
- Persistent postural perceptual dizziness • Neuropsychiatry • Biopsychosocial
- Treatment

KEY POINTS

- Functional neurological disorder (FND) is a "rule-in" diagnosis based on positive signs on examination and semiological features.
- Although the clinical history is generally nonspecific for an FND diagnosis, sensitively gathering a social history and performing a focused psychiatric screen aids the development of a biopsychosocial-informed clinical formulation.
- Following the communication of the diagnosis and affording the patient time to ask questions, consider a range of additional factors in real-time to help determine if the conversation should transition to discussing treatment recommendations.
- Developing a patient-centered treatment plan for FND is based on phenotype, the evidence-based literature, available clinical resources, and a work-in-progress biopsychosocial formulation.
- If treatment progress is suboptimal, revisit the biopsychosocial formulation to explore if there are perpetuating factors that are incompletely addressed.

INTRODUCTION

Functional neurological disorder (FND) is a condition at the intersection of neurology and psychiatry. The spectrum of FND includes hyperkinetic and hypokinetic movements

[a] Division of Behavioral Neurology, Functional Neurological Disorder Unit, Department of Neurology, Massachusetts General Hospital, Harvard Medical School, Boston, MA, USA;
[b] Department of Psychiatry, Massachusetts General Hospital, Harvard Medical School, 55 Fruit Street, Boston, MA, USA
* Corresponding author.
E-mail address: dlperez@nmr.mgh.harvard.edu

Neurol Clin 41 (2023) 681–693
https://doi.org/10.1016/j.ncl.2023.02.006
0733-8619/23/© 2023 Elsevier Inc. All rights reserved.

(including weakness), functional seizures, speech/voice difficulties, dizziness, sensory deficits, and cognitive symptoms—all diagnosed using positive examination signs and features of internal inconsistency.[1,2] Many individuals also experience other bodily symptoms, such as pain and fatigue, which negatively impact quality of life; psychiatric comorbidities including mood, anxiety, and trauma-related disorders are common although not universally present. FND treatments include physical rehabilitation and psychotherapy, albeit with variability in both patients' access and response to interventions. These factors underscore that diagnosis in isolation does not fully inform patient-centered treatment. Given this complexity, a precision medicine approach aims to deliver "the right treatment, for the right patient, at the right time."[3] In a few hospital-based settings, specialized FND clinics have been developed.[4] However, the high prevalence and chronicity of FND suggest that both expansion of such programs and continued engagement of community-based care will be needed.

This article aims to address knowledge and implementation gaps to help increase the number of neurologists and psychiatrists that feel equipped in managing adults with FND. First, the authors detail the components of an outpatient neuropsychiatric evaluation for referrals of suspected FND—modeled after the approach used in our subspecialty FND clinic and informed by expert opinion and the published literature.[1,5,6] Thereafter, the authors discuss how the information gathered and the real-time patient response to the communication of the diagnosis of FND informs the development of a work-in-progress biopsychosocial formulation that guides treatment (**Fig. 1**). Of note, an anticipated skillset needed to implement the approach put forth in this article is an element of both neurologic and psychiatric proficiency on the part of the physician (a.k.a. some shared expertise across neurology and psychiatry). This does not necessarily mean, however, that the physician must be dual-trained in neurology and psychiatry or fellowship-trained in neuropsychiatry; there are alternative pathways across health care systems through which such expertise can be obtained. However, a concrete requirement is that the physician making a diagnosis of FND must have neurologic expertise to develop an appropriate differential diagnosis and accurately appreciate positive findings supporting a diagnosis of FND. In addition, it is important to have access to outpatient physical rehabilitation treatments (ie, physical therapy [PT], occupational therapy [OT], speech and language therapy [SLT]) and psychotherapy (eg, cognitive behavioral therapy [CBT] referral pathways). The approach outlined here also supposes that there is already an index of suspicion for FND based on referral information/chart review—including that most referrals have previously undergone a general neurologic evaluation.

Preparing for the Encounter

In referrals for suspected FND, we use a 90-min intake appointment—allowing the clinician sufficient time to conduct an initial neuropsychiatric evaluation. Depending on the model of care at your center, this could alternatively be spread over two appointments in close succession.

Before the clinic visit, it is helpful to conduct a brief (∼5–10 minute) chart review of past neurologic/medical evaluations (and psychiatric/neuropsychological reports if available). Such efforts can give an initial understanding of the onset, severity, type, and trajectory of the neurologic symptoms (eg, seizure and tremor) and will help the provider in framing the appointment. As FND symptoms fluctuate, attention should be given to recorded neurologic examination findings—looking for "rule-in" signs that may have been identified (eg, Hoover's sign, tremor entrainment). For individuals with seizures, review notes to determine if a typical event has been observed by a neurologist (either in person or on video), and whether the described semiology is

Overview of a Patient-Centered (Precision Medicine) Approach to Functional Neurological Disorder Care

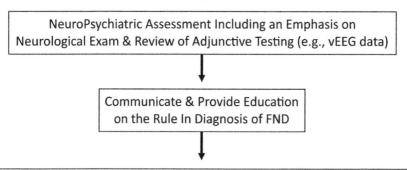

| NeuroPsychiatric Assessment Including an Emphasis on Neurological Exam & Review of Adjunctive Testing (e.g., vEEG data) |

↓

| Communicate & Provide Education on the Rule In Diagnosis of FND |

↓

| Proceed With Specific Treatment Recommendations After Benchmarks for Starting Treatment Are Met (e.g., General Agreement with Diagnosis) |

↓

| Develop a Treatment Plan Based on Phenotype, Research Evidence, Available Resources & a "Work in Progress" Biopsychosocial Formulation |

↓

| Monitor Clinical Progress & Use the Biopsychosocial Formulation to Refine Treatment Recommendations Longitudinally as Needed |

Fig. 1. Diagram outlining the general approach for how to develop a patient-centered treatment plan using in part the neuropsychiatric clinical assessment and work-in-progress biopsychosocial formulation. FND, functional neurologic disorder; vEEG, video-electroencephalography.

consistent with features supporting a functional seizure diagnosis (eg, asynchronous limb movements). Furthermore, for patients with functional seizures, note if an individual has undergone a video-electroencephalography (EEG) assessment to capture a typical event. As 1 in 5 individuals with functional seizures also has epilepsy, recording the absence or presence of interictal epileptiform activity can be a helpful pertinent negative or positive.[7] Furthermore, as a subset of individuals with FND will also have other neurologic conditions (eg, multiple sclerosis), the chart review can be used to consider the extent and results of available blood, neuroimaging, and electrophysiological tests.

Framing the Encounter
Once with the patient, set the frame (the context and expectation) for the visit. We do this by describing that our clinic specializes in evaluating individuals with neurologic symptoms that "live in between neurology and psychiatry." This can also be used as an opening to let the patient know that in addition to a neurologic assessment, you will also be doing a psychiatric screen (or vice versa, if you are a psychiatrist), so the patient has an understanding of what types of questions to expect during the appointment. We subsequently check in with the patient's understanding for referral.

Although the patient's response can be used to inform the trajectory of the encounter (eg, differences between a patient who comments that they are not sure why they have been referred vs another reporting that they are coming for FND treatment), it can be helpful to point out regardless that you have about 90-min together and that the physician would like to keep an open mind and start from the beginning of their symptom onset if agreeable.

Interview: Neurologic Symptoms First

As with other encounters, inquire about the chief complaint. In FND, this relates to motor abnormalities, seizures, speech/voice difficulties, dizziness, sensory deficits, and/or cognitive concerns. Determine when and how symptoms began, including the tempo of symptom onset (eg, gradual vs abrupt). In terms of onset, physical precipitants such as mild traumatic brain injury, limb injury, surgeries, infections, or vaccinations have been documented in the FND literature—suggesting that this can be an element to explore.[8] It is also important to understand how symptoms evolved over time, including asking about spontaneous resolutions. Ensure that some time is given to clarifying the list of *current* symptoms (ie, over the last 1–2 months) versus what has resolved. For those with paroxysmal symptoms, ask about *warning signs* (physical symptoms that signal to the patient that major symptoms are about to come on) and *symptom triggers*. For warning signs, if none are endorsed, consider exploring autonomic symptoms directly, as some individuals will subsequently report "panic attacks without panic" as part of the build-up for their functional neurologic events.[9] For triggers (experiences that bring about symptoms recurrently), ask open-endedly if any are appreciated and specifically inquire about connections to pain or physical sensations, other sensory stimuli (eg, bright lights, loud noises), level of arousal, and emotions.[10,11]

Given that many with FND have mixed symptoms (eg, tremor and stutter), regardless of the chief complaint, ask about other neurologic concerns. This can help prevent symptoms being brought up at later stages. For patients suspected of persistent postural-perceptual dizziness (3PD), specific questions should be posed based on established diagnostic criteria (eg, whether dizziness worsens with upright posture, active or passive motion without regard for head motion direction, and/or exposure to complex visual patterns).[2] Similarly, for patients with prominent cognitive symptoms, the interview requires some additional points of emphasis. For example, inquiring about the patient's perception of their memory abilities before a period of worsening can be helpful to gauge for possible memory perfectionism. In addition, the interview will offer opportunities to potentially identify features of internal inconsistency (criteria B for functional cognitive disorder [FCD]), such as when patients report severe memory symptoms yet are able to recount with accurate detail aspects of events/situations where they experienced significant memory difficulties.[12] Also, as criteria for FCD underscore that memory complaints are not better explained by another condition (or set of conditions), it is helpful to evaluate for symptom progression (or lack thereof) and the presence or absence of other neurocognitive/neuropsychiatric features as might be found in neurodegenerative conditions. Therefore, screening for factors known to contribute to cognitive difficulties (eg, psychotropic medications, insomnia, alcohol/drug use, depression, anxiety, and dissociation) is important.

In addition to "core" FND symptoms, many patients have other bodily concerns such as pain, fatigue, sleep problems, gastrointestinal, and genitourinary symptoms that are helpful to ask about specifically as such symptoms can require a medical workup of their own. Before transitioning to other portions of the interview, ask the patient open-endedly if there are any other physical symptoms that they are concerned about. Ensure that you understand the disability their symptoms confer, and what their functioning is like day-to-day. Throughout the assessment, take note of clinical details that might raise concern for an alternative diagnosis—pursuing evaluations for alternative diagnoses as needed.

Social and Psychiatric Screenings

Afterward, we recommend transitioning to social and psychiatric history screenings. It can help to be explicit in this transition, noting "Now I'd like to talk about a different topic for a bit of time, if that is okay. Help me understand you as a person. Where did you grow up and who was part of your family growing up?" Such a transition and opening sentence can help the clinician learn about what life was like for the individual as a child/adolescent. Inquiring about developmental trajectories, educational and work histories, current/past relationships, religious/cultural backgrounds, legal concerns (including pending litigation and/or disability claims), alcohol/substance use, social supports, and driving status are also important. In addition, a change of pace question around hobbies and activities enjoyed can identify potential goals of interest as well as aid rapport building. Assuming that there is sufficient time to ask sensitively, the latter stage of the social history offers an opportunity to ask about adverse life experiences. For some individuals, pertinent information may already be mentioned when asking the open-ended questions outlined above. If needed, the topic can be introduced as follows: "I'd like to ask you about other potentially challenging life experiences, if that is okay— have you ever experienced physical, sexual or emotional abuse (or neglect) as a child? What about as an adult, have you ever experienced an assault or another traumatic event?" When such experiences are endorsed, also mention that the patient does not have to share many details at this time to help limit potential emotional dysregulation. If a patient expresses a strong opinion to not discuss such topics, their wishes should be respected. However, such information can also aid the evaluation of possible comorbid post-traumatic stress disorder (PTSD) and related trauma symptoms (eg, dissociation),[13] and prior trauma can be a risk factor for developing FND.[14]

When transitioning to a mental health screening, it again can be helpful to do so transparently: "Now I'd like to switch topics again for a bit, and ask you some questions about how you are doing emotionally—would that be okay?" Here, the physician's familiarity with the diagnostic features of mood, anxiety, and trauma-related disorders is important. First, it is generally helpful to ask the patient how they have recently been feeling emotionally. Thereafter, inquire specifically about depressed mood, anhedonia, and suicidality among other mood symptoms. We typically ask if a patient has ever had a severe episode of depression lasting at least 2 weeks that impaired work or school performance and/or social functioning as a screening question for major depression. Similarly, as dysthymia (a.k.a. persistent depressive disorder) can be present in some patients with FND, asking if the individual feels that they have been depressed 50% of the time or more during the past 2 years is another useful question. Afterward, a few questions to rule out lifetime manic/hypomanic or psychotic symptoms can be succinctly asked. As a cautionary note, we have encountered referrals for suspected FND in somatically preoccupied individuals in the prodromal stages of a primary psychotic disorder. This highlights that there is a differential diagnosis across neurologic and psychiatric conditions to consider.

We subsequently generally transition to asking about anxiety. One way to begin is asking if the patient "struggles with worries," and if so, whether they have a specific worry or a range of different worries. Asking about health anxiety and illness beliefs is also important. In terms of anxiety disorders, a helpful question is whether the individual finds it hard to stop worrying. Similarly, asking if worries keep them up at night is another feature of pathologic anxiety. Such questions inform whether the patient may have a generalized anxiety disorder. Of note, some individuals during the interview will inquire about "what is anxiety or depression"—underscoring the possibility of alexithymia and related disturbances in emotion category construction.[15] We subsequently go on to ask about panic attacks (triggered and untriggered), agoraphobia, obsessive-compulsive disorder, PTSD, and abnormal eating behaviors. For PTSD, in addition to asking about intrusive recollections, hypervigilance, and avoidance, inquire about dissociative symptoms (eg, feeling disconnected from their body (depersonalization) or the outside world (derealization). For patients with prominent physical complaints (eg, pain, fatigue, and gastrointestinal distress), one should also consider the timing of screening for a possible somatic symptom disorder (SSD).[16] Some themes related to SSD may come up during the chief complaint portion of the interview, but the interviewer may consider deferring a detailed assessment for SSD comorbidity to follow-up (particularly as identifying "rule-in" psychological features of SSD can take time to explore and other factors may need to be prioritized at the initial encounter). It is also helpful to understand the acuity of past psychiatric symptoms and use of mental health services—including self-injurious behaviors, psychiatric hospitalizations, current/past psychiatric and psychotherapy care, and psychotropic medications used.

Although the use of transparent statements can help patients understand the direction of inquiry pertaining to social and psychiatric histories, a minority of individuals may express significant apprehension about answering such questions—inquiring about their relevance to their neurologic symptoms. In these instances, it can help to point out that these questions are asked to all patients coming into this clinic and that such topics can be, but are not always, relevant to treatment planning. Ultimately, if an individual has a strong preference to not answer that opinion should be respected, while nonjudgmentally noting that such omissions may leave potential gaps in your clinical assessment.

Before transitioning to the physical examination, complete the medical history, current medications and allergies, and family history (including neurologic and psychiatric conditions).

THE EXAMINATION

A mental status evaluation and an elemental neurologic examination should be performed—with "bedside" cognitive testing added based on the patient's symptom complex. Many of the mental status elements should have already been observed during the interview, with the need to only record those details (ie, appearance, behavior, speech pattern, mood, affect, and thought process). However, taking explicit account of the patient's thought content (eg, absence or presence of delusions), perceptions (eg, hallucinations), and abstraction abilities can provide useful information to expand or narrow the differential diagnosis. For individuals with prominent cognitive symptoms, we attempt to perform a Montreal Cognitive Assessment or the Mini Mental Status Examination (or targeted elements from these cognitive screenings)—the choice of which is based on the severity of the endorsed memory trouble. When considering the possibility of an FCD, a goal is to evaluate for features of internal inconsistency, leveraging the totality of the information gathered by history and bedside cognitive testing.[2]

The cranial nerve, motor/movement, sensory, reflexes, coordination, and gait assessments should be performed as one would for many other neurologic conditions. However, attention to a specific part or parts of the neurologic examination can also be tailored to the patient's presentation (eg, a more movement disorder-based examination for a patient with abnormal movements vs a more detailed speech and language evaluation for a patient with speech output difficulties). Of note, there are a growing number of "rule-in" signs that differentiate FND from other conditions, and the specific signs tested should be based on a patient's symptom complex. For example, in an individual with unilateral leg weakness, it is important to test for collapsing/giveway weakness, motor inconsistency, Hoover's sign, and the hip abductor sign. While beyond the scope of this article, the spectrum of "rule-in" motor, functional seizure, speech, and sensory signs has been reviewed elsewhere.[1,2,17] When functional neurologic signs are identified, share with the patient your observations in real time (eg, "I notice that your tremor seems to go away when I have you perform a motor task with your other hand. Can you appreciate that as well? Is this something you've noticed before?").[18] Such conversations can be revisited when discussing diagnostic impressions. It is also important to keep in mind that signs supporting an FND diagnosis should be robustly present, and take caution when apparent functional signs are only marginally appreciated.

For those with seizures, a subset will have events in the provider's office, allowing the clinician to appreciate the semiological features in real time. In addition, for seizures and other paroxysmal functional neurologic symptoms, inquire if videos are available and if not encourage that such videos be obtained if possible.

Adjunctive Testing

After conducting the interview and physical examination, consider taking a few minutes to revisit available test results. In a patient with functional seizures, review the details of prior epilepsy monitoring unit admission(s) to ensure that the semiology of the video-EEG captured event is consistent with the semiology discussed with the patient. If patients have one or more events per week and no prior attempts have been made to capture a typical event on EEG, consider doing so either via an ambulatory EEG or inpatient admission to allow for a clinically established or documented diagnosis. At a minimum, a routine EEG and head imaging should be performed. A subset of patients with 3PD develop symptoms following a vestibular system insult—as such, reviewing the results of a brain MRI with/without gadolinium is important to add clinical context. For those with prominent pain and fatigue, it can be helpful to ensure that an antinuclear antibody test has been performed (other tests to consider include a creatinine kinase, sedimentation rate, and c-reactive protein). For patients with fatigue and/or cognitive difficulties, ensure that a complete blood count, comprehensive metabolic panel including extended electrolytes, liver function tests, thyroid stimulating hormone, vitamin B12, and folate levels have been checked; in areas with high Lyme disease rates, a negative Lyme antibody test can be helpful. Consideration of additional brain and spine imaging, electrophysiological tests (eg, electromyography/nerve conduction studies), and other potential tests should be based on the index of suspicion for alternative or concurrent diagnoses. Of note, in our system, most individuals referred for a suspected FND evaluation have had prior brain imaging elsewhere, but if such imaging has not been obtained a low threshold should be used to gather these data. As much as is possible, try to arrange any adjunctive testing at the outset, avoiding repeated or sequential testing that will keep the patient in a state of diagnostic limbo.

COMMUNICATING THE DIAGNOSIS AND GAUGING RESPONSE

Assuming that it is clinically appropriate, the next step is to communicate the diagnosis of FND. Before providing your diagnostic impressions, ask the patient about what diagnosis, if any, they have previously received regarding their symptom complex—information that then can be used to personalize the discussion. The detailed descriptions of how to discuss the diagnosis have been published elsewhere.[19] In brief, it is generally helpful to lead with what the physician thinks is the diagnosis (not a long narrative of diagnoses not present). Although it is helpful to personalize discussions, we generally begin by pointing out that based on the examination and clinical history, symptoms are consistent with a "functional neurologic disorder." We go on to note that FND is real, common, and that treatments are available; we also explicitly point out that we do not think the patient is "crazy" or "making up their symptoms"—while also describing FND as a brain-based condition that "lies at the junction between neurology and psychiatry." It is important to avoid talking at the patient for prolonged amounts of time (eg, check in with the patient frequently about their understanding of what is being discussed). Ask the patient early on if they have ever heard of FND and what questions they have. If family members/care providers are present, involve them in the discussions and ensure that their questions are also answered.

Furthermore, although the interview is biopsychosocial-informed (to aid treatment planning detailed below), it is best to focus on "what" is causing the symptoms in early discussions. When patients ask "why" they have developed FND, it can be helpful to note that reasons are varied and complex, and that the patient may learn some of the "why" for themselves over the course of treatment. Another complementary approach is to use analogies such as relating FND to a "software rather than a hardware problem" or a form of "brain-mind-body overload"—pointing out that part of the rationale for psychotherapy (and other treatments overall) is to explore elements of "their personal equation" that trigger and/or worsen symptoms. For others that are readily drawing connections between biopsychosocial-informed risk factors, acute precipitants, and their FND symptoms, there is an opportunity to reflect back to the patient that some of what came up during the interview may represent part of their personal equation for FND. However, it is virtually impossible in one encounter to have a complete (and nuanced) appreciation of the various predisposing vulnerabilities, acute precipitants, and perpetuating factors, and detailed speculation at the first visit can often be incomplete and/or overtly rejected.

Once the diagnosis has been communicated, take inventory of how it went. Is the patient expressing major doubts or remaining fixated on an alternative diagnosis? If the latter, it is usually best to address that upfront (eg, why this is not Parkinson's disease or an epileptic seizure). Another scenario may be that the patient seemingly does not understand the diagnosis—or that discussions triggered dissociative and/or cognitive symptoms. In such situations (and other possibilities), it can be important to point out that the first step in treatment is understanding the diagnosis; providing other treatment recommendations at that juncture may be premature. One can point out that treatments such as physical rehabilitation and psychotherapy are available, but that such options can be discussed at follow-up. Providing educational materials, such as those available on www.neurosymptoms.org, and asking the patient to review them at home can be good suggestions (some individuals also find viewing patient testimonials online informative).

Another important consideration is whether it is the *right time* to engage in FND-specific treatment recommendations. Here, the clinician should consider if the information gathered has identified any obvious "road blocks" toward treatment initiation/engagement. For example, has the patient endorsed major financial, housing, and/or transportation difficulties that require social work/case management assistance before other interventions can be pursed. Similarly, are there any markedly destabilized medical/neurologic and/or psychiatric conditions that should be prioritized first? If an evaluation for a concurrent medical/neurologic problem is ongoing (eg, awaiting additional EEG testing for a possible comorbid epilepsy diagnosis or a dopamine transporter scan to clarify a comorbid Parkinson's disease diagnosis), such testing should generally be completed before initiation of FND-specific interventions. Pending litigation and/or disability claims are also frequent considerations. Our approach is to address these issues transparently, highlighting that the focus of the work is clinical care, and we ask the patient whether now is a good time to pursue FND treatment. Relatedly, we also ask the patient whether they would suspend disability claims and/or return to work if symptoms markedly improved. An affirmative answer to such questions can be helpful to ensure that the patient and clinical team are on the same page, whereas also allowing for patients to pursue litigation and disability claims as they think otherwise necessary.

In other instances, following the communication of the FND diagnosis, individuals will be inquiring about available treatments. In the context of the patient showing a reasonably good, early understanding of the diagnosis with no major "road blocks" identified, the physician can transition to discussing initial treatment recommendations.

Patient-Centered Treatment Planning

Developing a biopsychosocial-informed initial treatment plan based on the information gathered during the clinical assessment is a nuanced and collaborative task. There is likely not one ideal treatment package, but a range of potentially efficacious possibilities. Additional factors to consider include (1) the patient's symptom complex (core FND and other bodily symptoms such as pain and fatigue); (2) concurrent mental health concerns; (3) ongoing psychosocial challenges; and (4) access to treatments (including proximity to treatment sites). Some individuals may also have strong preferences for one treatment modality over another, and the patient's existing treatment team should also be factored in (eg, established psychotherapist).

Factoring in these principles, the physician can first consider what physical rehabilitation interventions might be needed. Consensus recommendations for PT, OT, and SLT have been published, aiding the dissemination of expert opinion on these treatments.[17,20,21] Tremor, jerks, limb weakness, gait difficulties, dystonia, and 3PD warrant consideration of PT; similarly, speech difficulties such as a functional stutter, foreign accent syndrome, and other functional communication symptoms warrant SLT consideration. For OT, there are several therapeutic considerations with some regional and health care system differences (eg, in the United States, some of the OT interventions detailed in the consensus recommendations fall more commonly in the domain of social work/case management—two other valuable services). While in need of prospective research, OT may anecdotally have a role in assessing and managing sensory processing difficulties that can be endorsed by some patients with FND.[10] In addition, for individuals with fixed dystonia, contractures, deconditioning and/or muscle wasting from prolonged limb underuse, early involvement of a physiatrist may be needed.

The other main treatment modality for FND is psychotherapy.[22] Although treatment response varies, psychotherapy is an emerging first-line treatment for functional seizures. Although the evidence basis is less substantial for other subtypes, we also consider psychotherapy an emerging first-line treatment for functional movement disorder and 3PD. There are a range of psychotherapy modalities studied in FND including psychodynamic psychotherapy, CBT, and other "second" and "third" wave skill-based psychotherapies (eg, dialectical behavioral therapy [DBT], mindfulness-based psychotherapy,[23] and prolonged exposure [PE]). As the evidence for CBT is most well-documented (and several manuals have been published), it can be prudent to consider an initial role for CBT. Alternatively, for others, there may be specific perpetuating factors that warrant consideration of an alternative modality (eg, prominent emotion dysregulation and self-injurious behaviors may favor DBT; overlap between PTSD and FND symptoms may suggest that a trauma-focused psychotherapy, eye movement desensitization and reprocessing, or PE could help). It is also possible that an initial course of CBT for FND may set the foundation for the use of another psychotherapy modality as relevant perpetuating factors become identified. Of note, physical rehabilitation and psychotherapy interventions can frequently be recommended together—in the context of multidisciplinary (team-based) care.

There are other patient-specific factors that can influence treatment planning including (1) pain and/or fatigue as the predominant symptom promoting disability; (2) concurrent cognitive symptoms; (3) intellectual disability; and (4) active psychiatric comorbidities warranting medication management (eg, major depression). For example, a subset of individuals with FND will endorse that pain is their primary issue. If this is coupled to a modest burden of core FND symptoms, an interdisciplinary pain treatment program can be considered. Cognitive symptoms are common in patients with other functional neurologic symptoms and can also occur in isolated FCD. Consensus recommendations for the management of FCD have not yet been developed, suggesting that this is a gap in the field. Potential therapeutic modalities to consider for functional cognitive symptoms include psychotherapy and/or SLT or OT-based cognitive interventions. A subset of individuals with FND have intellectual disability, and cognitive abilities should be factored into the suitability for manualized psychotherapies. For patients with active/decompensated depression, anxiety, and/or PTSD symptoms, it will be important to emphasize that optimizing treatment for those conditions may also aid their FND treatment. Point out that psychiatric comorbidities can potentially interrupt/limit clinical prognosis if left unaddressed (eg, contributing to their personal equation for "overload" or reasons why the "software" is crashing), while also noting that FND is distinct from these other psychiatric comorbidities. As such, if a patient does not currently have a psychiatrist or psychiatric medication prescriber, discussions should be had regarding the need for this intervention. For patients where there is no clear urgency to initiate and/or adjust psychiatric medications, we frequently suggest keeping medications stable, allowing patients time to engage in other treatments first. Part of the rationale for this is to ensure engagement in evidence-based FND treatments, as well as to model that the patient plays an important role in their own recovery (in other words, the agent of change is not an external factor such as a pill or surgical intervention).

In addition, although medications are generally not indicated for the specific treatment of FND symptoms *per se*, serotonergic medication initiation can be considered in 3PD.[2] Importantly, we find that two or three outpatient interventions (at most) should be prioritized upfront, as providers want to avoid overburdening the patient with too many treatments (and time commitments) all at once. Although getting the patient's feedback on treatment recommendations is important regardless, ask those with mixed FND which symptoms are most troubling as a way of guiding where to start. For example, a patient with functional tremor and functional speech may endorse that speech difficulties are most disabling, in which case SLT should be prioritized.

Other Considerations

The neuropsychiatric approach put forth here highlights general principles, prioritizing physical examination signs and semiological features to inform diagnostic clarification, while the biopsychosocial-informed interview allows for the development of a patient-centered treatment plan. However, considering the heterogeneity found in the range of possible predisposing vulnerabilities, acute precipitants, and perpetuating factors for a given patient with FND, there are undoubtedly many other clinical scenarios that are not covered in this article. As such, it is the overarching principles that we emphasize for the reader, cautioning against a formulaic approach to care. Furthermore, while beyond the scope of this article and detailed elsewhere, the biopsychosocial-informed interview can also guide longitudinal care—including triaging reasons for suboptimal treatment responses.[6]

In conclusion, the outpatient neuropsychiatric-informed clinical assessment for an individual suspected of FND can be used to provide both diagnostic clarification and personalized treatment recommendations. More research is needed to better operationalize this approach across health care systems.

CLINICS CARE POINTS

- When preparing for a referral of an individual suspected of having functional neurological disorder (FND), a brief chart review focused on clinical presentation, comorbidities, rationale for a suspected FND diagnosis, and prior workup are important data points.

- It is generally helpful to begin the clinical interview by setting the frame for the encounter and starting with the patient's neurologic chief complaint while also getting a good understanding of the patient's current overall symptom complex (including pain, fatigue, and cognitive complaints).

- When transitioning to the social history and psychiatric screenings, do so transparently so that the patient is kept informed.

- Rule-in examination signs and semiological features should be robustly present to guide the diagnosis of FND, taking caution if signs are only weakly (marginally) identified.

- While not considered definitive treatment when used in isolation, communicating the diagnosis to the patient and answering their questions is the first step in treatment.

DISCLOSURES

D.L Perez has received honoraria for continuing medical education lectures in functional neurologic disorder, royalties from Springer Nature for a textbook on functional movement disorder, is a paid senior journal editor at *Brain and Behavior*, is on the editorial board of *Epilepsy & Behavior* and *The Journal of Neuropsychiatry & Clinical Neurosciences*, and has received National Institutes of Health funding for work unrelated to this project. A. Saxena is a paid employee of Biogen for work unrelated to this project, and has received honoraria for continuing medical education lectures in epilepsy. S. Finkelstein has received honoraria continuing medical education lectures in functional neurologic disorder. C. Adams has no disclosures/conflicts of interest.

REFERENCES

1. Aybek S, Perez DL. Diagnosis and management of functional neurological disorder. BMJ 2022;376:o64.

2. Hallett M, Aybek S, Dworetzky BA, et al. Functional neurological disorder: new subtypes and shared mechanisms. Lancet Neurol 2022;21:537–50.

3. Saxena A, Paredes-Echeverri S, Michaelis R, et al. Using the Biopsychosocial Model to Guide Patient-Centered Neurological Treatments. Semin Neurol 2022. https://doi.org/10.1055/s-0041-1742145.

4. Aybek S, Lidstone SC, Nielsen G, et al. What Is the Role of a Specialist Assessment Clinic for FND? Lessons From Three National Referral Centers. J Neuropsychiatry Clin Neurosci. Winter 2020;32:79–84.

5. Finkelstein SA, Adams C, Tuttle M, et al. Neuropsychiatric Treatment Approaches for Functional Neurological Disorder: A How to Guide. Semin Neurol 2022. https://doi.org/10.1055/s-0042-1742773.

6. Adams C, Anderson J, Madva EN, et al. You've made the diagnosis of functional neurological disorder: now what? Pract Neurol 2018;18:323–30.

7. Kutlubaev MA, Xu Y, Hackett ML, et al. Dual diagnosis of epilepsy and psychogenic nonepileptic seizures: Systematic review and meta-analysis of frequency, correlates, and outcomes. Epilepsy Behav 2018;89:70–8.

8. Stone J, Carson A, Aditya H, et al. The role of physical injury in motor and sensory conversion symptoms: a systematic and narrative review. J Psychosom Res 2009;66:383–90.

9. Indranada AM, Mullen SA, Duncan R, et al. The association of panic and hyperventilation with psychogenic non-epileptic seizures: A systematic review and meta-analysis. Seizure 2018;59:108–15.

10. MacLean J, Finkelstein SA, Paredes-Echeverri S, et al. Sensory Processing Difficulties in Patients with Functional Neurological Disorder: Occupational Therapy Management Strategies and Two Cases. Semin Pediatr Neurol 2022;41:100951.

11. Geroin C, Stone J, Camozzi S, et al. Triggers in functional motor disorder: a clinical feature distinct from precipitating factors. J Neurol 2022;269:3892–8.

12. Ball HA, McWhirter L, Ballard C, et al. Functional cognitive disorder: dementia's blind spot. Brain 2020;143:2895–903.

13. Gray C, Calderbank A, Adewusi J, et al. Symptoms of posttraumatic stress disorder in patients with functional neurological symptom disorder. J Psychosom Res 2020;129:109907.

14. Ludwig L, Pasman JA, Nicholson T, et al. Stressful life events and maltreatment in conversion (functional neurological) disorder: a systematic review and meta-analysis of case-control studies. Lancet Psychiatry 2018;4:307–20.

15. Jungilligens J, Paredes-Echeverri S, Popkirov S, et al. A new science of emotion: implications for functional neurological disorder. Brain 2022. https://doi.org/10.1093/brain/awac204.

16. Lowe B, Levenson J, Depping M, et al. Somatic symptom disorder: a scoping review on the empirical evidence of a new diagnosis. Psychol Med 2021;15:1–17.

17. Baker J, Barnett C, Cavalli L, et al. Management of functional communication, swallowing, cough and related disorders: consensus recommendations for speech and language therapy. J Neurol Neurosurg Psychiatr 2021;92:1112–25.

18. Stone J, Edwards M. Trick or treat? Showing patients with functional (psychogenic) motor symptoms their physical signs. Neurology 2012;79:282–4.

19. Carson A, Lehn A, Ludwig L, et al. Explaining functional disorders in the neurology clinic: a photo story. Pract Neurol 2016;16:56–61.

20. Nielsen G, Stone J, Matthews A, et al. Physiotherapy for functional motor disorders: a consensus recommendation. J Neurol Neurosurg Psychiatr 2015;86:1113–9.

21. Nicholson C, Edwards MJ, Carson AJ, et al. Occupational therapy consensus recommendations for functional neurological disorder. J Neurol Neurosurg Psychiatr 2020;91:1037–45.

22. Gutkin M, McLean L, Brown R, et al. Systematic review of psychotherapy for adults with functional neurological disorder. J Neurol Neurosurg Psychiatr 2020. https://doi.org/10.1136/jnnp-2019-321926.

23. Baslet G, Ehlert A, Oser M, et al. Mindfulness-based therapy for psychogenic nonepileptic seizures. Epilepsy Behav 2020;103:106534.

Outpatient Approach to Occupational Therapy for Paroxysmal Functional Neurologic Symptoms

Sensory Modulation Training as an Emerging Treatment

Jessica Ranford, MS, OTR/L[a,b,*], Julie MacLean, OTR/L[a,b]

KEYWORDS

- Functional neurological disorder • Functional seizures • Dissociative seizures
- Functional movement disorder • Paroxysmal • Sensory processing
- Occupational therapy • Treatment

KEY POINTS

- Occupational therapists are an important part of the multidisciplinary approach to treatment of patients with functional neurological disorder.
- Some patients with functional neurological disorder endorse paroxysmal symptoms that may be triggered or exacerbated by sensory sensitivities (eg, symptom provocation or amplification in the setting of pain, bright lights, loud noises), and this population may benefit from a sensory-based treatment approach.
- More research (including prospective clinical trials) is needed to determine the potential efficacy of an occupational therapy-based sensory modulation treatment for individuals with functional neurological disorder.

INTRODUCTION

Occupational therapy (OT) is among the multidisciplinary treatments available for patients with functional neurological disorder (FND), with studies showing that inpatient or outpatient multidisciplinary therapy that includes OT is effective in treating FND both in the short-term and at medium- to long-term follow-up.[1–11] However, there

[a] Functional Neurological Disorder Unit and Research Group, Department of Neurology, Massachusetts General Hospital, Wang Ambulatory Care Center 8th Floor, Suite 835, 15 Parkman Street, Boston, MA, USA; [b] Department of Occupational Therapy, Massachusetts General Hospital, Wang Ambulatory Care Center 1st Floor, Suite 127, 15 Parkman Street, Boston, MA 02114, USA
* Corresponding author. Massachusetts General Hospital, 55 Fruit Street, White 1025i, Boston, MA 02114.
E-mail address: jranford@partners.org

Neurol Clin 41 (2023) 695–709
https://doi.org/10.1016/j.ncl.2023.02.008
0733-8619/23/© 2023 Elsevier Inc. All rights reserved.

is little detail in these studies regarding specific OT interventions used for treatment. OT consensus recommendations have recently been published, outlining interventions for the management of FND based on expert opinion.[12] Per these recommendations, occupational therapists are encouraged to focus on patient education, goal setting, symptom-specific treatment, patient engagement in task-specific training, and promoting positive health behaviors. In addition, the OT consensus recommendations highlight emerging strategies for quantifying and managing sensory processing difficulties as they can perpetuate symptoms, limit participation, and alter the pace of treatments. Patients with paroxysmal functional neurological symptoms often endorse sensory sensitivities that can induce or exacerbate symptoms of FND resulting in avoidance behaviors[13] as well as difficulty modulating responses to sensory experiences causing decreased participation in activities of daily living.[14]

Sensory-based interventions to treat sensory processing difficulties in neuropsychiatric conditions are an emerging area of OT practice that focus on education, increasing awareness of an individual's sensory processing preferences, use of sensory modalities for self-regulation, creating a sensory diet, forming healthy habits, and generalizing use of sensory modulation strategies across a range of activities and situations.[14] The Adolescent/Adult Sensory Profile (AASP) is a well-known 60-item self-report questionnaire used for ages 11+ to characterize the effect of sensory processing on performance of activities and translate patients' behavioral responses to everyday sensory experiences into a patient-specific sensory profile based on Winnie Dunn's Model of Sensory Processing[15] (**Fig. 1**).

OT's sensory-based approach to sensory processing difficulties in other neuropsychiatric conditions can likely be applied to patients with FND, as many patients with FND have comorbid psychiatric conditions and demonstrate sensory processing difficulties. A retrospective review of the sensory profiles of 44 patients with FND showed that they had, on average, extreme sensory processing patterns (ie, elevated low registration, sensory sensitivity, and sensory avoiding tendencies) compared with normative

NEUROLOGICAL THRESHOLD CONTINUUM		**BEHAVIORAL RESPONSE CONTINUUM**	
		PASSIVE	**ACTIVE**
HIGH		*LOW REGISTRATION* Disregard of and slow response to sensations. Require intense or variable stimuli to generate a response.	*SENSATION SEEKING* Enjoyment of stimuli characterized by engagement in behaviors that create strong sensory experiences.
LOW		*SENSORY SENSITIVITY* Characterized by distractibility, difficulty tuning out and discomfort with stimuli.	*SENSATION AVOIDING* Quantifies the extent to which an input is disfavored, resulting in behaviors that limit exposure to rich sensory environments.

Fig. 1. Four quadrant model of sensory processing. (*From* MacLean J, Finkelstein SA, Paredes-Echeverri S, Perez DL, Ranford J. Sensory Processing Difficulties in Patients with Functional Neurological Disorder: Occupational Therapy Management Strategies and Two Cases. Semin Pediatr Neurol. 2022;41:100951; with permission.)

population data.[16] In a meta-analysis of OT research examining the relationship between sensory processing abilities (using the AASP) and psychiatric/neuropsychiatric conditions — including anxiety, depression, post-traumatic stress disorder, and pathologic dissociation—adolescents and adults demonstrated extreme sensory processing patterns similar to the findings in patients with FND.[17] The sensory-based OT program for FND at the authors' institution incorporates the principles outlined in the OT consensus recommendations,[12] is rooted in the sensory-based OT approaches in mental health practice,[18–24] and has been previously briefly outlined.[25] This intervention is a part of an individualized, multidisciplinary treatment approach based on the clinical phenotype and the biopsychosocial formulation, which can also include physical therapy, speech and language pathology, and skill-based psychotherapy (all patients are provided education on FND).[26–28] This individualized treatment approach has demonstrated utility and feasibility as a transdiagnostic approach to management of patients with FND.[26,27] However, to date, the sensory-based OT program has not been systematically researched itself, including in prospective clinical trials. This article aims to operationalize the modules for this intervention to catalyze prospective clinical trial research aimed at further understanding the potential benefits and pitfalls of this treatment approach. The following overarching goals, adapted from the Sensory Modulation Treatment Program (SMTP)[20] and subsequent modules detailed below, are an in-depth description of our institution's outpatient OT sensory-based treatment program. This intervention is intended to be completed in approximately 1 to 6 months, encouraging one treatment session per week with the initial modules focused on education and subsequent modules allowing for practice in real-world situations that may be spread out over a few weeks (**Table 1** for additional details).

SENSORY MODULATION TREATMENT PROGRAM GOAL #1: FACILITATE SELF-AWARENESS OF SENSORY PROCESSING PATTERNS
Module 1: Sensory Assessment

The purpose of the first module is to gather information regarding the patient's sensory profile, their FND symptoms, current daily activity performance, and potential relationships between these factors. Assessment of an individual's sensory processing abilities includes identifying sensory processing strengths and areas of difficulty, as well as their influence on everyday activities, through the use of structured and unstructured clinical observations, a semi-structured interview, and administration of a self-report sensory processing questionnaire.[18] Our clinic uses the AASP, but several assessment options exist[29] — we suggest picking one that works well for your practice and using it consistently.

During the initial OT assessment, observe any behavioral or emotional responses to sensory stimuli in the natural environment (eg, ability to focus in a busy clinic, keeping sunglasses on indoors). Later, a more structured approach can be used by observing the patient in a sensory-rich environment tailored to elicit responses. The sensory history should gather information regarding the patient's overall responses to sensory stimuli (ie, movement, auditory, visual, olfactory, and tactile) including tolerability and whether stimuli are pleasant or unpleasant. Consider how these sensory symptoms may impact the patient's thoughts, feelings/emotions, and behaviors. If the patient endorses sensory sensitivities, identify whether this leads to avoidance behaviors, cognitive symptoms, or negative emotional responses such as feeling overwhelmed. It is important to assess if sensory processing abilities changed at FND onset and how they impact FND symptoms. Specifically, inquire about sensory stimuli that trigger or exacerbate FND symptoms (eg, flashing lights from emergency

Table 1
Overview of occupational therapy-based Sensory Modulation Treatment Program for functional neurological disorder

SMTP Goal	Module	Module Goals
# 1 Facilitate self-awareness of sensory processing patterns	1. Sensory assessment	Comprehensive sensory assessment; establish goals and an individualized, sensory-based treatment plan
	2. Providing education on sensory preferences and potential relationships to FND symptoms	Increase awareness of personal sensory processing tendencies and the impact on participation and FND symptoms
	3. Educate on arousal, self-regulation, and activities of daily living	Use of the arousal continuum as a reflection tool
	4. Identify sensory activities for self-regulation and FND symptom management	Develop a list of sensory-based activities for self-regulation and symptom management
# 2 Explore self-regulation strategies	5. Exploration and trial of sensory activities	Practice use of sensory-based activities to develop a patient-specific sensory toolkit
	6. Develop a personalized sensory diet	Create a sensory diet of activities used to achieve "just right" arousal state
# 3 Expand self-regulation strategies	7. Sensory diet modifications and application to daily schedule	Independent, consistent use of a sensory diet in routine, day-to-day activities
# 4 Repertoire expansion and skill enhancement	8. Application of sensory modulation strategies to daily life	Independent enhancements to sensory diet to accommodate increased participation in a variety of activities

vehicles set off seizure, unexpected loud sound induces tremor), as these have been shown to influence FND as perpetuating factors—often through increased avoidance behaviors.[13] In parallel, it is useful to also ask about warning signs (eg, muscle tension, cognitive clouding, and palpitations) that forecast an intense FND episode. It can be helpful to take note of any strategies, including sensory-based activities, currently used by the patient and if they could be improved on to aid relief. Review specifics regarding the patient's daily routine and what supports they have, with a focus on analyzing activities in relation to sensory processing.

Lastly, complete the AASP to gain additional understanding of the patient's sensory processing patterns. The questionnaire is completed together during the first session to allow an opportunity to educate the patient on their sensory processing patterns as defined in Winnie Dunn's Model of Sensory Processing[15] and how their sensory preferences may influence participation in activities at home, work/school, and the community.

Information from clinical observations, interview, and the AASP are collectively used to determine functional goals and treatment interventions specific to the patient's needs. Overall, the occupational therapist can aim to perform this initial assessment in the first session. If time is limited or the patient is actively symptomatic, the AASP can be provided to the patient to complete on their own.

Module 2: Providing Education on Sensory Preferences and Potential Relationships to Functional Neurological Disorder Symptoms

The purpose of Module 2 is to provide the patient with specific feedback regarding their sensory processing profile and begin to explore the relationship between their own sensory preferences and FND symptoms. The goals of providing this feedback are to help the patient understand their sensory processing tendencies, gain insight into how their sensory preferences may influence participation in daily activities, and develop awareness of how sensory stimuli may trigger or exacerbate FND symptoms.[30]

When scoring the AASP, it is important to note not just the scores within the sensory processing quadrants (eg, low registration, sensory sensitive, sensory avoiding more/ much more than others, and sensory seeking similar to/less than others), but if there are specific sensory stimuli that generate a more extreme response from the patient than others (eg, "almost always" or "almost never" responses to questions). Identifying extreme responses can increase the awareness of sensory preferences, improve the understanding of how their nervous system processes sensory information, and be used to start identifying what types of sensory stimuli may be useful for self-regulation. Based on initial pilot research, patients with FND who endorse sensory sensitivities that exacerbate or trigger their FND symptoms also report an extreme sensory processing pattern with elevated scores in low registration, sensory sensitivity, and sensory avoiding and typical or decreased scores in sensory seeking.[16] This pattern of sensory processing means that patients with FND can be highly sensitive to sensory information in some instances and are either passively responding with extreme emotional and/or behavioral responses that may trigger or exacerbate FND symptoms or are engaging in avoidance behaviors (eg, frequently wearing sunglasses in and out of the home). These sensory avoiding behaviors can create a lack of engagement with and exploration of sensory-rich environments. By limiting intense and variable sensory stimulation, the brain struggles to focus attention and process information.[31] These passive and maladaptive response patterns can impact an individual's participation in meaningful life activities as well as their perceived potential for recovery and overall quality of life.[30] Education that provides the patient some insight into their sensory processing profile and how it impacts participation will be the foundation for the subsequent modules in achieving the four goals of the SMTP. Although this education happens in the second session, this information is revisited throughout OT treatment.

Module 3: Education on Arousal, Self-Regulation, and Activities of Daily Living

The purpose of Module 3 is to introduce the concept of self-regulation and its impact on FND symptoms and daily life. Self-regulation is the ability to monitor and modify arousal levels to be comfortable and work well in a particular environment or situation. The goal of this module is for the patient to learn to use the arousal continuum as a self-reflection tool to accurately identify different arousal states and how they influence participation in daily activities. This is an important skill to develop, as many patients with paroxysmal FND have a nervous system that is on "high alert," where they may enter the extreme ends of the arousal continuum easily. In this situation, a patient may have a "fight, flight, or freeze" sympathetic response or experience dissociation while engaging in typical daily activities. A hyperarousal response may occur in reaction to sensory stimuli, such as bright lights or loud noises, which can then trigger FND symptoms (eg, a loud, unexpected noise may set a patient into full-body tremors).[32] Furthermore, when patients are living in the extreme ends of the arousal continuum, they can be at risk for unhelpful long-term behavioral responses to sensory stimuli that result in decreased participation in daily activities.

When introducing the arousal continuum, the patient is provided a handout that outlines arousal levels on a continuum from extreme hypoarousal to extreme hyperarousal with a window of "just right" in between (**Fig. 2**). Ask the patient to describe how they experience arousal states along this continuum. Patients may conceptualize high arousal as a change in physiologic (sensorimotor), cognitive, and/or emotional symptoms or may have difficulty describing this experience altogether.[33] It is important to note that although many patients can clearly identify extreme arousal states on the continuum and may have a vague idea of "just right," they can often lack the ability to register incremental changes to arousal, which can result in becoming shut down. The dysregulation that occurs in the extreme ends of arousal (ie, both hypo- and hyper-arousal) may trigger FND symptoms and can also decrease a person's cognitive/emotional flexibility. Having the patient provide their personal experience of arousal states gives the therapist insight into their ability to accurately self-reflect and identify these states.

Based on the patient's responses, the therapist may need to provide real-world examples that define arousal levels more clearly (eg, high arousal due to stress from

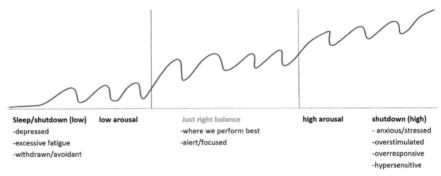

Sleep/shutdown (low)	low arousal	Just right balance	high arousal	shutdown (high)
-depressed		-where we perform best		- anxious/stressed
-excessive fatigue		-alert/focused		-overstimulated
-withdrawn/avoidant				-overresponsive
				-hypersensitive

Fig. 2. The arousal continuum is used as a self-reflection tool to help patients begin to recognize different arousal levels. Using sensory activities, patients work to achieve the "just right balance" necessary to perform optimally and complete daily tasks. Shut down can occur when extended time is spent in high or low arousal levels.

running late to an appointment may look like racing heart and feelings of anxiety; low arousal in the afternoon after eating lunch may be described as feeling groggy). Note that this exercise is also an opportunity to model self-reflection and help patients develop appropriate self-monitoring by providing structure of what to attend to (eg, less specific focus on bodily symptoms of FND and more focus on changes to arousal states in a variety of situations).

This education occurs during the second OT session, but patients who are finding it challenging to identify their arousal state and its fluctuations may need to be provided with homework to continue their self-reflection. Furthermore, as a catalyst for the work to be done in Module 4, patients are given the Sensory-Motor Preference Checklist[34] to complete at home; this is a self-report measure developed to help adults recognize how different activities influence their arousal levels.

Module 4: Identify Sensory Activities for Self-Regulation and Functional Neurological Disorder Symptom Management

The purpose of this module is to further improve the patient's self-awareness of their sensory processing patterns by helping them understand how different activities can influence their arousal levels. The goal is to identify a list of specific activities across sensory modalities that can be used to alter arousal levels for self-regulation and symptom management. It is important to emphasize that self-regulation can be achieved by choosing activities that modify arousal levels to match the demands of a task or situation (eg, low arousal at bedtime). The Sensory-Motor Preference Checklist, provided in Module 3, is reviewed in detail with the patient. Patients are asked to relate the sensory experiences in the checklist to a self-identified arousal response — calming, alerting, irritating, or a combination of such experiences (eg, yoga is calming, drinking ice water is alerting, listening to music is irritating). Discuss any patterns or themes within sensory modalities that elicit a consistent arousal response (eg, visual activities frequently identified as irritating) and how this may relate to their sensory processing profile and/or FND symptoms. Determine if, how, and when, they engage in these activities. Begin to categorize activities by arousal response, specifically calming and alerting, to create a list of activities the patient can trial to self-regulate. Explore activities identified as irritating to identify possible FND triggers as well as activities that may be used as a grounding technique (eg, an alerting or mildly irritating sensory activity that is not identified as a trigger can be used this way). Patterns, themes, and specific activity responses from the Sensory-Motor Preference Checklist inform clinical decisions regarding which activities to trial in Module 5.

Factors that may influence how quickly this module is completed depend on how well the patients have understood and completed the Sensory-Motor Preference Checklist before the session and their ability to grasp the concept of using activities to modify arousal levels. Patients are asked to select 1 to 2 activities from the checklist to trial at home and reflect on how they felt before and after the activity (ie, physically, emotionally, cognitively) to reinforce concepts discussed in this module and prepare for Module 5.

SENSORY MODULATION TREATMENT PROGRAM GOAL #2: EXPLORE SELF-REGULATION STRATEGIES
Module 5: Exploration and Trial of Sensory Activities

The purpose of Module 5 is to identify opportunities for patients to explore and trial a variety of sensory activities. Through a "trial and error" approach, the patient will practice and reflect on the use of sensory activities at different times of day and in a variety of situations to create a toolkit to achieve "just right" arousal levels. OT sessions should facilitate continued development of the reflection skills needed to self-regulate and increase participation in daily activities. Information gathered from the sensory assessment, Sensory-Motor Preference Checklist, patient's reflections on initial trial of sensory activities, and social history are used to guide clinicians and patients throughout this module.

First, the clinician and patient identify a combination of new and familiar sensory activities to trial (approximately three to five) considering how those activities influence their arousal levels. When guiding the patient in choosing sensory activities, the occupational therapist should incorporate their knowledge and understanding of how the characteristics of different sensory input may generally influence arousal levels[23] (**Table 2** for examples).

The occupational therapist should also consider the relationship between sensory processing, the patient's sensory preferences, the arousal continuum, and the properties (ie, amount, frequency, intensity, and/or duration) and type of sensory stimuli. For example, A.B. is hypersensitive to visual stimuli, so she would avoid going to the grocery store as she found the bright lights overwhelming. A.B. would use a Listerine strip as a coping strategy when she felt overwhelmed in the grocery store, but it was not effective in helping her self-regulate. Considering timing and intensity/duration of stimuli, the occupational therapist suggested that A.B. use a Listerine strip just before entering the grocery store and again as a grounding strategy when feeling her arousal level increasing.

Educate the patient as to why they may trial one sensory activity versus another. For instance, if the patient identifies they are at the high end of arousal, nearing "shut down," a calming activity may not be effective in lowering their arousal level. Rather, to achieve the desired result, they may need to trial a more intense sensory activity that has both calming and alerting properties before initiating a calming activity (eg, go for a brisk walk then come back and stretch). Emphasize that these activities are meant to facilitate self-regulation by helping them recognize and achieve the "just right" balance.

If the patient becomes symptomatic during the OT session, the therapist can use this time to introduce a new sensory experience (eg, putting a bag of ice on their

Table 2
General characteristics of sensory input

Type of Sensory Input	General Characteristics	Examples
Calming	Mild/soft	Natural or dim lighting
	Slow	Rocking chair
	Rhythmic	Ocean sounds
	Predictable	Heavy quilt or weighted blanket
	Familiar	Yoga/Tai Chi
	Soothing	Warm drink
	Low demands	Deep abdominal breathing
	Positive associations	Aromatherapy (eg, lavender)
Alerting	Strong	Bright colors or lighting
	Fast-paced	Jogging, dancing
	Nonrhythmic	Sound of hammer
	Unpredictable	Tickling feeling of feather
	Novel	Kickboxing/aerobics
	Irritating	Strong mints
	High demands	Doing a crossword puzzle
	Negative associations	Noxious odors (eg, skunk)

neck when they begin to feel warning signs of a seizure). The occupational therapist should then guide the patient through a self-reflection process to identify any changes in arousal level and/or FND symptoms.

An initial "tool kit" is typically developed in one session, with patients given homework to trial activities at home and come to the next OT session with feedback on what they tried, when they tried it, and how it made them feel—particularly in relation to their FND symptoms. They should identify arousal levels throughout the day as well as in response to specific sensory activities. The process of practicing, self-reflecting, providing feedback, and problem-solving occurs both at home and in OT sessions. If a patient grasps the concepts in Module 5 quickly, they may move on to Module 6 within two sessions, whereas others may need more time.

Module 6: Develop a Personalized Sensory Diet

The purpose of Module 6 is to develop an individualized "sensory diet" of scheduled daily activities to achieve and maintain the "just right" arousal level necessary to successfully engage in daily activities as well as identify strategies to help manage FND symptoms. A sensory diet is a personalized, balanced, and paced schedule of sensory-based activities, including sensory "meals," sensory "snacks," environmental supports, hideout spaces, and leisure activities (**Table 3**). The sensory activities identified in Module 5 as beneficial in managing FND symptoms and for self-regulation are used to develop an initial sensory diet, along with a sensory diet worksheet—we use the one provided by the Spiral Foundation.[35] Provide education on each section of the sensory diet, using examples from the patient's sensory preferences as well as your own personal examples to enhance understanding and activity selection.

Start with sensory meals, including helping patients recognize any activities they already engage in that can be considered a sensory meal (eg, showering to become

Table 3		
Overview of sensory diet		
Sensory Diet Strategies	**Explanation**	**Examples**
Sensory meals	Activities/tasks done as part of daily routine that provide large amounts of sensory input	Going for a walk or run Showering Meditating Use of weighted blanket
Sensory snacks	Quickly accessed activities used "as needed" during challenging situations to keep the body comfortable and/or focused	Diaphragmatic breathing Chewing gum Use of headphones/earplugs Use of fidget toys Wearing sunglasses
Environmental supports	Modest adaptations made to surroundings at home or work/school to enhance self-regulation	Changing lighting Decorating with plants Modifying room temperature
Hideout spaces	Physical places to access when alone or quiet time is needed during the day	Spare room Finished basement Garden Car
Leisure activities	Tasks done for enjoyment on a daily, weekly, or monthly basis that provide positive additional sensory input and facilitate well-being	Watching favorite TV show daily Visiting friends weekly Go to concert/theater monthly

more alert for a meeting, meditating in the evening to prepare for bed). If a patient is unable to identify specific meals, refer them back to the Sensory-Motor Preference Checklist to consider what alerting and calming activities they may want to trial.

Sensory snacks should only be used as needed—avoid overuse as this can cause a dependence on these strategies to engage in daily activities. Some patients have difficulty differentiating between a sensory meal and a sensory snack. Ensure understanding by providing individualized examples and encouraging the patient to trial specific activities as either a sensory meal or sensory snack to determine its effectiveness. If the patient continues to struggle, more time may need to be spent returning to Module 5 for practice and trialing additional activities with an eye to the type of sensory stimuli as well as intensity, duration, and frequency.

Finally, assist the patient in identifying specific strategies that can be written into their sensory diet in the areas of environmental supports, hideout spaces, and leisure activities. At the end of the session, the patient is given homework to further complete all sections of the sensory diet worksheet, begin to follow the sensory diet, and reflect on its effectiveness and impact on participation. Review completed homework at the next session and continue to evolve the sensory diet throughout OT treatment based on patient feedback.

SENSORY MODULATION TREATMENT PROGRAM GOAL #3: EXPAND SELF-REGULATION STRATEGIES AND FACILITATE POSITIVE CHANGE
Module 7: Sensory Diet Modifications and Applications to Daily Schedule

The purpose of Module 7 is to increase self-regulation skills for improved participation in daily activities and formation of healthy habits through independent, consistent use of a sensory diet for self-regulation. This module begins when the patient returns to OT with a completed sensory diet and reflections on the effectiveness of activities used outside of therapy. Unlike the other modules, Module 7 requires several sessions over a longer period of time. The process of assessing the effectiveness of the sensory diet, making modifications, and incorporating the next iteration of the sensory diet into a daily schedule is repeated until independence is achieved.

Refining the sensory diet: Review the sensory diet homework and assess the patient's understanding of foundational concepts from Modules 5 and 6. The occupational therapist should note the completeness of the sensory diet (eg, are there activities identified in all areas) as well as assessing the appropriateness of activities the patient identified as sensory meals and sensory snacks. If considering additional activities to include in the sensory diet, the occupational therapist may review previously identified arousal responses to activities in the Sensory-Motor Preference Checklist with the patient and facilitate their choice of alternative activities as needed. If the patient expresses difficulty recognizing when to use activities from the sensory diet, it may be helpful to guide the patient to trial a specific sensory meal or sensory snack considering the properties outlined in Module 5. It is also important to gain insight into the patient's ability to accurately reflect on their use of the sensory diet for management of FND symptoms and participation in daily activities. If the patient is unable to identify any positive changes in arousal levels when using their sensory diet, the occupational therapist should consider revisiting the arousal continuum in Module 2 for self-reflection. Once the sensory diet modifications are made, the patient is ready to apply the sensory diet to their day-to-day schedule.

Identifying and implementing a daily schedule: The occupational therapist should take time to educate the patient on the importance of creating balance in their daily schedule. Often, patients with FND symptoms will avoid activities when feeling symptomatic and over-extend themselves when feeling better. This can result in periods of "boom or bust" where a patient's ability to participate in daily activities fluctuates between two extremes (eg, avoidance and overextension) with little ability to modulate their participation over time.[36] Introduce the concepts of pacing and using brief rest breaks to reduce any "boom and bust" behaviors and help manage symptoms of FND. Explore ideas for what constitutes a rest break (eg, switch to a less demanding activity) with patients to ensure these activities provide respite and have the desired effect on arousal level. Developing a daily schedule should begin with capturing the patient's current daily roles and routine. The occupational therapist works with the patient to strategically insert sensory meals and rest breaks to create a more balanced routine of daily activities and maintain "just right" arousal levels for optimal performance in essential daily tasks. For instance, a patient may plan to go for a walk (sensory meal) to achieve the focus (arousal level) necessary to come home and pay bills (home management task). At the end of the session, patients should leave with a preliminary daily schedule that has incorporated their sensory diet into their daily routine. For homework, the patient is asked to follow the daily schedule for the next 1 to 2 weeks reflecting on its efficacy in improving participation in daily tasks and managing symptoms of FND.

Troubleshooting: When the patient returns to OT after 1 to 2 weeks of using their daily schedule, the session should focus on gathering the patient's reflections and troubleshooting any difficulties. The patient is asked to share reflections on their adherence to the daily schedule, success of the schedule in helping them modulate their arousal levels throughout the day, improvements in participation in daily activities, and any setbacks or challenges. Patients can often recognize what is not working, but may not know how to make modifications to improve success. The occupational therapist should troubleshoot with the patient as this is an important process for determining what modules may need to be revisited and if adjustments to the sensory diet or schedule are needed to help the patient achieve independence in their daily schedule. See **Table 4** for a range of potentially helpful troubleshooting questions and corresponding modules. Patients are then asked to follow their modified daily schedule and reflect on its efficacy in improving participation in daily tasks and managing symptoms of FND. The amount of time between home practice and the next OT session varies by patient. Some patients require little support and can take the foundational knowledge and insight they have developed to follow and modify the daily schedule as needed to achieve just-right balance and improved participation. These patients can typically follow up with OT once per month. Others continue to require frequent, ongoing check-ins with the occupational therapist to recognize challenges and make modifications. These patients may continue to follow-up every 1 to 2 weeks until they are more independent.

Goal Completion: As the patient achieves some success in using their sensory diet and daily schedule, they may notice positive changes in their ability to self-regulate and engage in daily tasks (as well as potential improvements in their functional neurologic symptoms). Their improved self-awareness and consistency result in feelings of competence and formation of healthy habits. As patients begin to master their daily schedule, they can add tasks over time. Module 7 is typically achieved over a period of 4 to 8 weeks. If the patient is not able to identify positive changes in symptom management and/or increased participation in daily activities after this timeframe, the OT may need to consider ending treatment.[12] Once the patient is following a balanced daily schedule consistently, they are ready to move on to the final module.

Table 4	
Troubleshooting use of the sensory diet in a daily schedule	
Targeted Skills	**Solutions to Consider**
Does the patient understand their sensory processing tendencies and how they may influence participation in daily activities and trigger or exacerbate FND symptoms?	• Revisit Module 2 to review neurologic threshold and behavioral response continuums in the Four Quadrant Model of Sensory Processing • Review patient's personalized sensory profile as determined by the AASP
Can the patient accurately self-reflect arousal levels using the arousal continuum?	• Review concepts in Module 3 • Guided self-reflection on patient's arousal states and fluctuations
Does the patient understand how different activities can influence their arousal levels and achieve a "just right" arousal level?	• Review concepts in Modules 4 and 5 • Provide personal experiences to facilitate ability to identify activities that are calming/alerting/irritating
Can the patient accurately self-identify changes in arousal level in response to sensory activities?	• Problem-solve barriers to skill acquisition in Module 5 • Increase time spent trialing sensory activities in clinic • Provide guided self-reflection on how these activities impact arousal level
Does the patient understand fundamental concepts of the sensory diet and incorporate these into daily routine?	• Revisit properties of sensory activities (eg, timing, intensity) from Module 5 and how to apply this to activity selection • Further explore concept of sensory meals and snacks from Module 6 and provide personal examples to enhance understanding and activity selection • Discuss feasibility of specific sensory meals and snacks in context of their daily routine

Abbreviation: AASP, adult/adolescent sensory profile.

SENSORY MODULATION TREATMENT PROGRAM GOAL #4: REPERTOIRE EXPANSION AND SKILL ENHANCEMENT
Module 8: Application of Sensory Modulation Strategies to Daily Life

The purpose of Module 8 is to provide patients with support to problem solve use of their sensory diet beyond the most essential tasks in their daily life. The goal of this module is for the patient to generalize use of their sensory diet across a variety of everyday life activities/situations and apply trained strategies in new situations. As the patient achieves independence and recognizes the value of their sensory diet (Goal #3/Module 7), they generally become more empowered to increase the types of activities they engage in (eg, increased pursuit of leisure or professional activities), which may result in changes to their daily schedule. As their daily schedule changes, the patient will need to make enhancements to how they incorporate their sensory diet into their day for continued balance and self-regulation. The ability to modify their sensory diet in the context of a changing schedule or setting, whether ongoing or for a finite period of time, can only be achieved if the patient is taking an active role in determining ways to expand their "toolkit" of sensory strategies and healthy habits. The occupational therapist's role at this stage is to facilitate the patient's feelings of mastery and empowerment to continue to enhance their lifestyle in preparation for discharge from OT. It is important to note that as patients challenge themselves more, they may experience the onset of new FND symptoms or a relapse in their recovery. Before discharge, a clear plan for managing any future symptom relapses should be discussed.

SUMMARY

Patients with FND can have significant sensory sensitivities that may trigger symptom onset and/or exacerbate existing symptoms. These sensitivities can lead to avoidance behaviors and hyperfocus on bodily symptoms that result in decreased participation in daily activities. This subset of patients has been shown to demonstrate extreme sensory processing patterns resulting in difficulty with self-regulation. Our experience has been that occupational therapists can help with FND symptom management by gaining an understanding of an individual's sensory processing patterns and implementing a sensory-based treatment approach. Prospective clinical trials examining the utility of this approach are now needed.

CLINICS CARE POINTS

- An assessment of sensory processing difficulties in patients with functional neurological disorder (FND) should include exploring the patient's sensory history through semi-structured interview, clinical observations, and administration of a self-report questionnaire such as the Adolescent and Adult Sensory Profile.
- Education is fundamental to treatment and should provide the patient some insight into their sensory processing profile, the role of the arousal continuum and sensory activities in self-regulation, and its relationship to improved function and FND symptoms.
- Treatment goals focus on facilitating self-awareness, exploring self-regulation strategies, expanding self-regulation to facilitate positive changes, and generalizing skills to a variety of everyday life activities/situations.

ACKNOWLEDGEMENTS

The authors thank Drs David L. Perez and Sara Finkelstein for their helpful article suggestions and edits.

DISCLOSURE

The authors do not report any disclosures or conflicts of interest.

REFERENCES

1. Czarnecki K, Thompson JM, Seime R, et al. Functional movement disorders: successful treatment with a physical therapy rehabilitation protocol. Parkinsonism Relat Disord 2012;18(3):247–51.
2. Demartini B, Batla A, Petrochilos P, et al. Multidisciplinary treatment for functional neurological symptoms: a prospective study. J Neurol 2014;261(12):2370–7.
3. Hebert C, Behel JM, Pal G, et al. Multidisciplinary inpatient rehabilitation for Functional Movement Disorders: A prospective study with long term follow up. Parkinsonism Relat Disord 2021;82:50–5.
4. Heruti RJ, Reznik J, Adunski A, et al. Conversion motor paralysis disorder: analysis of 34 consecutive referrals. Spinal Cord 2002;40(7):335–40.

5. Jordbru AA, Smedstad LM, Klungsoyr O, et al. Psychogenic gait disorder: a randomized controlled trial of physical rehabilitation with one-year follow-up. J Rehabil Med 2014;46(2):181–7.

6. McCormack R, Moriarty J, Mellers JD, et al. Specialist inpatient treatment for severe motor conversion disorder: a retrospective comparative study. J Neurol Neurosurg Psychiatry 2014;85(8):895–900.

7. Petrochilos P, Elmalem MS, Patel D, et al. Outcomes of a 5-week individualised MDT outpatient (day-patient) treatment programme for functional neurological symptom disorder (FNSD). J Neurol 2020;267(9):2655–66.

8. Saifee TA, Kassavetis P, Parees I, et al. Inpatient treatment of functional motor symptoms: a long-term follow-up study. J Neurol 2012;259(9):1958–63.

9. Speed J. Behavioral management of conversion disorder: retrospective study. Arch Phys Med Rehabil 1996;77(2):147–54.

10. Perez DL, Edwards MJ, Nielsen G, et al. Decade of progress in motor functional neurological disorder: continuing the momentum. J Neurol Neurosurg Psychiatry 2021;92:668–77.

11. Butz C, Iske C, Truba N, et al. Treatment of Functional Gait Abnormality in a Rehabilitation Setting: Emphasizing the Physical Interventions for Treating the Whole Child. Innov Clin Neurosci 2019;16(7–08):18–21.

12. Nicholson C, Edwards MJ, Carson AJ, et al. Occupational therapy consensus recommendations for functional neurological disorder. J Neurol Neurosurg Psychiatry 2020;91(10):1037–45.

13. Geroin C, Stone J, Camozzi S, et al. Triggers in functional motor disorder: a clinical feature distinct from precipitating factors. J Neurol 2022;269(7):3892–8.

14. Ranford J, Perez DL, MacLean J. Additional occupational therapy considerations for functional neurological disorders: a potential role for sensory processing. CNS Spectr 2018;23(3):194–5.

15. Brown C, Tollefson N, Dunn W, et al. The Adult Sensory Profile: measuring patterns of sensory processing. Am J Occup Ther 2001;55(1):75–82.

16. Ranford J, MacLean J, Alluri PR, et al. Sensory Processing Difficulties in Functional Neurological Disorder: A Possible Predisposing Vulnerability? Psychosomatics 2020;61(4):343–52.

17. van den Boogert F, Klein K, Spaan P, et al. Sensory processing difficulties in psychiatric disorders: A meta-analysis. J Psychiatr Res 2022;151:173–80.

18. Champagne TK. Evaluating sensory processing in mental health OT practice. OT Pract 2012;17(5).

19. Engel-Yeger B, Dunn W. The Relationship between Sensory Processing Difficulties and Anxiety Level of Healthy Adults. Br J Occup Ther 2011;74(5):210–6.

20. Champagne T. Sensory modulation and environment: essential elements of occupation: Handbook and reference. Sydney, NSW: Pearson Australia Group Pty Ltd.; 2011.

21. May-Benson TA, Kinnealey M. An Approach to Assessment of and Intervention for Adults With Sensory Processing Disorders. AOTA Continuing Education 2012;17(17). CE-1 - CE-8.

22. Pfeiffer B, Kinnealey M. Treatment of sensory defensiveness in adults. Occup Ther Int 2003;10(3):175–84.

23. Moore KM. The sensory Connection program self-regulation Workbook: Learning to use sensory activities to manage stress, anxiety, and emotional crisis. Framingham, MA: Therapro; 2008.

24. Ayres JA. Sensory Integration and the Child: understanding Hidden sensory challenges 25th Anniversary. Los Angeles: Western Psychological Services; 2005.

25. MacLean J, Finkelstein SA, Paredes-Echeverri S, et al. Sensory Processing Difficulties in Patients with Functional Neurological Disorder: Occupational Therapy Management Strategies and Two Cases. Semin Pediatr Neurol 2022;41:100951.

26. Glass SP, Matin N, Williams B, et al. Neuropsychiatric Factors Linked to Adherence and Short-Term Outcome in a U.S. Functional Neurological Disorders Clinic: A Retrospective Cohort Study. J Neuropsychiatry Clin Neurosciences 2018;30(2): 152–9.

27. Jalilianhasanpour R, Ospina JP, Williams B, et al. Secure Attachment and Depression Predict 6-Month Outcome in Motor Functional Neurological Disorders: A Prospective Pilot Study. Psychosomatics 2019;60(4):365–75.

28. Finkelstein SA, Adams C, Tuttle M, et al. Neuropsychiatric Treatment Approaches for Functional Neurological Disorder: A How to Guide. Semin Neurol 2022;42(2): 204–24.

29. DuBois D, Lymer E, Gibson BE, et al. Assessing Sensory Processing Dysfunction in Adults and Adolescents with Autism Spectrum Disorder: A Scoping Review. Brain Sci 2017;7(8).

30. Pfeiffer B, Brusilovskiy E, Bauer J, et al. Sensory processing, participation, and recovery in adults with serious mental illnesses. Psychiatr Rehabil J 2014;37(4): 289–96.

31. Dunn W. Living sensationally: understanding your senses. Philadelphia, PA: Jessica Kingsley Publishers; 2009.

32. Kozlowska K, Scher S, Helgeland H. The Autonomic Nervous System and Functional Somatic Symptoms. In: Functional Somatic symptoms in Children and adolescents.2020:119-136.

33. Jungilligens J, Paredes-Echeverri S, Popkirov S, et al. A new science of emotion: implications for functional neurological disorder. Brain 2022;145(8):2648–63.

34. Williams M, Shellenberger S. "How Does Your Engine Run?": A Leaders guide to the alert program for self regulation. Albuquerque, NM: Therapy Works, Inc.; 1996.

35. Guttadauro T. Sensory Diet Workseet. Worksheet. 2013. www.thespiralfoundation.org.

36. Maggio J, Kyle K, Stephen CD, et al. Lessons Learned in Outpatient Physical Therapy for Motor Functional Neurological Disorder. J Neurol Phys Ther 2023; 47(1):52–9.

Developing a Curriculum for Functional Neurological Disorder in Neurology Training: Questions and Answers

Sara A. Finkelstein, MD, MSc[a,1,*], M. Angela O'Neal, MD[b,1,*],
Gaston Baslet, MD[c], Barbara A. Dworetzky, MD[d],
Ellen Godena, EdM, MSW, LICSW[a], Julie Maggio, PT, DPT, NCS[a,e],
Daniel Millstein, PhD[a], Tracey Milligan, MD[f,2],
David L. Perez, MD, MMSc[a,g,2]

KEYWORDS

- Functional neurological disorder • Functional movement disorder
- Functional seizures • Psychogenic non-epileptic seizures • Dissociative seizures
- Education • Teaching • Neurology • Psychiatry

Continued

INTRODUCTION

Functional neurological disorder (FND) is a common condition in neurology across clinical settings,[1] and there is often high health care utilization among this population.[2,3] Reflecting this reality, the cost of emergency department and inpatient treatment alone for patients with FND was found to total more than $1.2 billion in the United States annually.[4] Etiology, diagnosis, and management of this disorder are active fields of research, with a growing body of evidence-based treatments

[a] Functional Neurological Disorder Unit, Division of Behavioral Neurology, Massachusetts General Hospital, Harvard Medical School, 55 Fruit Street, Boston, MA 02114, USA; [b] Division of General Neurology, Department of Neurology, Brigham and Women's Hospital, Harvard Medical School, 60 Fenwood Road, Boston, MA 02115, USA; [c] Division of Neuropsychiatry, Department of Psychiatry, Brigham and Women's Hospital, Harvard Medical School, 60 Fenwood Road, Boston, MA 02115, USA; [d] Division of Epilepsy, Department of Neurology, Brigham and Women's Hospital, Harvard Medical School, 60 Fenwood Road, Boston, MA 02115, USA; [e] Department of Physical Therapy, Massachusetts General Hospital, 55 Fruit Street, Boston, MA 02114, USA; [f] Department of Neurology, Westchester Medical Center Health Network, New York Medical College, Valhalla, NY, USA; [g] Division of Neuropsychiatry, Department of Psychiatry, Massachusetts General Hospital, Harvard Medical School, 55 Fruit Street, Boston, MA 02114, USA

[1] Co-first authors.
[2] Co-senior authors.
* Corresponding authors.
E-mail addresses: safinkelstein@mgh.harvard.edu (S.A.F.); maoneal@bwh.harvard.edu (M.A.O.)

Neurol Clin 41 (2023) 711–728
https://doi.org/10.1016/j.ncl.2023.02.007
0733-8619/23/© 2023 Elsevier Inc. All rights reserved.

neurologic.theclinics.com

Continued

KEY POINTS

- A structured curriculum for functional neurological disorder (FND) is needed as this is a common and potentially treatable disorder.
- Curricular content should encompass medical knowledge, clinical skills, and communication and collaboration.
- Teaching should be done through a combination of didactic lectures and clinical experiences.
- In the United States, curriculum development should align with current Accreditation Council for Graduate Medical Education Milestone structure and content.
- Energizing neurology trainees around this underserved population is important in the further development of the field and sustainability of care.

accrued over the past several decades.[5–7] Despite the fact that all general neurologists and many subspecialists in neurology are likely to encounter this disorder regularly throughout their careers, there remains little to no formal teaching (or established curriculum) regarding FND over the course of medical education.[8,9] Given this reliance on experiential learning alone, it is not surprising that a recent study showed that 40% of practicing neurologists do not feel as though they have good knowledge of FND.[10]

In this article, the authors seek to address this education gap by proposing a framework to guide the development of an FND curriculum for neurology residents, taking a question-and-answer approach. Over the course of responding to five timely questions, the authors discuss the rationale underlying a need for such a curriculum, provide a broad overview of the content that should be included, discuss methods for delivering curricular content, and consider how to better promote interest in neurology trainees around this disorder. This will be followed by a brief discussion regarding how this type of curriculum can be integrated into the current Accreditation Council for Graduate Medical Education (ACGME) framework for neurology training. Although this article is geared toward adult neurology residency

---

Box 1
Additional content considerations for pediatric neurology training programs

- Recognize that mixed symptom presentations are particularly common in pediatric populations, including patients experiencing several functional neurologic and/or functional somatic symptoms concurrently
- Understand the use of body-based language to ask and talk about symptoms
- Understanding of illness-promoting psychological processes
- Ability to perform a family assessment including psychosocial history, assessing family dynamics, and understanding possible predisposing, precipitating, and perpetuating factors for symptoms within the family context
- Ability to explain the diagnosis to both child/adolescent and their families in a developmentally appropriate way
- Working with patient and family to create a plan for reasonable accommodations for symptoms within the school system if needed

training programs, considerations regarding additional pediatric content can be found in **Box 1**.

QUESTION 1: WHY DO WE NEED A CURRICULUM FOR FUNCTIONAL NEUROLOGICAL DISORDER IN NEUROLOGY RESIDENCY?

Answer: FND is a commonly encountered disorder across inpatient, outpatient, and emergency department clinical neurology settings. In an outpatient general neurology setting, approximately 10% to 15% of patients have an FND diagnosis[1,11] and FND accounts for nearly 10% of all acute neurology admissions.[12] One could argue, given these statistics, that "learning through doing" is likely playing a role in neurology residents' learning to diagnose and manage this disorder. However, major gaps in understanding are likely to occur with a completely unstructured approach to this patient population—as reflected in a recent survey of French neurologists and neurology trainees reporting that only about one-third were familiar with a Hoover's sign.[13] Most programs would balk at providing neurology residents no formal teaching regarding multiple sclerosis or motor neuron disease—both of which are less common in a general neurology outpatient setting than FND[11]—and yet when it comes to FND this is the status quo.

Although ward teaching may cover some knowledge regarding the diagnosis of FND (eg, by providing instruction on rule-in examination signs and semiological features), it is not a sufficiently suitable setting for residents to learn about many of the nuanced issues that arise with longitudinal FND management (eg, patient-centered discussions about perpetuating factors). In addition, exclusively relying on clinical exposure-based teaching carries the risk of significant variability in the quality of training, given that misconceptions about FND still exist among many neurologists. Neurology curricula, in general, do not conventionally provide significant education about approaching patients from interdisciplinary and multidisciplinary perspectives, which is foundational to FND management. Given that FND is a condition at the intersection of neurology and psychiatry, the gap in FND education also parallels gaps in psychiatry education for neurology residents more broadly. A recent survey of early career neurologists highlighted that many thought they were underprepared to address psychiatric issues encountered in their patients.[14] Although research has demonstrated that multidisciplinary treatments can promote clinical improvements for patients with FND,[15] these approaches are most effective when there is a high level of understanding about what these treatments can offer as well as good communication skills among team members.[10] Residents may have exposure to physical therapy (PT) and occupational therapy (OT) approaches for other neurologic disorders, but the treatment approaches and strategies for FND tend to depart significantly from traditional PT and OT-based rehabilitation models.[16,17] For example, the use of assistive devices is generally discouraged for FND patients, while for a patient post-stroke, learning appropriate use of a walker may be integral to their care. Similarly, to manage patients with FND effectively, neurology trainees require an understanding of psychological principles beyond the recognition of major psychiatric disorders such as anxiety, mood, and trauma-related disorders. Nuanced recognition of psychological traits commonly associated with the disorder (such as perfectionism, somatic hypervigilance, dissociation, alexithymia, and poor distress tolerance) as well as cognitive and behavioral processes that play a role in symptom generation and maintenance (such as illness beliefs, attentional bias, prediction error, avoidance, and boom and bust patterns of behavior) can enhance clinical confidence and understanding of the underlying disease mechanisms.[5] As with PT and OT treatments for FND, current psychotherapeutic approaches have been tailored to the unique characteristics of these patients. For instance, in recent years, two manualized cognitive behavioral therapy treatments for FND have been adapted to address the specific psychological traits associated with the disorder.[18,19] Specialized knowledge gaps are only likely to be filled with a structured approach to FND education that incorporates interdisciplinary and multi-disciplinary perspectives not typically found elsewhere in the general neurology curriculum. Although aiming to become a transdisciplinary clinician for FND could be a goal for more advanced training and post-training stages (eg, cutting across the traditional boundaries of neurology, psychiatry, psychology, and rehabilitation specialties), neurology residents should nonetheless be encouraged to delve deeply into understanding psychological and rehabilitative components of FND care if motivated and appropriate supervision is available.

A recent study by Lehn and colleagues[10] found that neurologists may have relatively low levels of clinical interest in FND and be more likely to have a negative attitude toward these patients, when compared with other health care providers such as psychiatrists and physical therapists. In a systematic review looking at the perceptions of health care providers toward patients with functional seizures, significant findings were that the patients with FND were often considered frustrating and challenging, they had more volitional control over their symptoms than seemingly endorsed (despite symptoms in FND being involuntary as per diagnostic criteria), and functional seizures were considered less severe or disabling than epilepsy (a sentiment not supported by the quality of life literature).[20] Having an explicit and early FND curriculum may help to generate interest in treating this disorder and counteract some of the negative attitudes, misconceptions, and stigma that are often directed toward patients. Indeed, a recent qualitative study by Klinke and colleagues[21] demonstrated that among healthcare professionals providing care to patients with FND, negative perceptions of FND lessened with better education and comprehension of this disorder.

QUESTION 2: WHAT CURRICULAR CONTENT ON FUNCTIONAL NEUROLOGICAL DISORDER SHOULD BE INCLUDED AS PART OF NEUROLOGY RESIDENCY TRAINING?

Answer: Neurology residents should be exposed to similar curricular content regarding FND as with any other neurologic disorder, including pathophysiology, diagnostic signs and semiological features, differential diagnosis considerations, and management approaches. There are several issues that should additionally be covered with respect to FND. First, given that it is a clinical diagnosis, special attention should be paid to possible diagnostic pitfalls (see article in this issue[22]). Second, physicians have traditionally been poor at communicating an FND diagnosis[23] and explicit teaching on how to do so effectively should be included in curricular content. Finally, care for patients with FND is typically longitudinal and often involves a multidisciplinary team, and curricula should include the discussion of longitudinal care integration. Depending on the time allotted to teaching this topic, consideration could also be given to adding supplementary content covering overlapping or frequently comorbid disorders such as chronic pain disorders, other functional somatic disorders, and co-occurring psychiatric conditions as well as the intersection of FND with other neurologic conditions such as epilepsy, multiple sclerosis,[24] and Parkinson disease.[25] Indeed, FND-specific teaching should be complemented by enhanced educational initiatives to more effectively teach neurology residents how to perform psychiatric screenings and obtain developmental and social histories across a range of neuropsychiatric populations. In this section, we outline suggested curricular content divided into themes including

Table 1
Core content areas and educational resources for functional neurological disorder

Theme	Suggested Minimum Learning Objectives	Resources
Medical Knowledge	• Gain an understanding of pathophysiological and neuropsychological theories implicated in FND • Develop familiarity with diagnostic criteria for FND across subtypes • Develop a framework for case formulation using the biopsychosocial model, including consideration of predisposing, precipitating, and perpetuating factors • Develop a rationale and approach to ordering adjunctive testing • Gain an understanding of the principles, evidence for, and clinical implementation of PT, OT, speech language pathology (SLP), and psychotherapy for the treatment of FND • Be aware of common diagnostic pitfalls and neuropsychiatric differential diagnosis considerations	*Review papers:* Milligan et al.,[9] 2022 Finkelstein et al.,[15] 2022 Hallett et al., 2022[5] Perez et al.,[26] 2019 *Books:* *Functional Neurologic Disorders*[27] *Psychogenic Nonepileptic Seizures*[28] *Functional Movement Disorder*[29] *Web sites:* www.neurosymptoms.org www.fndsociety.org/fnd-education/past-webinar-topics www.nonepilepticseizures.com Basic Training Series: Psychogenic Nonepileptic Seizures (https://youtu.be/NIX-yNTX86w)
Clinical Skills	• Be able to perform a psychiatric and developmental/social history assessment, including a mental status examination and consideration of cultural-spiritual factors as potentially relevant • Recognition of psychological traits that increase risk of FND • Learn how to perform specific examination maneuvers and appreciate semiological features to evaluate for rule-in signs of FND • Learn how to formulate patient-centered, multidisciplinary treatment plans • Have an approach to longitudinal follow-up, including monitoring symptom progression or improvement	*Review papers:* Aybek & Perez,[6] 2022 Baslet et al.,[30] 2021 Espay et al.,[7] 2018 Adams et al.,[31] 2018

(continued on next page)

Table 1
(continued)

Theme	Suggested Minimum Learning Objectives	Resources
Communication and Collaboration	• Learn how to effectively convey a diagnosis of FND (including focusing on the "what" vs the "why" of diagnosis in early discussions) • Be able to provide education around the diagnosis and management suggestions to other team members • Discuss need, or lack of need, for further investigations following a diagnosis of FND with patients and their families • Discuss transparently questions or doubts regarding diagnosis with patients, families, or other members of care team • Understand the roles of and be able to collaborate with members of the multidisciplinary team around longitudinal care, including community-based providers	*Review papers:* Hall-Patch et al.,[32] 2010 Carson et al.,[33] 2016 *Web sites:* www.neurosymptoms.org https://www.hapyak.com/portal/experience/viewer/ dd61d430f5794103ab935740a3f02faf *Multidisciplinary Treatment:* Nielsen et al.,[16] 2015 Nicholson et al.,[17] 2020 Baker et al.,[34] 2021 Overcoming Functional Neurological Symptoms: A Five Area Approach (2011)[18]

"medical knowledge," "clinical skills," and "communication and collaboration." These themes, along with teaching resources, are summarized in **Table 1** (additional resources found in Supplemental Table 1).

Medical Knowledge

To effectively diagnose and manage patients with FND, neurology residents should be provided with knowledge regarding epidemiology and risk factors, an understanding of some of the prevailing neurobiological/neuropsychological theories for FND, be familiar with diagnostic criteria (and levels of diagnostic certainty), have a framework for case formulation, and understand current best practices for management.

As with many neurologic disorders, knowledge regarding FND-related etiological and mechanistic factors remains incomplete and continues to expand. FND can be conceptualized in part as a disorder of abnormal cross talk between brain networks. Understanding some of the pathways of brain dysfunction involved in this disorder can be helpful in both explaining FND to patients as well as enhancing both clinician and patient understanding regarding the utility of various therapeutic modalities. Residents should be especially familiar with how biased attention, predictive processing, self-agency, emotion processing, and dysregulated stress responses are thought to contribute to FND neurobiology (for recent reviews of these concepts, see Refs[5,35,36]).

The reasons for FND symptom generation and maintenance are often complex, and we would recommend providing learners with a framework that they can use to help with case formulation. Many experts in the field make use of the "biopsychosocial model." This model considers how biological, psychological, and sociocultural factors can predispose to, precipitate, and/or perpetuate FND symptoms. For a full review of this model, see Saxena and colleagues.[37]

Learners should be made aware of diagnostic criteria for FND across its subtypes. The Diagnostic and Statistical Manual of Mental Disorders, Fifth Edition (DSM-5), for example, emphasizes the need for rule-in signs to make a diagnosis of FND, and a preceding stressor is no longer required, both of which are departures from the previous DSM-IV version. Diagnostic criteria are also available for functional seizures,[38] functional movement disorder,[39] persistent postural perceptual dizziness (PPPD; a form of functional dizziness),[40] and functional cognitive disorder.[41]

Learners should also understand the role of adjunctive diagnostic testing in patients suspected of having FND. They should have an approach to ordering imaging, electroencephalogram (EEG), electromyography (EMG), or other potentially helpful investigations to ensure that any testing needed is ordered upfront, thus avoiding serial rounds of testing and reaching diagnostic clarity in a timely fashion. This should include the need to consider tests to evaluate causes for other commonly co-occurring bodily symptoms such as pain and fatigue—symptoms that are both prevalent and related to quality of life in this population.

Finally, learners should be made aware of management principles for FND and the data supporting use of various therapies. In particular, they should be familiar with how PT,[16] OT,[17] speech and language therapy,[34] psychotherapy modalities,[42] and multidisciplinary teams can be used in FND treatment. Further, they may benefit from understanding each discipline's role and the importance of communication across clinical team members. For a recent review of these therapeutic modalities for FND, see Finkelstein and colleagues.[15]

Clinical Skills

Residents should become familiar with how to look for rule-in signs or, in the case of functional seizures, semiological features consistent with the diagnosis of FND.

Several recent articles have reviewed these signs in detail and can be used as resources.[6,7,30] Residents should be able to confidently perform physical examination maneuvers to assess for functional motor disorders including limb weakness, movement disorders, and gait abnormalities. Consideration should also be given to including functional sensory disorders (eg, non-dermatomal sensory deficits, and functional vision loss), functional dizziness/PPPD, and functional cognitive disorder in the curriculum. As FND is a clinical diagnosis, learners should be made aware of common diagnostic pitfalls (eg, "pain-limited weakness" should not be confused with collapsing/give-way weakness found in functional limb weakness). A recent review of this topic by Perez and colleagues[26] provides further discussion. Another component of the FND assessment is being able to take screening psychiatric and developmental/social histories and document a detailed mental status examination, skills that should additionally be reviewed with neurology residents (and as discussed above are important skills that apply to a range of neuropsychiatric conditions cared for in neurology). For example, residents could be taught how to create a genogram or illness timeline as efficient methods for gathering social history.[43] Thorough assessment of social factors relevant to FND including family systems components, cultural frameworks within which a patient may be embedded, and economic and legal considerations are important to understanding how a patient will respond to the diagnosis and/or how treatment should be approached. Recognition of underlying psychological processes, either through administration of scales or based on clinical interview, can help further develop neurology trainees' confidence in an area in which they usually receive limited training. Cross-training with psychiatry, psychology, and social work faculty can facilitate this process and provide a model of interdisciplinary teaching and clinical collaboration.

Communication and Collaboration

FND is often a diagnosis unfamiliar to patients, their family members, and other care providers. It is still viewed by many as a purely "psychosomatic" illness and patients with FND may have experienced stigma, including negative health care experiences—for example, being made to think that it is "all in their head" or they are malingering. For these reasons, a thorough grasp of how to communicate the diagnosis and educate both patients/family members and health care professionals about this disorder is imperative. Residents should also be prepared to listen to and empathize with patients' past experiences and be able to communicate in a direct way designed to counteract stigma when delivering a diagnosis, such as by specifically making statements like "your symptoms are real." For an approach to communicating an FND diagnosis, see study by Hall-Patch and colleagues[32] as well as the vignette-based educational article by Carson and colleagues.[33] The use of supplementary materials (such as websites or animations) can reinforce the initial discussion and provide a framework for patients and family members to further understand the diagnosis.

Residents should feel confident discussing the need or lack of need for further investigations following diagnosis and fielding questions regarding the diagnosis with patients/families/health care team members. Finally, residents should have an approach to managing ongoing communication within an interdisciplinary and multidisciplinary team model, which is often used in FND care. This includes guidance on how to address out-of-scheduled visit clinical messages and phone calls, which is applicable to other neurology patient populations such as those with chronic migraine. In addition, focus on how the components of the clinical team can work together as a whole to integrate care should be emphasized, including incorporation of community-based providers into the care team who can reinforce the initial plan—a collaborative process that may require some orientation to and education around the FND diagnosis.

QUESTION 3: HOW SHOULD THE RECOMMENDED CURRICULAR CONTENT FOR FUNCTIONAL NEUROLOGICAL DISORDER BE TAUGHT AND EVALUATED DURING NEUROLOGY RESIDENCY?

Answer: The implementation of an FND curriculum should be grounded in the goals of educating neurology trainees about the diagnosis, mechanisms, etiologies, and management of this condition. The competencies of any educational process can be divided into three domains: (1) Knowledge about how to make the diagnosis, deliver it to the patient, and engage them in treatment; (2) Understand the attitudes/biases of both patients and providers that may hinder care; and (3) Develop the skills to care for this diverse and potentially challenging patient population. The optimal approach to teach such a curriculum depends on the patient population and available resources, including the need to tailor teaching to the specifics of the residency program and the health care system in which it is situated. Good teaching practices should provide a combination of didactic and clinical exposure opportunities that address themes relevant across inpatient and outpatient clinical settings (**Table 2**). The curriculum can be further enhanced by educational modules, case studies, simulation exercises, case presentations, and supervised clinical care,[9] and applying these competencies to a variety of training opportunities will help to consolidate learning. For example, simulation, use of standardized patients, or role-playing modules can provide residents the ability to practice individual and team-based clinical skills.

Topics for Didactic Learning

The basis on which to build clinical skills should start with a solid foundation in knowledge presented through didactic teaching sessions. These topics should include how to make the diagnosis based on "rule in" criteria, the pathophysiology of FND, appropriate adjunctive testing, case formulation using a biopsychosocial approach, and management principles. There is a need for cross-educational lectures in FND, given the wide range of symptoms and multidisciplinary management. Engaging a variety of neurology subspecialists to deliver lectures would provide residents the opportunity to learn from faculty with wide-ranging expertise about a disorder that cuts across many neurologic subspecialties. For example, teaching about how to make the rule in diagnosis of FND both can be taught independently as well as incorporated into lectures on movement disorders, epilepsy, syncope, dizziness, and neurocognitive disorders.[44–47] FND is a disorder where multidisciplinary care is often needed and should be modeled, including lectures delivered by physical therapists, occupational therapists, speech language pathologists, social workers, psychologists, and/or psychiatrists regarding their contribution to diagnosis and management whenever possible.[16,17,34,42] Supplemental didactics covering topics such as psychotherapeutic considerations for neurology populations, other functional somatic disorders, and factitious disorder/malingering could be considered.

Topics Best Modeled by Clinical Exposure

Elements of medical knowledge covered through didactic lectures that should be consolidated in a real-world clinical setting include history-taking, examination maneuvers to confirm a diagnosis of FND, an approach to using adjunctive testing, diagnostic pitfalls, and real-time case formulation using a biopsychosocial approach.

Table 2
Matching educational content to modalities of delivery and evaluation for a neurology residency curriculum in functional neurological disorder

Content Area	Competency	Method of Delivery	Method of Assessment
Pathophysiology	Medical knowledge	D	MCQ/short answer
Neuropsychiatric assessment	Medical knowledge; Patient care	D/CE/S	MCQ/short answer Direct clinical observation Simulation/standardized patient (OSCE)
Examination to "rule-in" diagnosis	Medical knowledge; Patient care	D/CE	MCQ/short answer Chart review Direct clinical observation Simulation/standardized patient (OSCE)
Adjunctive testing	Medical knowledge; Patient care; Communication skills	D/CE	MCQ/short answer Chart review Simulation/standardized patient (OSCE)
Diagnostic pitfalls	Medical knowledge; Patient care	D/CE	MCQ/short answer Direct clinical observation Simulation/standardized patient (OSCE)
Communicating the diagnosis	Medical knowledge; Patient care; Communication skills; Systems-based practice; Professionalism	D/CE	MCQ/short answer Direct clinical observation Simulation/standardized patient (OSCE) Patient experience survey
Longitudinal management and care integration	Patient care; Communication skills; Systems-based practice; Professionalism; Practice-based learning and improvement	CE/S	Chart review Simulation/standardized patient (OSCE) Patient experience survey Multisource feedback (360° feedback)

Abbreviations: CE, clinical exposure; D, didactic; MCQ, multiple choice question; OSCE, observed structured clinical evaluation; S, supplementary content.

The creation of a patient-centered management plan and an approach to patient follow-up, including addressing barriers to treatment, are best covered in clinical settings. Communication and team collaboration should also be a focus of the clinical teaching setting, including delivering a diagnosis, addressing patient questions and doubts, and promoting ongoing multidisciplinary team-based care during long-term management.[48,49] There are typically an abundant number of patients with FND, providing rich learning opportunities. Clinical exposure can also be supplemented or replaced by alternative practical skills sessions, such as medical simulation, role-play, or use of standardized patients if needed.

Limitations to initiating any curriculum are resources, including providers with the knowledge and experience in the content area, and time limitations in the residency educational agenda.[50] However, given the prevalence with which FND is encountered by neurologists, these challenges need to be overcome. There are multiple resources available that can aid in dealing with these challenges including educational websites (www.neurosymptoms.org; https://fndaustralia.com.au/resources/educational-videos.html; www.fndsociety.org), comprehensive review articles,[5-7,51] and authoritative textbooks.[27-29]

If there is limited time for didactics, then other teaching modalities such as simulation learning can be used. In the situation where there is a lack of local expertise, expert faculty from other institutions in remote didactic teaching, grand round presentations, or teaching modules can be used to fill this gap. A broader way to address the issue would be to establish a teaching curriculum at a national or international level, such as through the FND Society, American Academy of Neurology, and/or American Neuropsychiatric Association (eg, e-learning modules on FND diagnosis and management exist through e-Brain, hosted by the European Academy of Neurology[52]).

Having measurable objectives that can be evaluated once the curriculum is implemented will be important (see **Table 1**). Consideration should be given to providing residents with the opportunity to practice and assess clinical skills pertinent to FND.[31] Trainee evaluation, surveys, and feedback are critical to improving the curriculum[53] and a "plan-do-check-adjust" design could aid in curriculum improvement once initiated. The ACGME outlines a number of methods for neurology resident knowledge assessment, and the preferred method of assessment will vary depending on the skill in question.[54] Broadly, the material provided in didactic lectures can be tested using written tests (multiple choice or short answer), whereas the application of this knowledge in a clinical setting, as well as skills learned through clinical exposure, can be tested using real-world direct observation with faculty/patient feedback or standardized testing scenarios, such as through simulation or standardized patients (observed structured clinical evaluation). See **Table 2** for suggested methods of evaluation by content area.

QUESTION 4: CAN WE OPERATIONALIZE MILESTONES IN LINE WITH OTHER ACCREDITATION COUNCIL FOR GRADUATE MEDICAL EDUCATION CONTENT?

The ACGME sets standards for medical residency and fellowship programs within the United States. Milestones for knowledge and skill acquisition are published by specialty and are structured in a graded fashion. Milestones start with basic skills and progress through to a high level of proficiency which includes serving as a leader, teacher, and mentor for others, and endeavors to cover several themes, including medical knowledge, patient care, system-based practice, interpersonal and communication skills, and practice-based learning and improvement.[55]

There seems to be opportunities to expand and improve milestones focused on cross-disciplinary skills between neurology and psychiatry. The ACGME Neurology Milestones currently include a patient care milestone focused on achievement of skills pertaining to "psychiatric and functional aspects of neurology," in which senior residents are expected to be able to "Develop a shared management plan that addresses the psychiatric or functional contribution to neurologic symptoms."[55] The Psychiatry ACGME milestones also include the consideration of neurologic and medical contributions to clinical presentation and treatment planning.[56] As FND is a prototypical neuropsychiatric disorder (ie, a condition at the intersection of neurology and psychiatry), consideration of what a set of milestones for FND might look like helps to inform how both neurology and psychiatry milestones could be updated throughout the milestone curriculum to incorporate acquisition of a "neuropsychiatric" skillset. In **Table 3**, we propose what milestones for acquiring skills around FND diagnosis and management might include, using the ACGME format. Broadly, at a junior resident level, learners should recognize common presentations of FND and understand the principles of diagnosis communication. As they move through training, residents should be able to diagnose and manage more complex cases (eg, with multiple functional neurologic symptoms), use a biopsychosocial approach to guide a patient-centered treatment plan, and have an approach to longitudinal management.

QUESTION 5: HOW DO WE BETTER ENGAGE AND ENERGIZE NEUROLOGY TRAINEES AROUND THIS UNDERSERVED YET CHALLENGING PATIENT POPULATION?

Answer: As FND is a common condition seen in ambulatory neurology,[11,57] there is ample opportunity in both the inpatient and outpatient arenas to teach residents how to learn the needed skill set through appropriate modeling by faculty. Furthermore, this is a skill set readily translatable to other neurologic conditions: migraine, chronic pain, and post-concussive syndrome.[58] These are common neurologic disorders where there is a need for neurology residents to have a more integrated physical and mental health (neuropsychiatric) approach, leveraging multidisciplinary patient-centered care. Framing the FND-related skill set as valuable in the care of many neurologic patients will also help support the need to prioritize education in this content area. Programs where such an approach already exists but for a different patient population should try to consolidate efforts across subspecialties. This is an opportunity for programs to demonstrate that principles of care in FND do not differ substantially from what trainees may have already learned in other subspecialty clinics.

Listening to patient testimonials about how FND has affected their life, as well as following patients longitudinally, would allow trainees to understand care needs and gaps and experience the rewarding robust clinical improvement that can occur in a subset of patients (the effect sizes of which rivals any other improvement trajectories seen in neurology).

From a career development perspective, FND is markedly underdeveloped compared with other areas of neurology, providing significant academic opportunities across multiple domains to explore, such as educational and programmatic initiatives and research questions about pathophysiology, clinical outcomes, and novel treatment paradigms among other topics. For example, given the prevalence of FND, enrolling patients in studies may be less daunting than those for rarer neurologic conditions. The lack of expertise and research in FND leaves fertile ground for young clinician–scientists hoping to establish an academic niche. Overall, there are myriad

Table 3
Work-in-progress Accreditation Council for Graduate Medical Education milestones for diagnosis and management of functional neurological disorder

A. Understands the pathophysiology, diagnosis, and management of FND
B. Educates patients about the diagnosis and treatment of FND
C. Monitors patient response to treatment and adjust appropriately

Level 1	Level 2	Level 3	Level 4	Level 5
Identifies commonly encountered FND types (motor FND, functional seizures) based on rule-in signs	Diagnoses common FND types with easily elicitable and robustly appreciated rule-in signs	Diagnoses presentations of FND by incorporating clinical signs, semiological features, and adjunctive testing such as EEG data	In addition to motor FND and functional seizures, able to diagnose other manifestations of FND	Serves as a role model in diagnosis and management of patients with FND
Demonstrates understanding of basic components of communicating diagnosis	Identifies diagnostic pitfalls for FND	Able to complete a screen for potentially relevant psychological and social factors	Recognizes biological, psychological, and social contributions to FND symptom generation and maintenance	Able to diagnose all symptom types of FND, as well as include noncore FND symptoms (eg, chronic pain, and fatigue) into diagnostic formulation
	Able to communicate diagnosis and discuss basics of pathophysiology	Able to communicate diagnosis, including discussion of pathophysiology, and address patient questions and concerns	Able to communicate diagnosis and explain treatment principles to patient	Able to have ongoing discussions with patients throughout the course of treatment that explore a nuanced biopsychosocial formulation and predisposing, precipitating, and perpetuating factors
		Identifies core components of a management plan including need for multidisciplinary care where appropriate	Individualizes management and follow-up plan for commonly encountered FND conditions, considering risks, benefits, and non-pharmacologic strategies	Adapts management plan based on patient outcomes and other factors such as potential nonadherence
				Initiates and maintains interdisciplinary communication and collaboration to advance management

opportunities in this long-neglected field for trainees to make significant impacts across clinical care, educational initiatives, and research.

SUMMARY

Given how commonly FND is encountered in neurologic practice, a dedicated curriculum to appropriately train residents is needed. The aim of such a curriculum should be to provide knowledge, clinical acumen, communication skills, and effective use of team-based collaboration in treatment. In the United States, the methods for teaching and evaluating this knowledge and associated clinical skills should be linked to current ACGME neurology milestones.

CLINICS CARE POINTS

- There is an educational need to develop a FND curriculum which should be incorporated into neurology training.
- Medical knowledge, clinical and communication skills need to be taught.
- Residents would best learn this information by utilizing both didactics as well as clinical exposure.

FUNDING

None.

CONFLICTS OF INTERESTS/DISCLOSURES

S.A. Finkelstein has received honoraria from continuing medical education lectures in functional neurological disorder. D.L. Perez has received honoraria for continuing medical education lectures in functional neurological disorder, royalties from Springer Nature for a functional movement disorder textbook, is a paid senior editor at Brain and Behavior, is on the editorial board of Epilepsy & Behavior and The Journal of Neuropsychiatry & Clinical Neurosciences, and has received funding from the National Institute of Health (NIH) and Sidney R. Baer Jr Foundation unrelated to this work. M.A. O'Neal receives publishing royalties from Springer and Oxford Press, serves as a consultant for Best Doctors and CRICO, where she has provided expert medicolegal testimony in defense of physicians involved in cases of alleged neurologic injury. B.A. Dworetzky is on the executive board of the Functional Neurological Disorders Society, editorial board of Epilepsy & Behavior Reports, receives publishing royalties from Oxford University Press, and serves as a consultant for Bioserenity and Best Doctors provided EEG interpretation and expert second opinion for clinical care. G. Baslet has received honoraria for continuing medical education lectures in functional neurological disorder and receives royalties from Oxford University Press. J. Maggio has received honoraria for physical therapy continuing education and has received funding from the Sidney R. Baer Jr Foundation.

ACKNOWLEDGEMENTS

None.

SUPPLEMENTARY DATA

Supplementary data related to this article can be found online at https://doi.org/10.1016/j.ncl.2023.02.007.

REFERENCES

1. Stone J, Carson A, Duncan R, et al. Who is referred to neurology clinics?—The diagnoses made in 3781 new patients. Clin Neurol Neurosurg 2010;112(9): 747–51.
2. Merkler AE, Parikh NS, Chaudhry S, et al. Hospital revisit rate after a diagnosis of conversion disorder. J Neurol Neurosurg Psychiatr 2016;87(4):363–6.
3. Barsky AJ, Orav EJ, Bates DW. Somatization increases medical utilization and costs independent of psychiatric and medical comorbidity. Arch Gen Psychiatry 2005;62(8):903–10.
4. Stephen C, Fung V, Lungu C, et al. Assessment of emergency department and inpatient use and costs in adult and pediatric functional neurological disorders. JAMA Neurol 2021;78(1):88–101.
5. Hallett M, Aybek S, Dworetzky BA, et al. Functional neurological disorder: new subtypes and shared mechanisms. Lancet Neurol 2022;21(6):537–50.
6. Aybek S, Perez DL. Diagnosis and management of functional neurological disorder. BMJ 2022;376. https://doi.org/10.1136/BMJ.O64.
7. Espay AJ, Aybek S, Carson A, et al. Current concepts in diagnosis and treatment of functional neurological disorders. JAMA Neurol 2018;75(9):1132–41.
8. Hutchinson G, Linden SC. The challenge of functional neurological disorder – views of patients, doctors and medical students. J Ment Health Train Educ Pract 2021;16(2):123–38.
9. Milligan TA, Yun A, LaFrance WC, et al. Neurology residents' education in functional seizures. Epilepsy Behav Rep 2022;18. https://doi.org/10.1016/J.EBR.2021.100517.
10. Lehn A, Bullock-Saxton J, Newcombe P, et al. Survey of the perceptions of health practitioners regarding Functional Neurological Disorders in Australia. J Clin Neurosci 2019;67:114–23.
11. Ahmad O, Ahmad KE. Functional neurological disorders in outpatient practice: an Australian cohort. J Clin Neurosci 2016;28:93–6.
12. Beharry J, Palmer D, Wu T, et al. Functional neurological disorders presenting as emergencies to secondary care. Eur J Neurol 2021;28(5):1441–5.
13. de Liège A, Carle G, Hingray C, et al. Functional Neurological Disorders in the medical education: An urgent need to fill the gaps. Rev Neurol (Paris) 2022. https://doi.org/10.1016/J.NEUROL.2022.03.018.
14. Juul D, Gutmann L, Adams HP, et al. Training in neurology: feedback from graduates about the psychiatry component of residency training. Neurology 2021; 96(5):233–6.
15. Finkelstein SA, Adams C, Tuttle M, et al. Neuropsychiatric treatment approaches for functional neurological disorder: a how to guide. Semin Neurol 2022;42(2): 204–24.
16. Nielsen G, Stone J, Matthews A, et al. Physiotherapy for functional motor disorders: a consensus recommendation. J Neurol Neurosurg Psychiatr 2015; 86(10):1113–9.
17. Nicholson C, Edwards MJ, Carson AJ, et al. Occupational therapy consensus recommendations for functional neurological disorder. J Neurol Neurosurg Psychiatr 2020;91(10):1037–45.

18. Williams C, Carson A, Smith S, et al. Overcoming functional neurological symptoms: a five areas approach. Oxfordshire, England, UK: Routledge; 2011.
19. Reiter JM, Andrews D, Reiter C, et al. Taking control of your seizures: workbook. taking control of your seizures. Oxford Academic; 2015. https://doi.org/10.1093/MED:PSYCH/9780199335015.001.0001.
20. Rawlings GH, Reuber M. Health care practitioners ' perceptions of psychogenic nonepileptic seizures : a systematic review of qualitative and quantitative studies. Epilepsia 2018;(April):1–15. https://doi.org/10.1111/epi.14189.
21. Klinke ME, Hjartardóttir TE, Hauksdóttir A, et al. Moving from stigmatization toward competent interdisciplinary care of patients with functional neurological disorders: focus group interviews. Disabil Rehabil 2021;43(9):1237–46.
22. Finkelstein SA, Popkirov S. Functional neurological disorder: diagnostic pitfalls and differential diagnostic considerations. Neurol Clin 2023. in press.
23. Kanaan R, Armstrong D, Wessely S. Limits to truth-telling: neurologists' communication in conversion disorder. Patient Educ Couns 2009;77(2):296–301.
24. Walzl D, Solomon AJ, Stone J. Functional neurological disorder and multiple sclerosis: a systematic review of misdiagnosis and clinical overlap. J Neurol 2022; 269(2):654–63.
25. Hallett M. Patients with Parkinson disease are prone to functional neurological disorders. J Neurol Neurosurg Psychiatr 2018;89(6):557.
26. Perez DL, Hunt A, Sharma N, et al. Cautionary notes on diagnosing functional neurologic disorder as a neurologist-in-training. Neurol Clin Pract 2020;10(6): 484–7.
27. Hallett M, Stone J, Carson A. In: Functional neurologic disorders (handbook of clinical neurology, 139. Amsterdam, Netherlands: Elsevier BV; 2016.
28. Dworetzky B, Baslet G, editors. Psychogenic nonepileptic seizures: toward the integration of care. Oxford University Press; 2017. Available at: https://oxford medicine.com/view/10.1093/med/9780190265045.001.0001/med-9780190265045. Accessed July 4, 2022.
29. LaFaver K, Maurer CW, Nicholson TR, et al, editors. Functional movement disorder. Springer International Publishing; 2022. https://doi.org/10.1007/978-3-030-86495-8.
30. Baslet G, Bajestan SN, Aybek S, et al. Evidence-based practice for the clinical assessment of psychogenic nonepileptic seizures: a report from the American Neuropsychiatric Association Committee on Research. J Neuropsychiatry Clin Neurosci 2021;33(1):27–42.
31. Adams C, Anderson J, Madva EN, et al. You've made the diagnosis of functional neurological disorder: Now what? Practical Neurol 2018;18(4):323–30.
32. Hall-Patch L, Brown R, House A, et al. Acceptability and effectiveness of a strategy for the communication of the diagnosis of psychogenic nonepileptic seizures. Epilepsia 2010;51(1):70–8.
33. Carson A, Lehn A, Ludwig L, et al. Explaining functional disorders in the neurology clinic: a photo story. Practical Neurol 2016;16(1):56–61.
34. Baker J, Barnett C, Cavalli L, et al. Management of functional communication, swallowing, cough and related disorders: consensus recommendations for speech and language therapy. J Neurol Neurosurg Psychiatr 2021;92(10): 1112–25.
35. Jungilligens J, Paredes-Echeverri S, Popkirov S, et al. A new science of emotion: implications for functional neurological disorder. Brain 2022;145(8):2648–63.
36. Drane DL, Fani N, Hallett M, et al. A framework for understanding the pathophysiology of functional neurological disorder. CNS Spectr 2021;26(6):555–61.

37. Saxena A, Paredes-Echeverri S, Michaelis R, et al. Using the biopsychosocial model to guide patient-centered neurological treatments. Semin Neurol 2022; 42(2):80–7.

38. LaFrance W, Baker GA, Duncan R, et al. Minimum requirements for the diagnosis of psychogenic nonepileptic seizures : A staged approach: A report from the International League Against Epilepsy Nonepileptic Seizures Task Force. Epilepsia 2013;54(11):2005–18.

39. Gupta A, Lang AE. Psychogenic movement disorders. Curr Opin Neurol 2009; 22(4):430–6.

40. Staab JP, Eckhardt-Henn A, Horii A, et al. Diagnostic criteria for persistent postural-perceptual dizziness (PPPD): Consensus document of the committee for the Classification of Vestibular Disorders of the Bárány Society. J Vestib Res 2017;27(4):191–208.

41. Ball HA, McWhirter L, Ballard C, et al. Functional cognitive disorder: dementia's blind spot. Brain 2020;143(10):2895–903.

42. Gutkin M, McLean L, Brown R, et al. Systematic review of psychotherapy for adults with functional neurological disorder. J Neurol Neurosurg Psychiatr 2021; 92(1):36–44.

43. McDaniel SH, Doherty WJ, William J, et al. Medical family therapy and integrated care. 2nd ed. American Psychological Association; 2014. Available at: https://www.apa.org/pubs/books/4317314. Accessed October 20, 2022.

44. Lagrand T, Tuitert I, Klamer M, et al. Functional or not functional; that's the question: Can we predict the diagnosis functional movement disorder based on associated features? Eur J Neurol 2021;28(1):33–9.

45. Avbersek A, Sisodiya S. Does the primary literature provide support for clinical signs used to distinguish psychogenic nonepileptic seizures from epileptic seizures? J Neurol Neurosurg Psychiatr 2010;81(7):719–25.

46. Dieterich M, Staab JP. Functional dizziness: From phobic postural vertigo and chronic subjective dizziness to persistent postural-perceptual dizziness. Curr Opin Neurol 2017;30(1):107–13.

47. McWhirter L, Ritchie C, Stone J, et al. Functional cognitive disorders: a systematic review. Lancet Psychiatr 2020;7(2):191–207.

48. Sethi NK, Stone J, Edwards MJ. Trick or treat? Showing patients with functional (psychogenic) motor symptoms their physical signs. Neurology 2013;80(9):869.

49. Stone J, Carson A, Hallett M. Explanation as treatment for functional neurologic disorders. In: Hallett M, Stone J, Carson A, editors. Handbook of clinical neurology, vol 139. Elsevier B.V.; 2016. p. 543–53. https://doi.org/10.1016/B978-0-12-801772-2.00044-8.

50. Sell NM, Phitayakorn R. Developing and refining a surgical curriculum. Surgery 2020;167(3):528–31.

51. Stone J, Carson A. Functional neurologic disorders. Continuum 2015;21(3 Behavioral Neurology and Neuropsychiatry):818–37.

52. Finkelstein S, Stone J, Carson A. Functional neurological disorder: assessment. eBrain. 2020. Available at: www.ebrain.com.

53. Thomas PA, Kern DE, Hughes MT, et al. In: *Curriculum development for medical education: a six-step approach*. Baltimore, MD: Johns Hopkins University Press; 2015.

54. Holmboe ES, Iobst WF ACGME. Assessment guidebook. Chicago: Accreditation Council for Graduate and Medical Education; 2020.

55. Accreditation Council for Graduate Medical Education. Neurology Milestones. Available at: https://www.acgme.org/globalassets/pdfs/milestones/neurology milestones.pdf.

56. Accreditation Council for Graduate Medical Education. Psychiatry Milestones. Available at: https://www.acgme.org/globalassets/PDFs/Milestones/Psychiatry Milestones.pdf.

57. Carson AJ, Ringbauer B, Stone J, et al. Do medically unexplained symptoms matter? A prospective cohort study of 300 new referrals to neurology outpatient clinics. J Neurol Neurosurg Psychiatr 2000;68(2):207–10.

58. Clark CN, Edwards MJ, Ong BE, et al. Reframing postconcussional syndrome as an interface disorder of neurology, psychiatry and psychology. Brain 2022;145(6). https://doi.org/10.1093/BRAIN/AWAC149.

Setting up Functional Neurological Disorder Treatment Services

Questions and Answers

Sara A. Finkelstein, MD, MSc, FRCPC[a],*,
Alan Carson, MBChB, MPhil, MD, FRCPsych, FRCP[b],
Mark J. Edwards, MBBS, PhD[c], Kasia Kozlowska, MBBS, FRANZCP, PhD[d],
Sarah C. Lidstone, MD, PhD, FRCPC[e], David L. Perez, MD, MMSc[f],
Ginger Polich, MD, MS[g], Jon Stone, MBChB, FRCP, PhD[b],
Selma Aybek, MD[h]

KEYWORDS

- Functional neurological disorder • Functional movement disorder
- Functional seizures • Non-epileptic seizures • Functional cognitive disorder
- Persistent postural perceptual dizziness • Treatment

KEY POINTS

- In line with expanding evidence-based treatments and identified benefits from multidisciplinary care, there is an increasing need for services to treat functional neurological disorder (FND).
- When building a service, consideration should be given to the desired composition of the assessment and treatment teams, clinical setting, and duration and intensity of treatment being offered in the context of available resources.

Continued

[a] Department of Neurology, Massachusetts General Hospital, Harvard Medical School, 55 Fruit Street, Boston, MA, USA; [b] Department of Clinical Neurosciences, Centre for Clinical Brain Sciences, University of Edinburgh, Royal Infirmary of Edinburgh, 50 Little France Cres, Edinburgh EH16 4SA, UK; [c] Institute of Psychiatry, Psychology and Neuroscience, King's College 16 De Crespigny Park, London, SE5 8AF, UK; [d] Children's Hospital Westmead Clinical School, Faculty of Medicine and Health, University of Sydney, Westmead Institute for Medical Research, Psychological Medicine, The Children's Hospital at Westmead, Cn Hawkesbury Road, Hainsworth Street, Westmead, NSW 2145, Australia; [e] Integrated Movement Disorders Program, Toronto Rehabilitation Institute, University Centre, Room 3-131, 550 University Avenue, Toronto ON M5G 2A2, Canada; [f] Departments of Neurology and Psychiatry, Massachusetts General Hospital, Harvard Medical School, 55 Fruit Street, Boston, MA, 02114, USA; [g] Department of Physical Medicine and Rehabilitation, Spaulding Rehabilitation Hospital, Brigham and Women's Hospital, Harvard Medical School, 300 1st Avenue, Charlestown, MA 02129, USA; [h] Faculté des Sciences et de Médecine, Université de Fribourg, Bureau 2.106d, Chemin du Musée 5, 1700 Fribourg, Suisse
* Corresponding author. Massachusetts General Hospital, 55 Fruit Street, Boston, MA 02114.
E-mail address: safinkelstein@mgh.harvard.edu

Neurol Clin 41 (2023) 729–743
https://doi.org/10.1016/j.ncl.2023.04.002   neurologic.theclinics.com
0733-8619/23/© 2023 Elsevier Inc. All rights reserved.

Continued

- FND treatment services generally consist of 3 parts: assessment and triage, treatment (including monitoring), and chronic symptom/relapse management.
- Strict (and potentially narrow) referral criteria at the outset of service creation should be considered, in order to help ensure sustainability.
- Identifying and building connections with community partners, existing overlap services (eg, chronic pain clinic), and multidisciplinary health care practitioners with an interest in treating FND are necessary to sustainably grow the service over time.

INTRODUCTION

Specialized services for the diagnosis and management of functional neurological disorder (FND) have rapidly expanded over the last 2 decades. Nonetheless, most centers providing neurologic and neuropsychiatric care—across outpatient and inpatient settings—still lack established services in this area. This article brings together a panel of experts from North America, Europe, and Australia to share our perspectives regarding the rationale for the expansion of such services, along with providing a general blueprint for initial steps in developing FND programs for adults and children/adolescents. We address the types of services that can be included in an FND program and how to triage patient selection for these services. Finally, we discuss the sustainability of an FND treatment program given the logistical challenges that exist within health care systems.

Question 1: Why Do We Need a Functional Neurological Disorder Service?

Answer

FND is common in adult and pediatric neurology clinics, representing about 5% to 15% of patients,[1,2] and leads to a high rate of emergency department utilization.[3–5] Despite this, FND frequently finds itself without a medical "home" within a given health care system. The traditional model of care has been for neurologists to diagnose FND, given their expertise in interpreting the relevant physical examination signs and semiological features,[6] and then to refer on to psychiatrists—or in pediatrics a mental health team—to delve into etiologic factors and to provide treatment.[7] The difficulty with this unusual care model (where one specialty diagnoses and another treats) is that it does not easily allow for skill sharing between neurologists, psychiatrists, and allied health professionals or an integrated approach to diagnosis and management. An interdisciplinary approach is needed because FND symptoms can change over time (for example, initially presenting with functional seizures, then later developing functional limb weakness) and frequently are in part perpetuated by psychiatric comorbidities (eg, depression, anxiety, and posttraumatic stress disorder (PTSD)). Neurologic and psychiatric expertise is thus needed not only at initial diagnosis but also along the course of treatment. Without an integrated care model, patients run the risk of repeated referrals to both neurology and psychiatry each time new symptoms emerge—a cycle that contributes to unnecessary and prolonged "stops and starts" in care. Creating a program that houses both neurologic and psychiatric expertise can thus potentially save the patient and provider time, save the health care system resources, and improve care by allowing patients to be followed in a consistent and consolidated manner.

Many patients with FND—especially adults—have chronic symptoms, requiring longitudinal care.[8] Outcomes in children—when treated in specialist programs with a multidisciplinary approach – are often good.[9] Identifying and referring to appropriate allied health care providers is quickly becoming the standard of care for FND management, and having an FND service with a knowledgeable multidisciplinary team allows for appropriate access to patient-centered care. While participant numbers are typically small, randomized controlled trials and prospective cohort studies evaluating the efficacy of multidisciplinary teams in treating a range of FND subtypes have generally demonstrated patient improvement.[9,10] Expert consensus recommendations for physical therapy (PT), occupational therapy (OT), and speech and language therapy (SLT) treatment for FND—and for the treatment of children—have been published within the last several years.[9,11–14] There is also a growing body of evidence supporting the therapeutic role for psychotherapy, particularly skills-based interventions, in the treatment of patients with FND.[14,15]

Having an FND service can allow for better resource planning and may lead to decreased use of urgent/emergency care and need for hospitalization. Such programs may additionally help to normalize what is often a stigmatized diagnosis by health care providers.[16] Finally, such a service provides better opportunities for teaching future generations of physicians across the clinical neurosciences, as well as creating opportunities for more research in this population.

Question 2: What Kinds of Functional Neurological Disorder Services are There and How to Start Them? Grounding a Functional Neurological Disorder Service in Clinical Reality

Answer
When starting a service, it is important to ensure that admirable aims for a multidisciplinary team remain connected to the day-to-day reality for most people with FND and have the greatest reach. A service that has a very well-developed 6-week inpatient FND treatment program but a 2-year waiting list may not be using health care resources efficiently or serving the population as well as one that sees people quicker for less intensive treatment. The probable cost-effectiveness of helping many patients with milder symptoms return to work with briefer interventions needs to be balanced against the costs of devoting large amounts of time to people with more complex needs.

Inevitably there is no "one size fits all" approach and services are bound to vary according to health care systems—especially public versus private—and depend on what services already exist. A stepped care approach to services has often been advocated (**Fig. 1**), which emphasizes a graded approach based on patient needs.

Types of Functional Neurological Disorder Service

Primary point person/assessment team
Several models have been trialed regarding how best to initially assess a patient with FND and determine who follows and directs care over time. Neurologists should be cautious about setting out on their own to provide an FND service, especially if they have not had some psychiatric training. They may soon find themselves with a large cohort of patients with psychiatric or chronic somatic comorbidities for which the management and assessment are beyond their scope of expertise and their involvement alone may not improve patient outcomes.[17] A small randomized controlled trial of 23 patients involving neurologists and psychiatrists seeing patients together showed benefit in most cases, with improved occupational functioning and reduced health care usage at 1-year follow-up.[18] An expanded three-way model of FND care has been explored by author SL and colleagues where a neurologist, neuropsychiatrist, and physiotherapist all see the patient together. Many intensive multidisciplinary

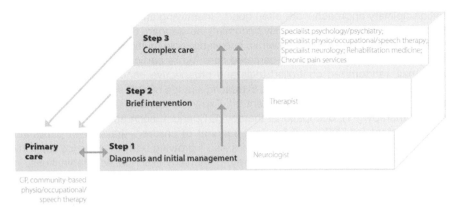

Fig. 1. Proposed model of stepped care for functional neurological symptoms. (*From* Stepped care for functional neurological symptoms: A new approach to improving outcomes for a common neurologic problem in Scotland. Report and recommendations" 2012, Health Improvement Scotland. Available at www.healthcareimprovementscotland.org/; with permission.)

clinics also involve physiatrists. These types of interdisciplinary/multidisciplinary care models will have a valuable cross-training benefit. Although expensive, it may be that such approaches are ultimately cost-effective.[19] An alternative model, which may avoid the issue of increased cost and simplify who acts as the primary provider, is for clinicians (such as a neurologist, neuropsychiatrist, or physiatrist) to pick up each other's skills enough to assess patients on their own, asking for help when required.[20]

Composition of the treatment team
Treatment may include psychotherapy, PT, OT, SLT, physiatry, and medication management of comorbidities (eg, migraines, insomnia, depression).[10,14,21] When working with children, concurrent family work and school-based interventions and collaboration with the school are additional treatment components.[9,14] Factors leading to FND symptom generation and perpetuation vary from patient to patient, leading to a need for an individualized, biopsychosocial-informed approach to care. For example, a patient presenting with functional seizures and functional stutter, who has a trauma history, may benefit from seeing a psychologist and SLT, while a patient with functional limb weakness and housing insecurity may benefit from PT, OT, and social work / case management. The optimal timing (sequential vs concurrent) and order of interventions can vary across patients.

Intensity/setting of therapy
Outpatient models, both standard and those with intensive daily treatment,[22,23] and inpatient models have been described.[24] Group therapies have also been studied, especially for patients with functional seizures.[20]

Duration of therapy
Brief 4 session 30-min psychotherapy, in conjunction with the use of a self-guided cognitive behavioral therapy workbook, has been explored for a range of FND symptoms and severity in a randomized controlled trial, showing some benefit (number needed to treat = 8).[25] There are undoubtedly patients with milder functional neurological symptoms for whom this approach may be sufficient, but experience suggests

that many with functional motor or seizure symptoms usually need more input. Many FND outpatient treatment programs opt for a "time-limited" approach (eg, an approximately 12-week program) to increase equitable access for all patients. The downside to adhering to a rigid timeline for all patients is that there are some who may benefit from shorter or longer duration of care.[26]

Building in education before treatment

There is a consensus among patients and clinicians that education is a key building block of treatment. Some services have explored enhanced ways of providing education in groups. One study of a single face-to-face education session in 193 patients and relatives with FND showed large effect sizes for improving the understanding of FND and is something to consider setting up alongside a clinical service.[26,27] Additionally, when treatment engagement is suspected to be sub-optimal upfront, consideration can be given to use of motivational interviewing strategies.[28]

Building a Team

Specialist FND services are undoubtedly needed, especially for complex cases, to do research and trickle-down expertise. However, FND is such a common problem that community-based solutions within existing services are needed. If neurologically- and psychologically-trained clinicians and therapists come to expect, through training and evidence-based practice, that FND is a disorder that they should be able to manage and treat to a reasonable degree, then there will be much better coverage for basic care aspects of the disorder. Indeed, author JS's FND service developed organically in this way, with a large set of local providers developing an FND-skillset through exposure over time.

It may not be possible to wait for local services to catch up, or some health systems may be too disjointed, for that approach to succeed. A business case for an FND service depends on the existing evidence for need, which is undoubted, but also cost-effectiveness, which is harder to prove. The National Neurosciences Advisory Group in the UK, a statutory body including health professionals and patient organizations, put together an "optimum clinical pathway for adults with FND" in 2022 (Available at https://www.nnag.org.uk/optimal-clinical-pathway-adults-fnd-functional-neurological-disorder) (**Fig. 2**). This aims to help clinicians in the UK navigate the different issues that need to be considered when setting up an FND service and may be helpful to those in different health care systems. The result suggests that simple stepped care models need to be updated to take into account the biopsychosocial complexity of patients with FND and the health care systems in which they are seen.

Question 3: Across Functional Neurological Disorder Services, How is a Treatment Course Developed and Monitored? How are Commonly Encountered Challenges Addressed?

Answer

Developing an FND treatment service is dependent upon many factors at the health system, provider, and patient levels (**Fig. 3**) and considers what treatment interventions offer a good likelihood of success. While what treatment can be offered first depends on system and provider factors, treatment success is incumbent upon the "match" between the patient's top concerns and the therapy offered addressing factors intrinsic to the maintenance of the patient's illness. Therapy cannot be simply applied "to the patient" in FND since recovery requires active participation, understanding, and engagement by the patient. In general, the basic components of an FND treatment service consist of 3 parts: assessment and triage, treatment (including

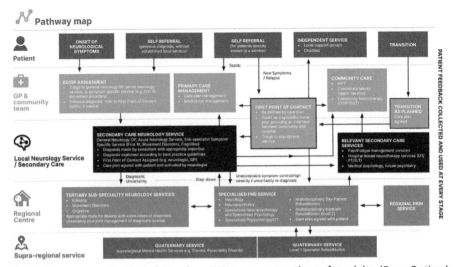

Fig. 2. A more complex United Kingdom FND treatment pathway for adults. (*From* Optimal clinical pathway for adults with Functional Neurological Disorder (FND) 2023, National Neurosciences Advisory Group - ■ Mark Edwards, Workstream clinical lead, Consultant Neurologist, St George's University Hospital NHS Foundation Trust. ■ Michael Dilley, Workstream clinical lead, Consultant Neuropsychiatrist, King's College Hospital NHS Foundation Trust. ■ Dawn Golder, Executive Director, FND Hope UK. Available at https://www.nnag.org.uk/optimal-clinical-pathway-adults-fnd-functional-neurological-disorder; with permission.)

monitoring and instruction on self-management strategies), and chronic symptom/relapse support.

1. Assessment and triage

Apart from diagnostic clarification, the purpose of the evaluation is to determine readiness for therapy and develop an initial formulation to help guide patient-centered

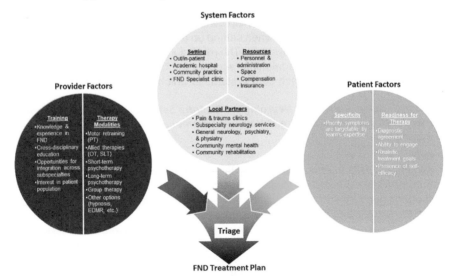

Fig. 3. Factors involved in developing a functional neurological disorder treatment program.

Box 1
Questions to determine readiness for engaging in treatment for functional neurological disorder

- Does the patient agree with the diagnosis?
- Are the patient's top concerns targetable by your team's expertise?
- Are there symptoms (eg, pain, fatigue, cognitive, anxiety,/low mood) or psychosocial circumstances (eg, major life stressors, secondary gain) that will limit treatment engagement?
- What are the patient's goals? Are they specific and/or realistic?
  - "I want to be able to prepare a meal for my family without any symptoms" versus "I want my old life back"
- What modality is the optimal introduction to treatment?
  - Consider what may have the best chance of initial uptake given your assessment

treatment planning. Not every patient is ready to embark on a treatment course at the time of assessment, and it is crucial to determine this at the initial or first few encounters to factor in allocation of finite resources. Diagnostic agreement, readiness to actively engage in treatment, and patient-reported improvement with other therapies tried may indicate good recovery potential. Conversely, prominent diagnostic ambivalence, an expectation to be "fixed" with treatment, overwhelming pain or fatigue, or a history of multiple failed treatments may indicate a more guarded prognosis (**Box 1**). If readiness for treatment is not clear at the initial assessment, consider providing some basic recommendations and assess the uptake/response at follow-up, such as providing educational resources to read and return with questions, noticing symptom inconsistency, or use of basic relaxation exercises. Equally important is to identify the patient's top concerns (not necessarily the same as the provider) and determine if they are targetable by your team's expertise. This requires an open and transparent discussion about what the team can and cannot offer. Treatment targets—including symptom reduction and functional goals—should ideally be developed in collaboration with the patient and include a combination of what symptoms most negatively impact quality of life and relevant perpetuating factors from the assessment (eg, anxiety). Once identified, the treatment targets can inform which therapeutic modalities may be most effective as a starting point.

2. Treatment and monitoring response
An FND treatment plan should begin with developing realistic goals with the patient that help to build self-efficacy (in itself a treatment target in FND) and promote a shared understanding about what is being targeted and why it is important for therapeutic success. Reaching those goals may encompass both physical and psychological therapies—for example, combining PT for gait difficulties, SLT for functional speech symptoms, and skills-based psychotherapy to connect thoughts, feelings, and behaviors to physical symptoms. The use of educational models for FND throughout the course of treatment that are tailored to patient symptom experience helps to create a shared language with the treatment team. Progress in therapy manifests with ongoing patient engagement, implementing symptom-management strategies between sessions, developing an awareness of brain-mind-body connections, understanding their FND symptom model, and slow and steady improvement. Symptom flare-ups, often in pain or fatigue, may occur as the functional neurological symptoms improve and often resolve in parallel as therapy progresses.

3. Self-management and chronic symptom/relapse support

Successful treatment of FND in many cases can be defined not by the absence of symptoms, but instead by the ability to effectively self-manage while re-engaging in activities. FND, while occasionally monophasic, often waxes and wanes over time. An understanding that FND is a vulnerability in the brain, that symptoms can arise depending on the degree of load on the nervous system, and that maintaining wellness actively requires lifestyle factor modification, avoiding triggers, and using learned strategies to treat symptoms confidently if they do arise, is key to improvement. Through the process of treating FND, patients may also be prompted to seek out treatment for comorbid conditions, such as long-term psychotherapy for trauma-related symptoms (eg, chronic PTSD with dissociation). Follow-up with whoever makes the diagnosis is likely to help in supporting treatment. Periodic visits if flare-ups or relapses do occur can be helpful to maintain self-management long-term.

Challenges can arise over the course of treatment, including treatment nonresponse, plateaus in improvement, or relapses. In these cases, ensuring that the diagnosis is correct, the modality is appropriate to the treatment target, and revisiting goals should be examined. If these are sound, then lack of treatment response may be related to strong perpetuating factors that maintain illness. The biopsychosocial formulation can help identify these factors, although they may not be initially obvious. In the clinical setting, common perpetuating factors limiting recovery include: (i) lack of access to evidence-based treatments; (ii) inadequacy or failure of the treatment available; (iii) poor care coordination across clinical providers; (iv) difficult to change psychosocial challenges; (v) deconditioning; (vi) avoidance patterns; (vii) a low sense of self-efficacy; (viii) decompensated psychiatric comorbidities including maladaptive personality traits such as help-seek-help-reject patterns; and/or (ix) comorbid medical conditions. Finally, it is also important to note that not all patients with FND require or benefit from therapy—a portion (typically with minimal, short-duration symptoms) can improve with diagnosis and education alone (**Fig. 4**).

Question 4: For Referral-Based Services (eg, Outpatient, Partial Hospital/Residential and/or Inpatient Programs), How is Patient Entry Triaged?

Answer

While it would be potentially beneficial to build comprehensive brain-mind-body assessment and treatment centers, resources are finite. In the authors' experiences, when advertising an FND service there is no shortage of patients. Services will help themselves by considering patient selection factors upfront in conjunction with resource availability. It is important to have clear inclusion and exclusion criteria for services, which will vary based on institutional and health care system resources, setting (eg, outpatient, partial hospital/residential, acute inpatient rehabilitation settings, and so forth), and treatment intensity.[29,30] Consider sending out department-wide emails and/or creating a program website covering what the service offers, the specific criteria for referral, and mechanism for referral. Recruiting appropriate referrals can also be aided by investing time in education and training sessions for referral sources, often times facilitated by visiting those clinics that are likely to refer a significant number of people.

As a general rule, prior to being evaluated in a specialized FND service, an evaluation should have previously been performed by a health care provider familiar with assessing for a potential FND diagnosis (eg, neurologist or neuropsychiatrist). Ideally, that prior evaluation should also include documentation of "rule-in" physical examination and/or semiological features supportive of the FND diagnosis.[6,14] In other instances (eg, inpatient programs), documentation that a diagnosis of FND has been

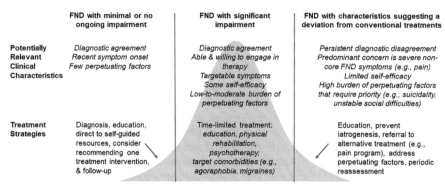

	FND with minimal or no ongoing impairment	FND with significant impairment	FND with characteristics suggesting a deviation from conventional treatments
Potentially Relevant Clinical Characteristics	*Diagnostic agreement* *Recent symptom onset* *Few perpetuating factors*	*Diagnostic agreement* *Able & willing to engage in therapy* *Targetable symptoms* *Some self-efficacy* *Low-to-moderate burden of perpetuating factors*	*Persistent diagnostic disagreement* *Predominant concern is severe non-core FND symptoms (e.g., pain)* *Limited self-efficacy* *High burden of perpetuating factors that require priority (e.g., suicidality, unstable social difficulties)*
Treatment Strategies	Diagnosis, education, direct to self-guided resources, consider recommending one treatment intervention, & follow-up	Time-limited treatment: *education, physical rehabilitation, psychotherapy, target comorbidities (e.g., agoraphobia, migraines)*	Education, prevent iatrogenesis, referral to alternative treatment (e.g., pain program), address perpetuating factors, periodic reassessment

Fig. 4. Work-in-progress consideration of functional neurological disorder (FND) treatment options. Here, graph displays the following factors: functional (activities of daily living, social, and occupational) impairment, other relevant clinical characteristics, appropriateness for FND-specific treatment, and treatment strategies more broadly. Note that list of clinical characteristics is not comprehensive, nor will all factors listed necessarily apply to a given individual. A minority of patients with FND have minimal or no impairment, potentially only requiring education, direction to self-guided care resources (eg, "Overcoming Functional Neurological Disorders: A Five Areas Approach" workbook, www.neurosymptoms.org) and follow-up; alternatively, a single time-limited intervention (eg, psychotherapy or physical therapy) could also be considered. Many patients will have at least moderate impairment of occupational or social abilities that can potentially improve with FND-specific treatment interventions, including multidisciplinary treatment. Additionally, a subset of individuals with FND may have a symptom complex and associated clinical (biopsychosocial) formulation suggesting the need for a deviation from FND-specific treatment (at least at a given time-point). Such factors include: 1) minimal or no response to recent, prior trials of evidence-based treatment, 2) other major factors that warrant prioritization over FND, or 3) basic benchmarks to proceed with FND treatment are not being met (eg, persistent fixation on alternative diagnosis). In such cases, focusing on education, addressing identifiable perpetuating factors (including directing to resources for the management of non-core FND symptoms such as chronic pain, insomnia, or psychiatric comorbidities), and providing follow-up may be the initial focus of care.

communicated to and generally agreed upon by the patient (and parents in cases of pediatric FND) may be required.[31] In medically complex cases being referred for short-term treatment, it will also be important to ensure clarity in the specific functional neurological symptoms that will be therapeutically targeted versus other neurologic comorbidities (eg, semiological differences between functional and epileptic seizures). Such an approach helps prevent FND services from being a referral center for diagnostically unclear cases where there is a broad differential diagnosis *and* the absence of rule-in diagnostic signs.

In terms of patient selection, some services may choose to take a transdiagnostic approach, providing care to the full spectrum of FND (eg, across functional movement disorder, functional seizures, persistent postural-perceptual dizziness, functional cognitive disorder, and so forth), while others may pursue a narrower focus (eg, limited to functional seizures). Given that many patients with FND—including children—can present with mixed symptoms, and others presenting with one cluster of symptoms can go on to develop distinct FND symptoms over the natural history of their condition, there is good support to consider developing a transdiagnostic service, particularly in the outpatient and pediatric settings.[14,32,33] This perspective needs to be balanced, however, with practical considerations (eg, an expanded patient population requires a greater set of available clinicians) and treatment differences based on symptom type (eg, psychotherapy in functional seizures vs a role for physical rehabilitation for those with functional motor symptoms).[15,34]

For short-term inpatient services (eg, 1–2-week interventions), there are other special considerations to highlight. The ability (or inability) to participate in multi-hour physical rehabilitation on consecutive days is an important consideration for inpatient rehabilitation. A general admission criterion for inpatient rehabilitation in the US is the ability of the patient to participate in 3 hours per day of physical interventions and require regular supervision from a rehabilitation physician; a general criterion for inpatient pediatric rehabilitation is the child's willingness and ability to participate in a therapeutic timetable, which in addition to the above-described elements, includes attendance at school.[9,14] Inpatient programs should also likely communicate with patients beforehand (for example, during a prehospitalization consultation) the anticipated length of stay, ensuring that the patient is in agreement (eg, including that discharge will occur in cases of suboptimal treatment response in order to avoid prolonged and futile rehabilitation stays).[31] Currently in the US, obtaining insurance approval from private or public payors can be a major barrier to admission to an inpatient rehabilitation facility.

Lastly, many of the factors discussed in the response to *Question 3* pertaining to readiness/appropriateness for treatment initiation are also important considerations when a provider is accepting a new patient referral for time-limited inpatient treatment services.

Question 5: How Do We Ensure the Sustainability of Functional Neurological Disorder Services?

Answer

Any FND service that establishes itself within a health system will be starting from a position of relative isolation and will also often be fragmented, as the service is unlikely to have all of the necessary types of services and personnel that are required by the heterogenous population of people with FND. Ideal services for FND cut across traditional service boundaries and, in particular, between physical (neurologic) and mental (psychiatric) health. FND is likely to be one of the conditions where there could be questions raised by both health professionals and political/government funders about its very legitimacy as a medical condition that deserves attention, with significant associated stigma.[16]

As illustrated in the sections above, conceptually and with reference to the literature, interdisciplinary and multidisciplinary care is most likely to meet the complex and heterogenous needs of patients with FND. However, this is often not well supported by health systems, is superficially more complex than siloed single specialty working, and runs into the sensitivities that often exist between health care specialist groups about what "bit" is theirs and theirs alone to manage.

Thus, FND services are subject to a series of threats and pressures challenging sustainability: isolation, fragmentation, traditional service boundaries, legitimacy, and need for interdisciplinary working. We consider some of these challenges in more detail and how they might be faced.

It is common for services to begin with a few interested and committed individuals who have recognized the clinical need to deliver better care to people with FND. Depending on their skillsets, they will be able to establish an aspect of an FND service, for example, a neurology- or psychiatry-led specialist FND clinic, a psychotherapy service for people with functional seizures, or a PT program to treat functional motor symptoms. Several problems may threaten the sustainability of these nascent services. First, services can become rapidly overwhelmed by demand due to the lack of any other services for FND. Second, services may receive referrals for people who have needs beyond those which the service can reasonably address. For example, a psychologist may be referred a person with significant physical disability who would be best treated in a multidisciplinary program. Third, services may be referred people who have primary symptoms of pain, fatigue, pathological health anxiety, or multiple somatic symptoms.[35]

Key strategies to ensure sustainability are to have clear inclusion and exclusion criteria for predefined services that can be offered and ensuring these are communicated early and effectively to referrers and patients/families (as discussed in the responses to *Question 3* and *4*). For example, patients with fibromyalgia may be alternatively redirected to a multidisciplinary chronic pain program. Thought should also be given to the geographic restriction of the service, as another way of limiting referrals to a manageable number. Outcome measures should be collected to support future service expansion, making sure these are aligned with those used by the health service within which the FND program is operating.[36] Time should be set aside as part of the weekly running of the service to support service development, in particular to reach out to other health professionals who could join the service to build a more comprehensive set of treatments and assessment services.

In this regard, there are often existing nonspecialist services who could (and maybe already do) see people with FND, but typically feel under-supported and under-skilled in managing people with FND. Such services can be useful to co-opt into the developing FND service by offering them, for example, training and support, access to FND expertise to manage more complex patients, or filtering of referrals by the FND specialist service to provide the nonspecialist service with appropriate patients. This can allow one to develop a larger service extending into, for example, community neurorehabilitation and mental health services, quite quickly and with limited investment. Patients can then step up and down through this service depending on need.

Sustainability of services also relies on building institutional support (locally, regionally, nationally) for FND service development (see response to Question 1 for supporting arguments). These arguments can be used at a local and national level to support investment in FND services. As the evidence base grows for specific FND treatments (and hopefully service pathways too), these will add to the case for the development of national frameworks for the delivery of FND services. National and international patient and health professional organizations can also be helpful to add political and reputational pressure to health services and health funders to invest in care pathways for people with FND.

It is often challenging to work in an interdisciplinary fashion and across traditional service boundaries (eg, physical and mental health). However, one potential solution comes from the realization that such interdisciplinary and cross-boundary services are actually those which most closely align with the needs of patients with all causes of neurologic symptoms, not just FND. The rate of psychiatric comorbidity is often very high with other neurologic illnesses. For example, more than 50% of people with neurologic illness have anxiety and depression or another psychiatric diagnosis, and such symptoms are often rated by patients, for example, with Parkinson's disease, as their most disabling symptoms, over and above their neurologic symptoms.[37] Holistic rehabilitation, sensitive to the specific needs of an individual patient and that is capable of managing neurologic, psychiatric, and social complexity is exactly what is needed for many people with neurologic conditions. The practices of supervision in psychology and psychiatry, which offer health care professionals a chance to discuss challenging patients and to manage associated emotional stress, could also be usefully leveraged into an integrated service to help reduce burnout and associated health problems in staff. Indeed, some centers have operationalized "FND Rounds" to discuss clinical challenges and success stories, as well as to support clinicians in their own therapeutic journeys with patients. Overall, the work in developing services for FND might in fact be an ideal model to improve services for people with neurologic symptoms in general and this could be a powerful argument for investment in such services.

Question 6: Are there Other Noteworthy Clinical and/or Research Considerations in the Initial Phases of Functional Neurological Disorder Service Development?

Answer

While the above sections address major themes in starting an FND service, numerous other challenges and opportunities are likely to arise throughout this process. Perhaps one of the most difficult components of putting together a program is recruiting staff, many of whom may be unfamiliar with FND and its treatment, to help manage patients. Consider education sessions for PT, OT, SLT, and psychotherapy providers at your institution. If an allied health provider is new to treating FND, you may need to start with referrals of less complex cases. This will allow colleagues to refine their skills and be more likely to see patients improve, thus energizing them further in providing care for this patient group. One way to engage these allied professionals is to prepare local guidelines in the local language based on published recommendations[11–13] (in English) and send it directly or through the patients themselves.

Many FND clinics are affiliated with a research program, in which patients are often keen to participate.[29] Research activities can help with ongoing support and funding for an FND program, as well as increase your referral rate. A successful research program can also increase departmental leadership's interest in FND initiatives overall, an important component of programmatic growth across clinical services and research efforts. For ease of research, even if to be done retrospectively, consider standardizing note templates across providers to aid data collection, aggregation, and outcome monitoring. In the case of prospective research, consider how recruitment could be integrated across multiple clinical providers.

SUMMARY

Just as there is no "one size fits all" treatment intervention for patients with FND, many models for FND services can potentially work well. Common themes that arise are deciding on which team members to include, how much to draw on resources already in place, and ensuring appropriate patient triage to services. While many challenges still exist with regard to providing care for this patient population, considering how challenges will be addressed at the outset will help to ensure the sustainability and success of any FND program.

CONFLICTS OF INTERESTS/DISCLOSURES

S.C. Lidstone receives royalties from UpToDate for the article "Functional Movement Disorders." D.L. Perez has received royalties from Springer Nature for a textbook on functional movement disorder, honoraria for continuing medical education lectures on functional neurological disorder, and is a paid senior editor at *Brain and Behavior*. A.J. Carson is an unpaid President of Functional Neurological Disorders society, paid editor of Journal of Neurology, Neurosurgery and Psychiatry and gives expert testimony in Court on a range of neuropsychiatric topics. J. Stone has received royalties from UpToDate. He is an unpaid secretary of the Functional Neurological Disorder

Society and gives expert testimony in court in relation to FND. M.J. Edwards receives royalties from the Oxford University Press, is a paid associate editor of the European Journal of Neurology and gives expert testimony in medicolegal cases including FND.

FUNDING

S. Aybek has received funding from the Swiss National Science Foundation grant PP00P3_210997.

REFERENCES

1. Ahmad O, Ahmad KE. Functional neurological disorders in outpatient practice: An Australian cohort. J Clin Neurosci 2016;28:93–6.
2. Stone J, Carson A, Duncan R, et al. Symptoms "unexplained by organic disease" in 1144 new neurology out-patients: How often does the diagnosis change at follow-up? Brain 2009;132(10):2878–88.
3. Stephen CD, Fung V, Lungu CI, et al. Assessment of emergency department and inpatient use and costs in adult and pediatric functional neurological disorders. JAMA Neurol 2021;78(1):88–101.
4. Williams ERL, Guthrie E, Mackway-Jones K, et al. Psychiatric status, somatisation, and health care utilization of frequent attenders at the emergency department: A comparison with routine attenders. J Psychosom Res 2001;50(3):161–7.
5. Dickson JM, Dudhill H, Shewan J, et al. Cross-sectional study of the hospital management of adult patients with a suspected seizure (EPIC2). BMJ Open 2017; 7(7):e015696.
6. Aybek S, Perez DL. Diagnosis and management of functional neurological disorder. BMJ 2022;376:o64.
7. Kanaan R, Armstrong D, Barnes P, et al. In the psychiatrist's chair: how neurologists understand conversion disorder. Brain 2009;132(Pt 10):2889–96.
8. Gelauff J, Stone J, Edwards M, et al. The prognosis of functional (psychogenic) motor symptoms: A systematic review. J Neurol Neurosurg Psychiatry 2014; 85(2):220–6.
9. Vassilopoulos A, Mohammad S, Dure L, et al. Treatment Approaches for Functional Neurological Disorders in Children. Curr Treat Options Neurol 2022; 24:77–9.
10. Finkelstein SA, Adams C, Tuttle M, et al. Neuropsychiatric Treatment Approaches for Functional Neurological Disorder: A How to Guide. Semin Neurol 2022;42(2): 204–24.
11. Nielsen G, Stone J, Matthews A, et al. Physiotherapy for functional motor disorders: A consensus recommendation. J Neurol Neurosurg Psychiatry 2015; 86(10):1113–9.
12. Nicholson C, Edwards MJ, Carson AJ, et al. Occupational therapy consensus recommendations for functional neurological disorder. J Neurol Neurosurg Psychiatry 2020;91(10):1037–45.
13. Baker J, Barnett C, Cavalli L, et al. Management of functional communication, swallowing, cough and related disorders: consensus recommendations for speech and language therapy. J Neurol Neurosurg Psychiatry 2021;92(10). https://doi.org/10.1136/jnnp-2021-326767. jnnp-2021-326767.
14. Kozlowska K, Chudleigh C, Savage B, et al. Evidence-Based Mind-Body Interventions for Children and Adolescents with Functional Neurological Disorder. Harv Rev Psychiatry 2023;31(2):60–82.

15. Gutkin M, McLean L, Brown R, et al. Systematic review of psychotherapy for adults with functional neurological disorder. J Neurol Neurosurg Psychiatry 2020;92(1):36–44.

16. Macduffie KE, Grubbs L, Best T, et al. Stigma and functional neurological disorder: a research agenda targeting the clinical encounter. CNS Spectr 2020;26(6): 587–92.

17. Pleizier M, De Haan RJ, Vermeulen M. Management of patients with functional neurological symptoms: a single-centre randomised controlled trial. J Neurol Neurosurg Psychiatry 2017;0:1–7.

18. Hubschmid M, Aybek S, Maccaferri GE, et al. Efficacy of brief interdisciplinary psychotherapeutic intervention for motor conversion disorder and nonepileptic attacks. Gen Hosp Psychiatry 2015;37(5):448–55.

19. Lidstone SC, MacGillivray L, Lang AE. Integrated Therapy for Functional Movement Disorders: Time for a Change. Mov Disord Clin Pract 2020;7(2):169–74.

20. Cope SR, Smith JG, King T, et al. Evaluation of a pilot innovative cognitive-behavioral therapy-based psychoeducation group treatment for functional non-epileptic attacks. Epilepsy Behav 2017;70:238–44.

21. Lafaver K, Lafrance WC, Price ME, et al. Treatment of functional neurological disorder: current state, future directions, and a research agenda. CNS Spectr 2020; 26(6):607–13.

22. Nielsen G, Buszewicz M, Stevenson F, et al. Randomised feasibility study of physiotherapy for patients with functional motor symptoms. J Neurol Neurosurg Psychiatry 2017;88(6):484–90.

23. Polich G, Thompson J, Molton I, et al. Intensive rehabilitation for functional motor disorders (FMD) in the United States: A review. NeuroRehabilitation 2022;50(2): 245–54.

24. Gilmour GS, Jenkins JD. Inpatient Treatment of Functional Neurological Disorder: A Scoping Review. Can J Neurol Sci/J Can Sci Neurol 2021;48(2):204–17.

25. Sharpe M, Walker J, Williams C, et al. Guided self-help for functional (psychogenic) symptoms A randomized controlled efficacy trial. Neurology 2011;77(6): 564–72.

26. Godena EJ, Perez DL, Crain LD, et al. Psychotherapy for Functional Neurological (Conversion) Disorder: A Case Bridging Mind, Brain, and Body. J Clin Psychiatry 2021;82(6):21ct14246.

27. Cope SR, Smith JG, Edwards MJ, et al. Enhancing the communication of functional neurological disorder diagnosis: a multidisciplinary education session. Eur J Neurol 2021;28(1):40–7.

28. Tolchin B, Baslet G, Martino S, et al. Motivational interviewing techniques to improve psychotherapy adherence and outcomes for patients with psychogenic nonepileptic seizures. Journal of Neuropsychiatry and Clinical Neurosciences 2020;32(2):125–31.

29. Aybek S, Lidstone SC, Nielsen G, et al. What Is the Role of a Specialist Assessment Clinic for FND? Lessons From Three National Referral Centers. J Neuropsychiatry Clin Neurosci 2020;32(1):79–84.

30. Jacob AE, Kaelin DL, Roach AR, et al. Motor Retraining (MoRe) for Functional Movement Disorders: Outcomes From a 1-Week Multidisciplinary Rehabilitation Program. PM and R 2018;10(11):1164–72.

31. Polich G, Zalanowski S, Maney J, et al. Development of an inpatient rehabilitation pathway for motor functional neurological disorders: Initial reflections. NeuroRehabilitation 2022;50(2):231–43.

32. Tinazzi M, Morgante F, Marcuzzo E, et al. Clinical Correlates of Functional Motor Disorders: An Italian Multicenter Study. Mov Disord Clin Pract 2020;7(8):920–9.
33. McKenzie PS, Oto M, Graham CD, et al. Do patients whose psychogenic non-epileptic seizures resolve, "replace" them with other medically unexplained symptoms? Medically unexplained symptoms arising after a diagnosis of psychogenic non-epileptic seizures. J Neurol Neurosurg Psychiatry 2011;82(9):967–9.
34. Perez DL, Edwards MJ, Nielsen G, et al. Decade of progress in motor functional neurological disorder: continuing the momentum. J Neurol Neurosurg Psychiatry 2021;92(6):668–77.
35. Löwe B, Levenson J, Depping M, et al. Somatic symptom disorder: a scoping review on the empirical evidence of a new diagnosis. Psychol Med 2021;52(4):632–48.
36. Pick S, Anderson DG, Asadi-Pooya AA, et al. Outcome measurement in functional neurological disorder: a systematic review and recommendations. J Neurol Neurosurg Psychiatry 2020;91(6):638–49.
37. The Neurological Alliance. Together for the 1 in 6: UK Findings from My Neuro Survey. 2022. Available at: https://www.neural.org.uk/wp-content/uploads/2022/05/Together-for-the-1-in-6-UK-Findings-from-My-Neuro-Survey-v6.pdf. Accessed April 3, 2023.

Somatic Symptom Disorder and Health Anxiety

Assessment and Management

Karoline S. Sauer[a],*, Michael Witthöft, PhD[a], Winfried Rief, PhD[b]

KEYWORDS

- Somatic symptom disorder • Functional somatic syndromes
- Illness anxiety disorder • Hypochondriasis • Health anxiety
- Pathological health anxiety

KEY POINTS

- The newly introduced somatic symptom disorder (SSD) requires the presence of at least one distressing somatic symptom during 6 months, which is accompanied by excessive symptom-related thoughts, feelings, and behaviors.
- The specification that symptoms must be (at least partly) medically unexplained was abandoned in SSD. People with pathological health anxiety can be diagnosed with SSD or with Illness Anxiety Disorder (IAD) in case of absent or only mild somatic symptoms.
- Epidemiological data on SSD and IAD are yet limited; previous studies on related mental health disorders, though, suggest a high prevalence of somatic symptoms with a medically unclear genesis and of (subclinical) health anxiety in the general population and in medical settings.
- A combination of measures that assess symptom severity and the excessiveness of symptom-related thoughts, feelings, and behaviors is most suitable for screening of SSD and IAD.
- Cognitive-behavioral therapy (CBT) approaches are best-studied for SSD and IAD treatment.

DEFINITION AND HISTORY

The "Somatic Symptom and Related Disorder" category of the fifth edition of the Diagnostic and Statistical Manual of Mental Disorders (DSM-5[1]) comprises mental health disorders, in which the perception of somatic sensations and/or of worries in relation

[a] Department of Clinical Psychology, Psychotherapy, and Experimental Psychopathology, Johannes Gutenberg-University of Mainz, Wallstraße 3, Mainz 55122, Germany; [b] Department of Clinical Psychology and Psychotherapy, Philipps-University Marburg, Gutenbergstraße 18, 35032 Marburg, Germany
* Corresponding author.
E-mail address: karsauer@uni-mainz.de

Neurol Clin 41 (2023) 745–758
https://doi.org/10.1016/j.ncl.2023.02.009
0733-8619/23/© 2023 Elsevier Inc. All rights reserved.

to health/illness is the prominent feature. Three diagnoses included in this category are "somatic symptom disorder" (SSD), "illness anxiety disorder" (IAD), and "functional neurological symptom disorder (conversion disorder)" (FND). The mentioning and studying of the symptoms of these diagnoses dates back to early Egyptian and Roman times.[2] In the history of somatic symptom perception and somatization, the concept of "hysteria,"[3] a term which changed its meaning from sexual dysfunction in Greek antiquity to a neurological disorder in the nineteenth century, and the definition of "dissociation" and "conversion" are considered as important milestones.[4] The terms "dissociation" and "conversion" were introduced by Sigmund Freud and his pupil Pierre Janet and were/are seen as defense mechanisms in psychoanalytic theories. Nowadays, dissociation is defined as "a disruption of and/or discontinuity in the normal, subjective integration of one or more aspects of psychological functioning, including–but not limited to–memory, identity, consciousness, perception, and motor control."[5] Current terms that refer to the concept of somatization include somatic symptoms with a medically unclear genesis, functional somatic symptoms and syndromes (eg, chronic fatigue syndrome, fibromyalgia, and irritable bowel syndrome), or somatoform symptoms.

Regarding health anxiety, the term "hypochondriasis," which dates back to the ancient Greek word "hypochondrium" (referring to a body part, which should be related to mental disorders), was long predominant and even taken up by literature (eg, drama "Le Malade imaginaire" [the imaginary sick person] by Molière). Because it is increasingly perceived as stigmatizing by affected people, the terms "pathological health anxiety" or "pathological illness anxiety" are preferred to describe the pathologically heightened anxiety to have (or get) a severe disease (eg, cancer). As people with pathologically heightened health worries can now be diagnosed both with DSM-5[1] SSD and IAD (as described in detail in the preceding paragraph), the term "pathological health anxiety" can be seen as an umbrella term for pathologically heightened health worries.

CLASSIFICATION

The DSM-5[1] SSD, IAD, FND replace the former category of "somatoform disorders" (including hypochondriasis and conversion disorder) of the fourth edition of the Diagnostic and Statistical Manual of Mental Disorders (DSM-IV[6]) but substantially differ in relation to some criteria. Most importantly, although in somatoform disorders according to DSM-IV,[6] the perceived somatic symptoms cannot be fully explained by a medical condition, reflecting the "somatization" or "somatoform" concept, in DSM-5,[1] this criterion was dropped. Instead, SSD demands the presence of at least one distressing symptom during a period of 6 months (symptoms are allowed to change in that period) but also includes fully (or partially) medically explained symptoms or symptoms within a medical condition. Diagnosis requires excessive cognitive (ie, persistent thoughts about the seriousness of symptom(s)), behavioral (eg, symptom-related avoidance behavior, body checking, doctor visits), and affective (ie, exaggerated distress or anxiety about symptom(s)) features in relation to symptoms (B-Criterion: at least one excessive feature must be fulfilled), independent of the "origin" of symptoms. It can be specified if pain symptoms are predominant, if the disorder is persistent (over 6 months), and if severity can be considered as mild, moderate, or severe (1, 2, or 3 symptoms of criterion B are fulfilled, respectively).

The SSD category, therefore, can also apply to people with pathological health anxiety, if distressing somatic symptoms are present. If somatic symptoms are absent or only mild, people with pathological health anxiety (of at least 6 months with possibly varying feared diseases) are better classified as having IAD. IAD is—similar to SSD—further characterized by excessive health-related behavior (eg, body checking, doctor visits), and/or illness-related avoidance behavior (eg, avoidance of doctor visits). A care-avoidant and care-seeking type can be differentiated.

The diagnosis of DSM-5[1] FND, which is prominently featured in the other articles of this collection and thus not in the focus of this article, requires the presence of at least one distressing and impairing symptom of an altered motor or sensory function, which is not sufficiently explained by or at least partly incompatible with a medical, especially a neurological, condition. Thus, a notable addition to the DSM-5 FND diagnosis was the emphasis of clinical findings providing evidence of incompatibility with other medical/neurological conditions (ie, internal inconsistency). People, therefore, can fulfill criteria for both SSD and FND, if distressing/impairing motor/sensory function (with no sufficient alternative medical explanation) and other somatic (including medically explained) symptoms simultaneously are present.[1]

The changes due to the introduction of the DSM-5[1] SSD and IAD categories are still a subject of discussion. Former DSM-IV[6] hypochondriasis was assigned to 2 diagnoses in DSM-5[1]: SSD and IAD, separated by the intensity of somatic symptoms. Because most people with former DSM-IV[6] hypochondriasis suffer from somatic symptoms, people with pathological health anxiety will be more often diagnosed with SSD than IAD.[7] The validity of this separation is debatable, although people with pathological health anxiety now diagnosed with SSD report higher levels of health anxiety and health care use than people who fulfill the criteria of IAD.[7] Giving up the differentiation between medically explained and unexplained symptoms in DSM-5,[1] SSD expands the former too restrictive concept of somatoform disorders.[7,8] Still, it is not yet clear if medically explained and unexplained symptoms completely underlie the same mechanisms.[8] However, the change from DSM-IV[6] somatoform disorders to DSM-5[1] SSD and IAD responds to criticism about a missing psychological component in the former diagnoses. The new diagnostic entities increasingly focus on maladaptive coping with somatic symptoms and/or health anxiety on different levels (affective, behavioral, and cognitive), which can be considered as indicative of the disorders.[9]

The Hierarchical Taxonomy of Psychopathology (HiTOP) system,[10] which arranges symptoms and syndromes in a dimensional and hierarchical manner based on their covariance, includes both SSD and IAD based on limited data in the somatoform spectrum.[10] Due to considerable overlap between the somatoform and the internalizing spectrum[11] (consisting of, eg, distress-related and fear-related symptoms), the existence of a common higher order emotional dysfunction superspectrum has recently been proposed.[12] This superspectrum should reflect differences in negative affect/neuroticism (including shared genetic, neural, behavioral, and cognitive-affective correlates), which are observed both in the somatoform and the internalizing spectrum.[12]

EPIDEMIOLOGY

Somatic symptoms with a medically not fully explained genesis are common in the general population (eg, 81.6% report to suffer from at least one distressing symptom[13]). The prevalence of SSD, IAD, or their predecessor diagnoses (according to DSM-IV[6]) seems considerable and comparable to affective disorders and anxiety disorders (eg, 12-month prevalence of 11% for somatoform disorders according to DSM-IV[6,14]). About 13% of the general population reports some illness worry.[15] Nevertheless, the point prevalence of DSM-IV[6] hypochondriasis "only" fluctuates around 0.4%.[16] Although no substantial gender differences are observed regarding pathological health anxiety, body sensations with a medically unclear genesis seem to be more frequently reported in female sex,[17] although biased observations cannot be fully excluded. Both pathological health anxiety as well as other somatoform disorders (and DSM-5[1] diagnoses SSD and IAD) can be considered as quite stable,[17,18] indicating that people mostly suffer longer times from these respective mental health disorders.

Considering the new diagnoses SSD and IAD, thus far, epidemiological data are partly based on self-report measures and clinical judgement but not on structured interviews. Estimates on SSD prevalence range from 12.9% in the general population up to 22.3% in medical settings,[19] thus being similar to the prevalence of DSM-IV somatoform disorders[14] (including the previously most frequently diagnosed unspecified somatoform disorder). Regarding IAD, epidemiological studies in the general population are missing completely. However, it is estimated that between 70% and 80% of patients who were formerly diagnosed with DSM-IV[6] hypochondriasis now fulfill the criteria of DSM-5[1] SSD due to the presence of distressing somatic sensations.[7,20] Furthermore, people with pathological health anxiety who fall in the range of the DSM-5[1] SSD were reported to seek more reassurance from doctors, to be more strongly impaired, and to have to a higher proportion a comorbid panic or generalized anxiety disorder.[20]

In relation to comorbidities, again, only limited data on DSM-5[1] SSD and IAD exist. As observed in relation to former diagnostic criteria (eg, DSM-IV[6]),[17] a high comorbidity with depressive disorders and anxiety disorders is expected. According to the HiTOP framework, this high comorbidity is attributable to the existence of a higher order emotional dysfunctional superspectrum.[12]

ASSESSMENT

The Structured Clinical Interview for DSM-5[1] Disorders (SCID-5[21]) only includes DSM-5[1] SSD and IAD in their research version and additional modules (referred to by single screening questions), nevertheless indicating to sufficiently support the diagnostic process.[22]

For pathological health anxiety (and respective diagnosis of SSD [with predominant health worries] and IAD) several reliable and validated self-administered and clinician-administered questionnaires and interviews exist. In particular, the 14-item Whiteley-Index (WI), which exists as a dichotomous[23] and as a 5-point Likert-scale version (coded 1–5),[24] and the 18-item multiple-choice (coded 0–3) Short Health Anxiety Inventory[25] (SHAI) are briefly administered self-report measures that are widely used to screen for an indication of pathologically heightened levels of health anxiety. The items of the SHAI can be aggregated to 2 factors: "Health Anxiety" (item 1–14) and "Negative Consequences of Illness" (item 15–18). Both cutoff scores of 5[26] and of 8[27] in the dichotomous WI are discussed as possible optimal (in relation to sensitivity and specificity) cutoffs to differentiate between people with pathological health anxiety (DSM-IV[6] hypochondriasis) and people with no mental disorders[26,27] and/or patients with other somatoform disorders.[27] Regarding the SHAI, data on cutoff scores are limited to one study by Abramowitz and colleagues,[28] who identified a cutoff of 45 in a 1-to-4-coded version of the SHAI (resembling a cutoff of 27 in a 0-to-3-coded version of the SHAI[29]) as being best to differentiate between people with pathological health anxiety (DSM-IV[6] hypochondriasis) and people with anxiety disorders. The Hypochondriasis Yale-Brown Obsessive-Compulsive Scale[30] (H-YBOCS), a clinician-administered, semistructured interview, additionally allows for an assessment of the severity of health anxiety.

Regarding DSM-5[1] SSD, a combination between an instrument that assesses symptom burden and a measure that examines the new B-criterion of SSD (excessive thoughts, feelings, or behaviors related to the somatic symptoms or associated health concerns) has proven to work well for screening purposes.[31] In particular, the combination of several self-report instruments, that is, the Patient Health Questionnaire-15[32] (PHQ-15), or the Somatic Symptom Scale-8[33] (SSS-8), with the Somatic Symptom Disorder–B Criteria Scale[34] (SSD-12)[31] and/or the dichotomous 7-item WI[35] is considered to be valid for screening. The PHQ-15 is a 15-item scale that assesses the presence of 15 somatic symptoms during the past 4 weeks on a 3-point scale from 0 to 2. Cutoffs of 5, 10, and 15 are reported to differentiate between mild, moderate, and severe somatic symptom burden.[32] In the 8-item SSS-8,[33] the severity of 8 somatic symptoms in the past week can be rated on a 5-point scale (coded 0–4). Sum scores of 0 to 3, 4 to 7, 8 to 11, 12 to 15, and 16 to 32 are considered to reflect minimal, low, medium, high, and very-high somatic symptom severity.[36] The SSD-12,[34] however, enables an assessment of the B-criterion of SSD and comprises 12 items (coded on a 5-point scale from 0 to 4), which can be aggregated to 3 sum scores, reflecting the affective, cognitive, and behavioral components of SSD. The SSD-12,[34] developed as a new instrument after the introduction of DSM-5[1] SSD, has proven to be reliable and valid both in the general population[37] and clinical populations.[34] **Table 1** gives an overview of the described interviews and questionnaires for the assessment of DSM-5[1] SSD and IAD, whereas **Table 2** highlights potential screening questions during clinical assessment.

ETIOLOGY AND PATHOGENESIS

Although the exact etiology of SSD and IAD is still unknown, current etiological perspectives on SSD and IAD, or on somatic symptoms and pathological health anxiety in general, overlap in some relevant points. They focus on interactions between psychological, that is, cognitive, behavioral, and affective, factors and processes, potentially predisposing and triggering experiences (ie, social factors), and biological variables, thus forming a biopsychosocial perspective.

The integrative model on medically unexplained symptoms by Brown (2004)[38] and the model on pathological health anxiety by Warwick and Salkovskis (1990)[39] propose that critical experiences, including, for example, traumatic experiences or experiences with disease, can form somatic representations or health-related/illness-related schemata, which can be activated and lead (potentially in the combination with acute stressors/triggers, eg, critical life incidences or daily hassles) to salient somatic sensations and/or health-related/illness-related thoughts via automatic (bottom–up) and intentional (top–down) attention processes. Somatosensory amplification, that is, the tendency to catastrophize potentially benign somatic sensations,[40] represents a further cognitive factor next to other cognitive biases, such as attention and somatic interpretation biases,[41,42] affecting the perception and interpretation of somatic sensations and/or health-related/illness-related information.

The predictive processing framework, which was adapted to somatic symptom perception by Van den Bergh, Witthöft, and Petersen (2017),[43] also proposes a cognitive and inference-based process, which both includes bottom–up (sensory input: somatic sensations with varying precision) and top–down ("prior": specific expectations and predictions on symptoms) information, which are combined in an iterative way to form a "posterior," for example, a somatic complaint. In SSD and IAD, highly precise priors (ie, predictions about symptoms) probably meet with often imprecise sensory input, which leads to a biased symptom perception.

Table 1
Reliable and validated interviews and questionnaires for the assessment of DSM-5[1] somatic symptom disorder and illness anxiety disorder

Name	Type	Field of Application	Further Information
SCID-5[21]	Semistructured interview	SSD IAD	SSD and IAD can be assessed through the research version and the additional modules of the SCID-5
H-YBOCS[30]	Semistructured interview	(Pathological) health anxiety	The H-YBOCS can help to assess the severity of health anxiety
SHAI[25]	Self-report questionnaire	(Pathological) health anxiety	• Two factors: "Health Anxiety" and "Negative Consequences of Illness" • Cutoff of 45 (in 1-to-4-coded version) and 27 (in 0-to-3-coded version) optimal
WI[23,24]	Self-report questionnaire	(Pathological) health anxiety	Cutoff of 5 or 8 (in dichotomous version) optimal
PHQ-15[32]	Self-report questionnaire	Somatic symptom burden	Cutoff of 5 (mild), 10 (moderate), and 15 (severe)
SSS-8[33]	Self-report questionnaire	Somatic symptom burden	Sum Scores of 0–3 (minimal), 4–7 (low), 8–11 (medium), 12–15 (high), 16–32 (very high)
SSD-12[34]	Self-report questionnaire	B-criterion of SSD	Three subcriteria: affective, cognitive, behavioral

Table 2
Potential screening questions for DSM-5[1] somatic symptom disorder and illness anxiety disorder during clinical assessment

Diagnostic Entity	Questions

SSD	• "In the last 6 months, did you suffer from any distressing body-related (somatic) symptom(s)?"
	• "Do you worry about your health and/or about the seriousness of this symptom/these symptoms? Are you afraid the symptom(s) could indicate a severe physical disease?"
	• "What do you do to cope with the symptom(s)?";
	Additional further questions that may be helpful:
	  ○ "Do you avoid anything (eg, physical exercise) because of your symptom(s)?"
	  ○ "Do you repeatedly check your body for the symptom(s)?"
	  ○ "Do you check the Internet for information on your symptom(s)?"
	  ○ "Do you often consult medical personnel on your symptom(s)?"

IAD	• "In the last 6 months, were you afraid of having and/or acquiring a serious illness? Is there any reason (preexisting medical condition, family history) why you should have and/or acquire this illness?"
	• "Are your health worries triggered and/or accompanied by any body-related (somatic) symptoms?"
	• "What do you do to cope with health worries?"
	Additional further questions that may be helpful:
	  ○ "Do you avoid anything (eg, health-/illness-related media information, hospitals) because of your health worries?"
	  ○ "Do you repeatedly check your body for signs of illnesses?"
	  ○ "Do you check the Internet for information on health-related/illness-related content?"
	  ○ "Do you seek reassurance with medical personnel or your personal contacts, when you are afraid of having a serious illness? If you are reassured, how long does your certainty of not having that illness last?"

Learning processes such as the classical conditioning of somatic sensations as conditioned reactions to negative affective triggers (eg, negative images or thoughts),[44] as well as operant learning processes as seen in chronic pain, where the catastrophic interpretation of somatic sensations lead to fear and avoidance behavior (fear-avoidance model of pain[45]), are considered as further relevant pathogenetic factors.[46] The latter, furthermore, points to the importance of behavioral variables in SSD and IAD. This includes—in addition to avoidance and resting behavior—safety-seeking behavior, comprising body checking, reassurance behavior (with professional personnel [eg, doctors] or in private surroundings [eg, family, friends]), as well as a general withdrawal from social and positive activities. All behaviors can produce short-term relief but over the long term can intensify health worries and the perception of somatic sensations.[47] Affective variables, that is, negative affect and emotion regulation processes, are listed as further relevant factors. In particular, negative affect(ivity) was found to be associated with somatic symptom perception.[48] Regarding emotion regulation, both for somatic symptom perception as well as for (pathological) health anxiety, a significant correlation was found with reported difficulties to identify feelings (a facet of alexithymia) and to (flexibly) access and use emotion regulation strategies, as well as partly with a suppressive regulation style.[49,50] These results must be interpreted with some caution as only limited experimental and causal data exist.[51] Furthermore, some studies also report conflicting results, which only partly confirm the proposed emotional impairments in experimental settings in people with SSD and/or pathological health anxiety.[52]

Regarding psychophysiology, an involvement of the hypothalamic-pituitary-adrenal (HPA) axis, probably reflected by a hypocortisolism, has been repeatedly suggested as one etiological factor in somatic symptom perception.[53] Further studies point to immunological processes and to a potential role of the serotonergic system; research on these facets, however, is limited[53] (**Fig. 1** for a model of pathogenesis and maintenance of somatic symptom perception and pathological health anxiety).

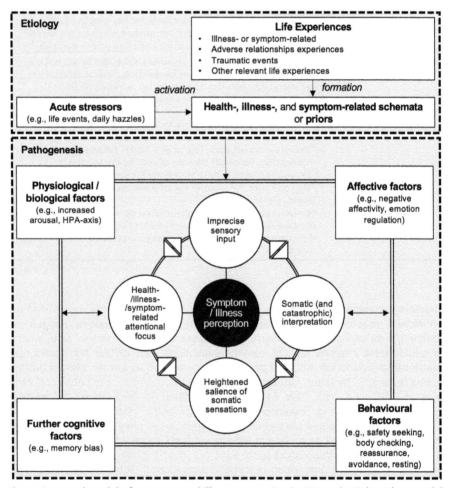

Fig. 1. Proposed model of symptom and illness perception in SSD and IAD based on models by Brown (2004)[38], Van den Bergh and colleagues (2017)[43], and Warwick and Salkovskis (1990)[39]: life experiences contribute to the formation of health-related, illness-related, and symptom-related schemata/priors, which are activated by acute stressors and trigger a vicious circle of a health-related/illness-related/symptom-related attentional focus, a somatic and catastrophic interpretation of imprecise sensory input, and further affective, behavioral, cognitive, and biological/physiological factors.

THERAPEUTIC OPTIONS

Regarding psychotherapeutic interventions, several meta-analyses and reviews point to cognitive-behavioral therapy (CBT) for SSD and IAD. CBT is highly effective in reducing health anxiety in people with pathological health anxiety (Hedges' $g = 0.79$, 95% CI [0.57, 1.01],[54] Cohen's $d = 1.01$, 95% CI [0.77, 1.25],[55] Hedge's $g = 0.95$, 95% CI [0.66, 1.22][56]), and still moderately but undoubtedly minorly effective in decreasing somatic symptom intensity in people with SSD and/or functional somatic symptoms (Cohen's $d = 0.25$, 95% CI [0.12, 0.38][57]; standardized mean difference $= -0.37$ [-0.69, -0.05][58]), both in comparison with control conditions (eg, waitlist-control, usual care).

CBT for SSD and IAD comprises several joint interventions, which target common mechanisms (for a more detailed description of the cognitive-behavioral treatment of medically unexplained symptoms and/or pathological health anxiety see, eg, Creed at al. (2011)[59] and Hedman-Lagerlöf (2019)[60]). Especially for people with SSD, an intensive psychoeducation on the diagnosis should be implemented before other interventions. Previous treatment attempts and experiences with the health-care system should be discussed because they often cause a skepticism toward psychological approaches, which is further increased by an often-present somatic disease model. Practitioners should avoid arguing against this model but rather focus on expanding it to a biopsychosocial framework by establishing further factors for symptom and/or illness perception. Joint cognitive interventions include, but are not limited to, attention retraining to reduce a partly maladaptively heightened symptom focus and the identification and questioning of the somatic and catastrophic interpretation biases regarding somatic sensations and/or illness-related/health-related information via cognitive restructuring. The effect of stress on symptom perception and subsequent stress management techniques (eg, relaxation techniques, such as progressive muscle relaxation), as well as approaches to reduce stress in daily life (eg, via identification and removal of stressors), are established. Thereafter, maladaptive behaviors (eg, body checking, doctor visits, health-related/illness-related Internet search) should be diminished by, for example, establishing alternative strategies to body checking or time-contingent instead of symptom-contingent doctor consultations. Similarly, another focus of CBT for SSD and IAD is on the reduction of excessive resting or avoidance behavior (eg, avoidance of somatic sensations by avoiding physical activity). Physical activity is gradually increased, which should be accompanied by interoceptive exposure exercises to examine fears around somatic sensations and/or physical activity. In particular, for pathological health anxiety additional in vivo (real-life; eg, confrontation with health-/illness-related information, such as documentaries on diseases) and in sensu (in imagination; eg, worst-case confrontation with most feared disease) exposure exercises are recommended.[61–63]

Thus far, studies indicate that selective serotonin reuptake inhibitors (SSRIs) could be a treatment option for pathological health anxiety, both as a monotreatment and as a combined treatment with CBT.[64–66] Regarding somatoform disorders, a very limited amount of studies point to minor positive effects of natural products, SSRIs, and selective noradrenalin reuptake inhibitors (sometimes in combination with antipsychotic medication) for medically unexplained somatic symptoms,[67] although these results should be taken with caution, as data is fairly limited and mainly of low quality. Furthermore, a higher risk of medication withdrawal due to unpleasant side effects (especially further somatic sensations) should be considered for SSD and IAD when deciding on a psychopharmacological medication.

DISCUSSION

Somatic symptoms with a medically unclear genesis are widely reported in the general population and in medical settings.[14,19] Health worries, that is, fears of having a severe disease, in its subclinical form also represent an often-declared phenomenon.[15] Somatoform disorders (according to DSM-IV[6]) and SSD and/or IAD (according to DSM-5[1]), thus, (should) belong to the most prevalent mental health disorders, although this area is drastically underrepresented in large epidemiological studies due to nosological debates. The newly introduced SSD, IAD, and FND diagnoses in DSM-5[1] replace the former DSM-IV[6] diagnoses of somatoform disorders, including hypochondriasis and conversion disorder. DSM-5[1] SSD abandons the empirically and theoretically problematic distinction between "medically explained" and "medically unexplained" and focuses on related excessive affects, thoughts, and behaviors. People with pathological health anxiety now can be diagnosed with IAD, if somatic symptoms are absent or only mild, or with SSD, if at least moderate somatic symptoms are reported. As most people with pathological health anxiety tend to report distressing somatic symptoms, DSM-5[1] SSD will probably be more often assigned.[7,20] There is still some debate regarding the validity of the separation between SSD and IAD for pathological health anxiety and regarding the inclusion of somatic symptoms with a medically clear genesis in SSD. Nevertheless, especially the latter can be interpreted as a necessary step toward breaking-up the mind-body dualism, which is no longer supported by research. Furthermore, both diagnostic entities (SSD and IAD) include maladaptive affective, cognitive, and behavioral responses to somatic symptoms and/or health-related/illness-related information.

A screening for SSD, therefore, should include an assessment of symptom severity (eg, with the PHQ-15[32]) and of the B-criterion of SSD (ie, excessive symptom-related thoughts, feelings, and behaviors; eg, with the SSD-12[34]). Regarding pathological health anxiety (no matter if diagnosed as SSD or IAD), further measures (eg, the WI[23,24] and/or SHAI[25]) to specifically assess health worries are recommended.

Current etiological and pathogenetic models point to a multifactorial genesis and maintenance of SSD and IAD, including psychological and biological processes and factors.[38–42,43–53] Future research should focus on further elucidating basic processes of somatic symptom perception (eg, predictive processing[43]) and on their therapeutic modification.

Due to questionable efficacy, possible side effects, and a high-withdrawal rate, a pharmacological approach to the treatment of SSD and IAD is currently less recommended. To date, CBT, which comprises cognitive (eg, reduction of the body-related attention bias and the somatic and catastrophic interpretation bias) and behavioral (eg, reduction of maladaptive behaviors, such as body checking, and avoidance, gradual increase of physical activity) interventions, is the psychotherapeutic treatment of choice. In relation to SSD and somatic symptoms with a medically unclear genesis, there is still much to be learned regarding treatment efficacy.

SUMMARY

The DSM-5[1] diagnoses of SSD and IAD more strongly emphasize maladaptive affective, cognitive, and behavioral responses to distressing symptoms and/or health-related/illness-related information. Because distressing somatic symptoms and related worries are widely reported in the general population and in primary and specialist care settings,[14,19] the improvement of the assessment and treatment of SSD and IAD should be in the focus of professional contact partners (eg, practitioners). Easy-to-access and easy-to-implement screening instruments exist for both SSD and IAD. CBT approaches are currently most suitable for treating patients with SSD and IAD.

CLINICS CARE POINTS

- DSM-5[1] SSD, IAD, and FND have replaced the DSM-IV[6] diagnoses of somatoform disorders, including hypochondriasis and conversion disorder.
- In particular, DSM-5[1] SSD is highly prevalent in the general population and should therefore be considered routinely by clinicians, particularly in patients with comorbid anxiety or affective disorder.
- Screening for SSD should include an assessment of both symptom severity and of symptom-related excessive thoughts, feelings, and behaviors. Pathological health anxiety (diagnosed as SSD or IAD) can be screened for with well-validated self-report instruments and a clinician-administered interview.
- Pharmacological approaches should not be considered as a first-line treatment. Rather, CBT represents the treatment of choice for SSD and IAD.

DECLARATION OF INTERESTS

None.

FUNDING

This research did not receive any specific grant from funding agencies in the public, commercial, or not-for-profit sectors.

REFERENCES

1. American Psychiatric Association. Diagnostic and statistical manual of mental disorders. 5th ed. Washington: APA Publishing; 2013.
2. Morschitzky H. Somatoforme Störungen: Diagnostik, Konzepte und Therapie bei Körpersymptomen ohne Organbefund. Springer; 2007. Wien.
3. Pilowsky I. From conversion hysteria to somatisation to abnormal illness behaviour? J Psychosom Res 1996;40(4):345–50.
4. Kapfhammer HP. Somatoforme Störungen. Nervenarzt 2001;72(7):487–500.
5. Spiegel D, Loewenstein RJ, Lewis-Fernández R, et al. Dissociative disorders in DSM-5. Depress Anxiety 2011;28(9):824–52.
6. American Psychiatric Association. Diagnostic and statistical manual of mental disorders. 4th Ed. Washington: APA Publishing; 2000.
7. Newby JM, Hobbs MJ, Mahoney AEJ, et al. DSM-5 illness anxiety disorder and somatic symptom disorder: Comorbidity, correlates, and overlap with DSM-IV hypochondriasis. J Psychosom Res 2017;101:31–7.
8. Rief W, Martin A. How to use the new DSM-5 somatic symptom disorder diagnosis in research and practice: a critical evaluation and a proposal for modifications. Annu Rev Clin Psychol 2014;10(1):339–67.
9. Toussaint A, Hüsing P, Kohlmann S, et al. Excessiveness in symptom-related thoughts, feelings, and behaviors: an investigation of somatic symptom disorders in the general population. Psychosom Med 2021;83(2):164–70.
10. Kotov R, Krueger RF, Watson D, et al. The hierarchical taxonomy of psychopathology (HiTOP): a dimensional alternative to traditional nosologies. J Abnorm Psychol 2017;126(4):454–77.

11. Krueger RF, Chentsova-Dutton YE, Markon KE, et al. A cross-cultural study of the structure of comorbidity among common psychopathological syndromes in the general health care setting. J Abnorm Psychol 2003;112(3):437–47.

12. Watson D, Levin-Aspenson HF, Waszczuk MA, et al. Validity and utility of hierarchical taxonomy of psychopathology (HiTOP): III. Emotional dysfunction superspectrum. World Psychiatr 2022;21(1):26–54.

13. Hiller W, Rief W, Brähler E. Somatization in the population: from mild bodily misperceptions to disabling symptoms. Soc Psychiatry Psychiatr Epidemiol 2006; 41(9):704–12.

14. Jacobi F, Wittchen H-U, Hölting C, et al. Prevalence, co-morbidity and correlates of mental disorders in the general population: Results from the German health interview and examination survey (GHS). Psychol Med 2004;34(4):597–611.

15. Noyes R, Carney CP, Hillis SL, et al. Prevalence and correlates of illness worry in the general population. Psychosomatics 2005;46(6):529–39.

16. Weck F, Richtberg S, Neng J. Epidemiology of hypochondriasis and health anxiety: Comparison of different diagnostic criteria. Curr Psychiatry Rev 2014;10(1): 14–23.

17. Creed F, Barsky AJ. A systematic review of the epidemiology of somatisation disorder and hypochondriasis. J Psychosom Res 2004;56(4):391–408.

18. Behm AC, Hüsing P, Löwe B, et al. Persistence rate of DSM-5 somatic symptom disorder: 4-year follow-up in patients from a psychosomatic outpatient clinic. Compr Psychiatry 2021;110:152265.

19. Löwe B, Levenson J, Depping M, et al. Somatic symptom disorder: a scoping review on the empirical evidence of a new diagnosis. Psychol Med 2022;52(4): 632–48.

20. Bailer J, Kerstner T, Witthöft M, et al. Health anxiety and hypochondriasis in the light of DSM-5. Hist Philos Logic 2016;29(2):219–39.

21. First MB, Williams JBW, Karg RS. Structured clinical interview for DSM-5(R) disorders - clinician version (SCID-5-CV). Arlington: APA Publisher; 2015.

22. Jiang Y, Wei J, Fritzsche K, et al. Assessment of the structured clinical interview (SCID) for DSM-5 for somatic symptom disorder in general hospital outpatient clinics in China. BMC Psychiatry 2021;21(1):144.

23. Pilowsky I. Dimensions of hypochondriasis. Br J Psychiatry 1967;113(494):89–93.

24. Welch PG, Carleton RN, Asmundson GJG. Measuring health anxiety: moving past the dichotomous response option of the original whiteley index. J Anxiety Disord 2009;23(7):1002–7.

25. Salkovskis P, Rimes KA, Warwick HMC, et al. The health anxiety inventory: Development and validation of scales for the measurement of health anxiety and hypochondriasis. Psychol Med 2002;32(5):843–53.

26. Hedman E, Lekander M, Ljótsson B, et al. Optimal cut-off points on the Health Anxiety Inventory, Illness Attitude Scales and Whiteley Index to identify severe health anxiety. PLoS One 2015;10(4):e0123412.

27. Hiller W, Rief W, Fichter MM. Dimensional and categorical approaches to hypochondriasis. Psychol Med 2002;32(4):707–18.

28. Abramowitz JS, Olatunji BO, Deacon BJ. Health anxiety, hypochondriasis, and the anxiety disorders. Behav Ther 2007;38(1):86–94.

29. Alberts NM, Hadjistavropoulos HD, Jones SL, et al. The short health anxiety inventory: a systematic review and meta-analysis. J Anxiety Disord 2013;27(1): 68–78.

30. Greeven A, Spinhoven P, van Balkom AJLM. Hypochondriasis Y-BOCS: a study of the psychometric properties of a clinician-administered semi-structured interview

to assess hypochondriacal thoughts and behaviours. Clin Psychol Psychother 2009;16(5):431–43.

31. Toussaint A, Hüsing P, Kohlmann S, et al. Detecting DSM-5 somatic symptom disorder: criterion validity of the Patient Health Questionnaire-15 (PHQ-15) and the Somatic Symptom Scale-8 (SSS-8) in combination with the Somatic Symptom Disorder – B Criteria Scale (SSD-12). Psychol Med 2020;50(2):324–33.

32. Kroenke K, Spitzer RL, Williams JBW. The PHQ-15: validity of a new measure for evaluating the severity of somatic symptoms. Psychosom Med 2002;64(2): 258–66.

33. Gierk B, Kohlmann S, Toussaint A, et al. Assessing somatic symptom burden: a psychometric comparison of the Patient Health Questionnaire-15 (PHQ-15) and the Somatic Symptom Scale-8 (SSS-8). J Psychosom Res 2015;78(4):352–5.

34. Toussaint A, Murray AM, Voigt K, et al. Development and validation of the somatic symptom disorder-B criteria scale (SSD-12). Psychosom Med 2016;78(1):5–12.

35. Laferton JAC, Stenzel NM, Rief W, et al. Screening for DSM-5 somatic symptom disorder: diagnostic accuracy of self-report measures within a population sample. Psychosom Med 2017;79(9):974–81.

36. Gierk B, Kohlmann S, Kroenke K, et al. The somatic symptom scale–8 (SSS-8). JAMA Intern Med 2014;174(3):399.

37. Toussaint A, Löwe B, Brähler E, et al. The somatic symptom disorder - B criteria scale (SSD-12): factorial structure, validity and population-based norms. J Psychosom Res 2017;97:9–17.

38. Brown RJ. Psychological Mechanisms of medically unexplained symptoms: an integrative conceptual model. Psychol Bull 2004;130(5):793–812.

39. Warwick HMC, Salkovskis P. Hypochondriasis. Behav Res Ther 1990;28(2): 105–17.

40. Barsky AJ, Wyshak G. Hypochondriasis and somatosensory amplification. Br J Psychiatry 1990;157(3):404–9.

41. Shi C, Taylor S, Witthöft M, et al. Attentional bias toward health-threat in health anxiety: a systematic review and three-level meta-analysis. Psychol Med 2022;1–10.

42. Witthöft M, Kerstner T, Ofer J, et al. Cognitive biases in pathological health anxiety. Clin Psychol Sci 2016;4(3):464–79.

43. Van den Bergh O, Witthöft M, Petersen S, et al. Symptoms and the body: taking the inferential leap. Neurosci Biobehav Rev 2017;74(Pt A):185–203.

44. Van den Bergh O, Winters W, Devriese S, et al. Learning subjective health complaints. Scand J Psychol 2002;43(2):147–52.

45. Vlaeyen JWS, Crombez G, Linton SJ. The fear-avoidance model of pain. Pain 2016;157(8):1588–9.

46. Carson A, Ludwig L, Welch K. Psychologic theories in functional neurologic disorders. Handb Clin Neurol 2016;139:105–20.

47. Olatunji BO, Etzel EN, Tomarken AJ, et al. The effects of safety behaviors on health anxiety: an experimental investigation. Behav Res Ther 2011;49(11): 719–28.

48. Schenk HM, Bos EH, Slaets JPJ, et al. Differential association between affect and somatic symptoms at the between- and within-individual level. Br J Health Psychol 2017;22(2):270–80.

49. Görgen SM, Hiller W, Witthöft M. Health anxiety, cognitive coping, and emotion regulation: A latent variable approach. Int J Behav Med 2014;21(2):364–74.

50. Okur Güney ZE, Sattel H, Witthöft M, et al. Emotion regulation in patients with so-matic symptom and related disorders: A systematic review. PLoS One 2019; 14(6):e0217277.
51. Schnabel K, Petzke TM, Witthöft M. The emotion regulation process in somatic symptom disorders and related conditions - A systematic narrative review. Clin Psychol Rev 2022;102196.
52. Schnabel K, Schulz SM, Witthöft M. Emotional reactivity, emotion regulation, and regulatory choice in somatic symptom disorder. Psychosom Med 2022;84(9): 1077–86.
53. Rief W, Barsky AJ. Psychobiological perspectives on somatoform disorders. Psy-choneuroendocrinology 2005;30(10):996–1002.
54. Axelsson E, Hedman-Lagerlöf E. Cognitive behavior therapy for health anxiety: Systematic review and meta-analysis of clinical efficacy and health economic out-comes. Expert Rev Pharmacoecon Outcomes Res 2019;19(6):663–76.
55. Cooper K, Gregory JD, Walker I, et al. Cognitive behaviour therapy for health anx-iety: a systematic review and meta-analysis. Behav Cogn Psychother 2017;45(2): 110–23.
56. Olatunji BO, Kauffman BY, Meltzer S, et al. Cognitive-behavioral therapy for hypo-chondriasis/health anxiety: a meta-analysis of treatment outcome and modera-tors. Behav Res Ther 2014;47(1):33–41.
57. Kleinstäuber M, Witthöft M, Hiller W. Efficacy of short-term psychotherapy for mul-tiple medically unexplained physical symptoms: a meta-analysis. Clin Psychol Rev 2011;31(1):146–60.
58. van Dessel N, den Boeft M, van der Wouden JC, et al. Non-pharmacological in-terventions for somatoform disorders and medically unexplained physical symp-toms (MUPS) in adults. Cochrane Database Syst Rev 2014;(11).
59. Creed F, Henningsen P, Fink P. In: *Medically unexplained symptoms, somatisa-tion, and bodily distress : developing better clinical services.* 1st edition. Cam-bridge: Cambridge University Press; 2011.
60. Hedman-Lagerlöf E. In: *The clinician's guide to treating health anxiety : diagnosis, mechanisms, and effective treatment.* 1st edition. London: Academic Press; 2019.
61. Weck F, Neng JMBB, Richtberg S, et al. Cognitive therapy versus exposure ther-apy for hypochondriasis (health anxiety): a randomized controlled trial. J Consult Clin Psychol 2015;83(4):665–76.
62. Myers L, Sarudiansky M, Korman G, et al. Using evidence-based psychotherapy to tailor treatment for patients with functional neurological disorders. Epilepsy Be-hav Reports 2021;16:100478.
63. Liu J, Gill NS, Teodorczuk A, et al. The efficacy of cognitive behavioural therapy in somatoform disorders and medically unexplained physical symptoms: A meta-analysis of randomized controlled trials. J Affect Disord 2019;245:98–112.
64. Greeven A, van Balkom AJLM, Visser S, et al. Cognitive behavior therapy and paroxetine in the treatment of hypochondriasis: a randomized controlled trial. Am J Psychiatry 2007;164(1):91–9.
65. Fallon BA, Ahern DK, Pavlicova M, et al. A randomized controlled trial of medica-tion and cognitive-behavioral therapy for hypochondriasis. Am J Psychiatry 2017; 174(8):756–64.
66. Schweitzer PJ, Zafar U, Pavlicova M, et al. Long-term follow-up of hypochondria-sis after selective serotonin reuptake inhibitor treatment. J Clin Psychopharmacol 2011;31(3):365–8.
67. Kleinstäuber M, Witthöft M, Steffanowski A, et al. Pharmacological interventions for somatoform disorders in adults. Cochrane Database Syst Rev 2014;(11).

Functional Neurological Disorder Among Sexual and Gender Minority People

Mackenzie P. Lerario, MD, NYS, CRPA/CPS-p[a,b,*],
Nicole Rosendale, MD[c,d], Jeff L. Waugh, MD, PhD[e],
Jack Turban, MD, MHS[f], Tina Maschi, PhD, LCSW[a,b]

KEYWORDS

- LGBTQ healthcare • Sexual and gender minority • Transgender
- Functional neurological disorder • Functional seizures
- Psychogenic nonepileptic seizures • Functional movement disorder
- Conversion disorder

KEY POINTS

- Some studies suggest a higher prevalence of functional neurological disorder and other brain-mind-body conditions among sexual and gender minority (SGM) people; however, the data are limited, particularly in studies of clinical phenotype and treatment trials.
- There are unique stressors associated with the process of concealment, societal rejection, stigmatization, and systemic discrimination that a sexual or gender minority person faces. Such stressors can contribute to the generation and maintenance of neuropsychiatric symptoms, including functional neurological disorder.
- Treatment of functional neurological disorder in the SGM community is similar to that of cisgender, heterosexual people and includes education, physical rehabilitation, and psychotherapy; other additional considerations include developing enhanced resiliency mechanisms, building psychosocial support networks, and providing affirming health care in inclusive environments.
- Involving social services and community agencies for appropriate referrals to resources is important to address social determinants of health.

[a] Fordham Graduate School of Social Service, New York, NY, USA; [b] Greenburgh Pride, Greenburgh, NY, USA; [c] Department of Neurology, University of California San Francisco; [d] Weill Institute for Neurosciences, University of California San Francisco; [e] Department of Pediatrics, UT Southwestern Medical School, Dallas, TX, USA; [f] Division of Child & Adolescent Psychiatry, University of California San Francisco
* Corresponding author. Fordham Graduate School of Social Service, 113 West 60th Street, New York, NY 10023.
E-mail address: mackenzie.lerario@greenburghpride.org

Neurol Clin 41 (2023) 759–781
https://doi.org/10.1016/j.ncl.2023.02.010
0733-8619/23/© 2023 Elsevier Inc. All rights reserved.

INTRODUCTION

Functional neurological disorder (FND) is a multinetwork brain disorder that exists at the intersection between neurology and psychiatry.[1] It is one of the more common outpatient neurological diagnoses,[1] and is a disabling, costly condition with a poor prognosis in some patients.[2,3] Patients with FND have reduced health-related quality of life similar to patients with Parkinson disease, epilepsy, or limb weakness,[4,5] and individuals with this condition can experience substantial health-care-related stigma.[6]

"Sexual and gender minority (SGM)" is an umbrella term used in the medical literature to describe a diverse range of identities inclusive of lesbian, gay, bisexual, transgender, and queer (LGBTQ) people. The percentage of the population self-identifying as part of the SGM community is higher among younger generations.[7] More than 1 in 5 members of generation Z (born 1997–2003) identify as LGBTQ, and 1 in 50 identify as transgender alone.[7] Although female sex—in the context of other biopsychosocial considerations—is a risk factor for developing FND, there may be disparities in the care and outcomes of FND across sexuality and gender, including among individuals who identify within the SGM community.[8,9] Although earlier FND research detailed the sex of participants (with a number of articles conflating sex and gender), they have not reported the SGM status of people with FND in a standardized fashion. However, limited reports suggest that rates of FND may be higher in the SGM community.[10,11]

The objective of this article is to describe differences in FND across sex, gender, and sexuality, with particular focus on the SGM community. We will explore how minority stress theory is one model that may be used to understand some of the biological and sociocultural factors contributing to FND in some SGM people. Finally, we address the treatment of functional neurological symptoms in the SGM community, with particular attention to resiliency building, community collaboration, and creating affirming health-care environments.

TERMINOLOGY: "SEXUAL AND GENDER MINORITY" DEFINED

The SGM community encompasses a diverse range of identities, which differ from heteronormative, binary standards of sex, sexual orientation, and gender identity. More than half of the individuals in the SGM community are bisexual.[7] Although now accepted as normal variations of gender and sexuality, the medical and psychiatric professions classified SGM identities as pathological and "disordered" in earlier versions of the Diagnostic and Statistical Manual of Mental Disorders (DSM) and the International Classification of Diseases.[12] The use of inclusive language in clinical and research settings is important for the development of affirming environments, which have been shown to improve neuropsychiatric outcomes in patients with SGM.[13,14] **Table 1** presents a list of definitions for widely accepted terminology describing the SGM community.

SEX DIFFERENCES IN ASSUMED CISGENDER FUNCTIONAL NEUROLOGICAL DISORDER SAMPLES

Most of the available research directly comparing epidemiology and phenotypes of FND in males versus females did not attempt to identify SGM status.[8,9,16–38] Virtually all of these studies conflate sex and gender (**Table 2**), and none specify participant sexual orientation and/or gender identity. Half of these studies (11/22) were performed in the United States and included small numbers of subjects (N < 300); larger cohorts (400–4000+), developed through multinational collaboration[35] and meta-analysis,[8] also had limited or no characterization of SGM status. This literature predominantly

Table 1
Lexicon of sexual and gender minority terminology

Term	Definition
Sex	Referring to the sex assigned at birth as declared by a medical professional, usually based on the appearance of external genitalia. Individuals are commonly categorized as "male," "female," or "intersex" at birth. Sex is a multidimensional construct that can include observable characteristics of external genitalia, gonads, and sex chromosomes, among other variables
Intersex	Refers to those whose sex-defining characteristics or reproductive anatomy does not fit into binary standards of male or female. Intersex conditions are often referred to as "disorders of sex development" or "differences of sexual development." Intersex conditions include complete or partial androgen insensitivity syndrome, mixed gonadal dysgenesis, 5-alpha-reductase deficiency, penile agenesis, and congenital adrenal hyperplasia
Gender/gender identity	A person's internal sense of their gender, which includes cisgender, transgender, gender nonconforming, and nonbinary identities, among others
Gender expression	The diverse, contextual, and malleable range of social, cultural, physical, and behavioral cues that a person uses to display their gender, including clothing, pronouns, and physical embodiment
Transgender	Someone whose gender identity differs from their sex assigned at birth
Cisgender	Someone whose gender identity aligns with their sex assigned at birth
Nonbinary	Someone whose gender identity is not within the binary of man or woman. Someone who is gender nonbinary may identify as both man and woman (bigender), as having no gender (agender), as having a gender identity, which changes in expression or intensity over time (genderfluid or genderflux), among other gender identities
Genderqueer/gender nonconforming	Refers to people who display nonnormative gender roles, expressions, and identities as defined by cultural expectations for sex assigned at birth
Two-spirit	A culturally specific term used in some North American Indigenous populations, which refers to someone who embodies both a masculine and feminine spirit
Gender dysphoria	Refers to psychological distress due to the incongruence between sex assigned at birth and gender identity. Not all transgender people experience gender dysphoria. Often a DSM-5-TR diagnosis of gender dysphoria is required for health-care insurers to reimburse transition-related care for transgender people
Gender affirmation	Refers to practices aimed at supporting a person's authentic gender identity, which may include mental health, medical, legal, and surgical aspects of care. Some refer to this process as a gender transition
Sexual orientation	Distinct from gender. Refers to the gender(s) of the individual(s) toward whom someone is attracted, including asexual (a heterogenous sexual orientation defined by having limited or no sexual attraction to others). The SGM community generally

(*continued on next page*)

Table 1 (continued)	
Term	**Definition**
	uses gender identity, and not sex, as the reference point for someone's sexual orientation
Gay, lesbian	Refers to someone who is attracted to the same sex or gender, such as women who are primarily attracted to women and men who are primarily attracted to men
Straight	Refers to someone who is attracted to a different sex or gender, such as women who are primarily attracted to men and men who are primarily attracted to women
Bisexual	Historically refers to someone who is attracted to more than one sex or gender. More recently, the term pansexual has been used to be more inclusive of transgender and nonbinary identities
Queer	A reclaimed slur for a sexual orientation or gender identity outside of culturally dominant and historically binary definitions of gender and sexuality. This word may be considered offensive to some in the SGM community and should only be used if someone self-identifies as such
Coming Out	The process of accepting and disclosing an SGM identity to others

Components of sex, sexual orientation, and gender identity are described.[15] Sexual and gender minorities represent a diverse range of identities outside of binary standards of cisgender-heteronormativity.

Abbreviation: DSM-5-TR, diagnostic and statistical manual of mental disorders, fifth edition text revision.

focused on functional seizures before 2016, when sex differences in mixed phenotypes and functional movement disorder began to be evaluated.

The female:male ratio in adult FND is approximately 3:1.[8,19,39,40] Most people with FND are young to middle-aged adults, with less data available on pediatric and elderly populations. Female predominance in FND is highest from adolescence to middle age, with data from 2 large cohorts showing female:male parity in prepubescent and postmenopausal patients. The reasons for this are unknown but could be due to diverse factors such as a contribution of sex hormones or gender-specific abuse—along with other biopsychosocial considerations.[8,32] Although some data suggest that FND onset is earlier in women,[8] this is not found universally.[23,38] Although FND is more common in women, an FND diagnosis should not be made or excluded based on sex or gender because this heuristic can lead to misdiagnoses and perpetuate implicit biases in clinical care and research.

Although some studies report sex-related differences in FND semiology,[17,18,27,29,31,35,36,41] others demonstrate no significant differences in clinical phenotypes of FND between men and women,[8,21–23,30,34,37,38] including in the largest cohort (N = 4905) of patients with FND.[8] More consistent findings in the literature include that women are more likely to weep during functional seizures[18,21] and FND-related unemployment is more common among men.[21,34] Women are more likely to have disclosed history of sexual or physical trauma,[9,16,20–22,33,35,41] and this finding has been associated with higher rates of FND observed in women.[9,16] One study found that men were more likely to have an indeterminate diagnosis after referral for characterization of predicted functional seizures.[28] Cultural differences between cohorts may also have influenced the expression of FND. The lack of data collection regarding SGM status in FND research reflects the assumption that subjects were cisgender, a significant limitation in our understanding of the influence of SGM identity on FND.

Table 2
Literature review on sex differences in functional neurological disorder

Author(s), Year	Location	FND Type	Study Design	N	Mean Age (Diagnosis), years	Male (%)	Reported Sex-Related Associations	Other Findings of Interest
Van Merode et al,[41] 1997	Netherlands	FS	Systematic review (1947–1993, Medline)	62	NR: Age ranged from 14 to 77	24	Women: sexual abuse Men: tonic-clonic	Semiology in sexual abuse victims did not differ from total cohort
Rosenbaum[24] 2000	United States	FS	Case series	2	28	50	Women: rage, fear, helplessness, low assertiveness	Implicit bias: sexism
Holmes et al,[25] 2001	United States	FS	Retrospective, epilepsy control group	84	Men: 36 Women: 33	32	Men: higher education, worse emotional adjustment (based on MMPI [Minnesota Multiphasic Personality Inventory] scales)	Later onset of FS compared with epilepsy controls
Oto et al,[39] 2005	United Kingdom	FS	Prospective	160	Men: 41 Women: 35	26	Men: higher unemployment, lower family acceptance of diagnosis Women: self-harm, sexual abuse, weeping Similar semiology between sexes	

(continued on next page)

Table 2
(continued)

Author(s), Year	Location	FND Type	Study Design	N	Mean Age (Diagnosis), years	Male (%)	Reported Sex-Related Associations	Other Findings of Interest
Noe et al,[28] 2012	United States	FS	Retrospective, physiologic and indeterminate diagnosis control group	184	43	23	Men: higher likelihood of indeterminate diagnosis after evaluation for predicted FND	
Thomas et al,[22] 2013	United States	FS	Retrospective	86	40	31	Women: physical and sexual abuse, psychiatric comorbidity, chronic pain. Similar semiology between sexes	
Asadi-Pooya et al,[30] 2013	Iran	FS	Prospective	222	Men: 28 Women: 28	31	Similar semiology between sexes	
Gale et al,[27] 2015	United States	FS	Prospective, epilepsy control group	205	39	28	Men: antisocial features, somatic complaints, motor seizures. Women: depressive symptoms	
Say et al,[31] 2015	Turkey	FS	Retrospective	62	14	29	Men: tonic-clonic, lower academic achievement, ADHD	Tremor was most prevalent ictal motor sign in

Study	Country	Type	Design	No.	No.	No.	Sex differences	Additional findings
Kamble et al,[29] 2016	India	FMD	Prospective	73	29 (30% were ≤18 y of age)	49 (64% in ≤18 y cohort)	[Attention-deficit/hyperactivity disorder] Women: atonic falls, longer episodes, depression; Women: tremors	both men and women; Adults: tremor Children: myoclonus 43% required admission 58% improved after treatment
Del Bene et al,[26] 2017	United States	FNS	Retrospective, epilepsy control group	77	28	14	Women: higher emotional distress, higher suicidal ideation	FS: Higher MMPI-2-RF scores (particularly somatic and mood)
Matin et al,[33] 2017	United States	Mixed Motor FND	Retrospective	100	40	21	Men: cognitive complaints, functional weakness Women: physical and sexual trauma	Illness duration correlated with number of self-reported medication allergies
Myers et al,[20] 2018	United States	FS	Retrospective	148	Men: 34 Women: 37	35	Men: avoidance, depression Women: sexual trauma, dissociation,	

(continued on next page)

Table 2
(continued)

Author(s), Year	Location	FND Type	Study Design	N	Mean Age (Diagnosis), years	Male (%)	Reported Sex-Related Associations	Other Findings of Interest
							sexual disturbances	
Korucuk et al,[23] 2018	Turkey	FS	Retrospective, epilepsy control group	41	27 (Range: 16–65)	24	Women: older age of onset, longer median FND duration Similar semiology between sexes	Forced eye closure common in both sexes
Türe et al,[18] 2019	Turkey	FS	Retrospective	155	34 (Range: 13–67)	41	Men: major motor activity, lateralizing motor activity, opisthotonic posture, pelvic thrust motion Women: weeping Similar rates of concomitant epilepsy and family history between sexes	23% confirmed concomitant epilepsy
Asadi-Pooya et al,[35] 2019	Multinational	FS	Retrospective	451	Men: 25 Women: 27	32	Women: sexual and physical abuse, presence of auras	
Raper et al,[38] 2019	United Kingdom	Mixed FND	Retrospective	124	Range: 4–19	44	Women: Longer time to diagnosis No significant	FND Incidence: 6 per 100,000 children

Reference	Country	FND type	Study design	N	Age		association between symptom presentation group and sex	Long-term outcomes
Baizabal-Carvallo & Jankovic[17] 2020	United States	FMD	Prospective	196	Men: 44 Women: 38	30	Men: functional gait disorder Women: functional dystonia	23% had symptoms lasting into adulthood
Kletenik et al,[16] 2020	United States	FMD	Retrospective, general neurology control group	199	46	25	Women: sexual abuse	
Asadi-Pooya & Homayoun[32] 2020	Iran	FS	Retrospective	275	29 (Range: 10–67)	36	Female:Male sex ratio of FND is lowest in prepuberty and postmenopause, and highest in adulthood	Suggests sex hormones influence higher rates of FND in females
Tinazzi et al,[37] 2020	Italy	Motor FND	Prospective	410	47	29	No sex-related differences in presentation with isolated motor FND vs mixed FND symptoms	1 person had gender dysphoria diagnosed by a psychiatrist
Garcin et al,[34] 2021	France	Motor FND	Prospective	482	40 (median at TMS treatment)	76	Similar semiology between sexes	58% were unemployed 66% had psychiatric comorbidity 83% reported trauma.

(continued on next page)

Table 2
(continued)

Author(s), Year	Location	FND Type	Study Design	N	Mean Age (Diagnosis), years	Male (%)	Reported Sex-Related Associations	Other Findings of Interest
Lidstone et al,[8] 2022	International Collaboration	Mixed Motor FND	Meta-analysis (1968–2022)	4905	40 (symptom onset) 8% pediatric onset 11% onset over age 60	27	Women: earlier age of onset. Similar semiology between sexes	Mixed FMD (23%), tremor (22%) and weakness (18%) most common semiology FMD peaks in midlife
Delgado et al,[36] 2022	Italy	FMD	Retrospective	100	40.9	37	Men: longer FND symptom duration	19/21 (90%) patients with joint hypermobility were women
Kletenik et al,[9] 2022	United States	FMD	Retrospective, case-control	696	45	26	Women: sexual and physical abuse	

Literature search performed in the PubMed.gov database maintained by the United States National Library of Medicine at the National Institutes of Health. Search terms included ("sex" or "gender") AND ("functional neurological disorder" or "conversion disorder" or "functional seizure" or "psychogenic nonepileptic seizure" or "pseudoseizure" or "functional movement disorder"). Titles and abstracts (as well as citations from included articles) were screened for inclusion based on relevance by a single board-certified neurologist (MPL). Articles not reporting sex differences in the title or abstract were excluded. Peer-reviewed publications in English language were included from inception to June 20, 2022.

Abbreviations: FMD, functional movement disorder; FND, functional neurological disorder; FS, functional seizures; NR, not reported; TMS, transcranial magnetic stimulation.

FUNCTIONAL NEUROLOGICAL DISORDER IN SEXUAL MINORITY PEOPLE

There are limited data on the effect of sexual orientation on the prevalence and semiology of FND, and the existing publications are outdated in terms of our current understanding of the complex biopsychosocial mechanisms underlying FND.[42–44] There is some early indication from case reports that the development of FND in some individuals may be linked to unique stressors observed in sexual minority communities, such as concealment of one's sexual orientation, the coming out process, and real or perceived societal rejection. For example, a report from India describes a 20-year-old gay man (presumed cisgender) who experienced functional seizures attributed to feelings of guilt and shame surrounding his identity.[43] His symptoms resolved following intensive psychotherapy addressing parental attachment wounds. A second case report, from the United States, described a 17-year-old boy with multiple somatic complaints and behavioral disturbances following a brief, self-limited febrile illness, associated with fear of rejection from family and peers regarding his sexual orientation.[42] His symptoms resolved after disclosing same-sex attractions to his treating pediatrician. Interestingly, although the specific sociocultural factors contributing to shame may be different across patients (and in some pertain to themes related to SGM identity), shame has been identified as a relevant psychological factor in FND across a range of circumstances.[45]

FUNCTIONAL NEUROLOGICAL DISORDER IN GENDER MINORITY PEOPLE

Two epidemiological studies suggest the prevalence of brain-mind-body (functional) disorders is higher among the gender minority (GM) community compared with cisgender populations.[10,11] A study of 535 GM patients and age-matched cisgender controls in Germany showed that somatoform disorders and severe stress reactions were 67% more prevalent in the GM cohort.[11] A retrospective study of patients presenting to a FND clinic in Australia found that GM patients were overrepresented compared with expected prevalence based on Australian census data.[10] These analyses did not adjust for sexual orientation of the participants. One prospective, Italian multicenter study of 410 patients with motor FND found that 1 (0.2%) patient had gender dysphoria diagnosed by a psychiatrist; however, the gender identities of patients within this cohort were not reported.[37]

A study of 50 self-identified members of the Hijra community, a GM identity indigenous to some Indian communities, found that the prevalence of lifetime somatoform disorders was 6%.[46] No comparison group was provided in this study. There were negative correlations between the experience of discrimination or physical violence and quality of life. A case series of 3 transmasculine patients with postural orthostatic tachycardia syndrome and multiple somatic complaints was reported from the United States.[47] Notably, all patients were treated with gender affirming hormone therapy with improvement in their symptoms.

Three case reports of GM patients with FND exist in the literature.[48–50] The authors theorized that stressors related to GM identity may be contributing factors to the patients' presentation with FND. From these reports, prognosis seems favorable if the GM person can come out and receive affirming medical care as safe, appropriate, and part of the overall treatment approach.

There is a single case report of FND misdiagnosis describing a transgender woman presenting with pain and paralysis who was ultimately found to have a spinal cord injury.[51–59]

MINORITY STRESS MODELS

Normativity of cisgender heterosexual roles in society has at times excluded patients with SGM from clinical care, research, and professional practice. Unfortunately, SGM

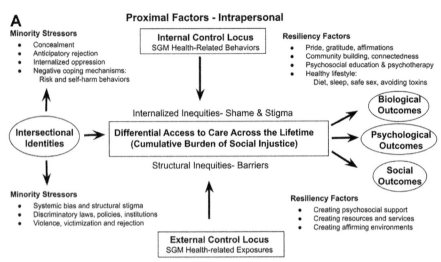

A

Proximal Factors - Intrapersonal

Minority Stressors
- Concealment
- Anticipatory rejection
- Internalized oppression
- Negative coping mechanisms:
  Risk and self-harm behaviors

Internal Control Locus
SGM Health-Related Behaviors

Resiliency Factors
- Pride, gratitude, affirmations
- Community building, connectedness
- Psychosocial education & psychotherapy
- Healthy lifestyle:
  Diet, sleep, safe sex, avoiding toxins

Internalized Inequities- Shame & Stigma

Biological Outcomes

Intersectional Identities

Differential Access to Care Across the Lifetime (Cumulative Burden of Social Injustice)

Psychological Outcomes

Structural Inequities- Barriers

Social Outcomes

Minority Stressors
- Systemic bias and structural stigma
- Discriminatory laws, policies, institutions
- Violence, victimization and rejection

Resiliency Factors
- Creating psychosocial support
- Creating resources and services
- Creating affirming environments

External Control Locus
SGM Health-related Exposures

Distal Factors - Environmental, Institutional & Interpersonal

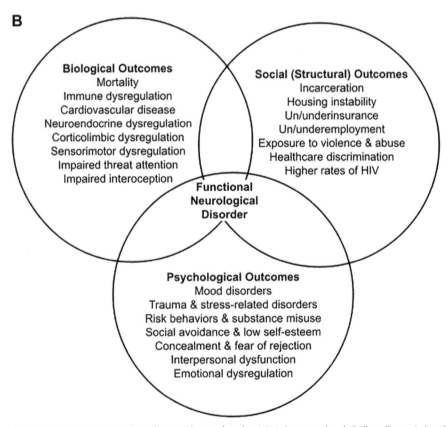

B

Biological Outcomes
Mortality
Immune dysregulation
Cardiovascular disease
Neuroendocrine dysregulation
Corticolimbic dysregulation
Sensorimotor dysregulation
Impaired threat attention
Impaired interoception

Social (Structural) Outcomes
Incarceration
Housing instability
Un/underinsurance
Un/underemployment
Exposure to violence & abuse
Healthcare discrimination
Higher rates of HIV

Functional Neurological Disorder

Psychological Outcomes
Mood disorders
Trauma & stress-related disorders
Risk behaviors & substance misuse
Social avoidance & low self-esteem
Concealment & fear of rejection
Interpersonal dysfunction
Emotional dysregulation

Fig. 1. Minority Stress and Resiliency Theory for the SGM Community. (*A*) The allostatic load model (within a stress-diathesis framework) suggests the cumulative disadvantage of social injustice and protective resiliency factors can modulate risk for the development of

people face high rates of discrimination, health-care disparities, and other systemic inequities at all levels of society.[60] These social injustices range from microaggressions to violence, including verbal harassment and physical assault. Minority stress models describe oppression against patients with SGM as intersecting with other forms of discrimination, including racism and socioeconomic disadvantage, and together are responsible for structural pathways leading to systemic health-care inequities (**Fig. 1**).[61,62]

Although FND is etiologically and mechanistically heterogeneous, there is an overlap of the neural mechanisms underlying trauma/stress-related disorders and FND.[6,65] Allostatic load, or the cumulative burden of stress over a lifetime, can explain some of the increased rates of neuropsychiatric conditions observed in the SGM community.[65,66] Current minority stress models propose that patients with SGM may engage in risk behaviors as negative coping mechanisms to systemic stressors.[67] The rates of these systemic stressors are more often experienced by SGM communities of color[68] and in those with co-occurring mental health disorders,[69] suggesting the importance of intersectionality in minority stress theory.[61] A combination of both risk and protective factors likely influence a person's lifetime susceptibility to FND.[62,65] More recent data evaluate the SGM community's resiliency through the building of positive coping skills and psychosocial support.[58,62] Resiliency factors include community building, advocacy, role modeling, and other expressions of pride, self-worth, and self-acceptance.

TREATMENT

The treatments for FND in SGM communities overlap with FND treatment options in cisgender, heterosexual people. These treatments include a combination of education, psychotherapy, physical rehabilitation (eg, physical therapy), and building psychosocial support systems.[39] Development of resiliency, empowerment, and a sense of agency are important in the treatment of FND for all people. Although stress and trauma are potential predisposing or precipitating factors for FND symptoms in some patients, specific psychosocial stressors are unique to the SGM community. Treatment of patients within the SGM community with FND should address the sources and consequences of these stressors and the trauma sustained because of structural discrimination and other forms of historical oppression, as part of an overall biopsychosocial formulation and approach to care.

FND clinics should take a multidisciplinary, biopsychosocial-oriented, patient-centered, and team-based approach to addressing the various interpersonal, intrapersonal, and systemic misalignments that may occur in patients with SGM presenting with FND.[6] Gains in physical and mental health can often be made when the treatment team addresses diseases and the social conditions that may contribute to or cause them (ie, the social determinants of health).[70] A horizontally distributed therapeutic team promotes shared leadership and empowers all providers with the freedom to provide the highest level of culturally inclusive, patient-centered care. Treatment teams should ideally represent the diversity of the patients they treat, and therapeutic

---

neuropsychiatric symptoms.[63] Social attribution theory relates the perception of control to outcomes.[64] (*B*) The biopsychosocial outcomes experienced by SGM individuals in response to allostatic load. There is overlap in the neurobiological mechanisms behind trauma/stress-related disorders and stress-related disorders and FND. HIV, human immunodeficiency virus; SGM, sexual and gender minorities.

approaches should be affirming and address the intersectionality of SGM status with other historically oppressed identities, such as race, ethnicity, disability, or neurodivergence. Because the development of FND in patients with SGM may be in part related to stigma, concealment, and rejection of their identities, important therapeutic modalities may include disclosure of shared identities, promotion of resiliency factors, and building community support.

Both individual counseling and group therapy are important to consider in treating SGM people with FND. Gender affirming medical providers, including individual psychotherapists, can be found through the World Professional Association For Transgender Health.[71] Other important resources, such as community forums and family or school support materials can be found online.[72,73] Additionally, telemedicine has allowed for expanded access to group therapy and SGM-affirming individual therapy in remote areas. Trauma-informed psychotherapy, when there is a disclosed history, and appropriate pharmacological treatment of trauma-related disorders and psychiatric comorbidities can be critical parallels to FND treatment. Incorporating certified peer specialists into practice is a promising recent innovation.[74] If present, referrals should be made for co-occurring housing instability, underemployment, underinsurance, substance misuse, sexual health screening, and eating disorders because these stressors may interplay with onset or persistence of FND symptoms.[60,75]

Local community agencies can be allies in developing a treatment plan for SGM people with FND. These agencies offer a wide variety of SGM-specific services and resources, including peer support groups, educational materials, social events, and inclusivity trainings. When interested, providers should encourage patients to build psychosocial support structures and facilitate patient involvement in community events, which have been shown to increase resiliency in SGM people.[58,62,76]

There is little available evidence on specific treatments for FND in SGM people. Dialectical behavioral therapy may improve emotional dysregulation and interpersonal dysfunction caused by gender dysphoria and minority stress.[77,78] A study of 57 GM patients reported improved psychological distress and somatization symptoms through the Symptom Checklist-90 when receiving gender affirming services and medical care.[75] The largest decrease in neuropsychological distress occurred after the initiation of gender affirming hormone therapy, after which time the Symptom Checklist-90 scores resembled those of the general population. Safe and affirming environments to express thoughts and feelings related to SGM identity are important to the exploration process and to building resiliency against shame. In a study of 62 cisgender gay men, social avoidance and somatic symptoms improved with expressive writing as a venue to discuss and explore sexual orientation.[79]

The social environments in clinical offices, hospitals, and research settings are critical to the health and well-being of patients with SGM.[13,60,80] Nonaffirming health-care environments create barriers to care, preventing patients with SGM from receiving health-care services of adequate quality.[81,82] In contrast, recent data have demonstrated that affirming environments, including social and medical transition for those who require it, are associated with better mental health outcomes (depression, suicidality, and substance addiction) for patients with SGM.[13,80,83] Affirming clinical environments establish psychotherapeutic rapport, create trust between patient and provider, and promote patient engagement with the treatment process.[6,84,85]

Neurologists can design clinical and research environments that support their patients with SGM with FND by adopting good practices (**Table 3**) that affirm their patients' identities.[84–86] Patients should feel safe to give feedback to the provider when the provider does not produce an affirming patient experience. In these situations, the provider's response should be transparent and timely. Representation of

Table 3
Recommendations to create affirming clinical and research spaces for sexual and gender minorities

Category	Action	Examples
Language	Use noninvasive, respectful, affirming, and empowering language	• Document and use patients' chosen/preferred name and pronouns. Include sexual orientation and gender identity data in clinical intake and EHR forms • If not sure, ask. Do not assume. Use gender-neutral language if unsure. Avoid unnecessarily gendered language • If a provider makes a mistake, immediately apologize once, explain this is something being worked on, then move on. Improve by practicing with allies or researching implicit bias. The patient should not be expected to comfort the provider for emotions behind the mistake. Do not assume an apology is excusive of transphobic language • Ask the patient's preference as to what terms are used for their genitals, as relevant
Boundaries	Have appropriate boundaries, and respect patients' boundaries	• Avoid invasive questions out of curiosity. Ask only what is needed and think how these questions can be asked most sensitively. Not every patient desires social, legal, medical, and/or surgical transition • Do not assume the patient's SGM identity is related to their FND diagnosis • Do not assume a person's current anatomy or future transition plans. Ask only if it is appropriate to do so (and relevant to the clinical care or research) • Consider disclosing shared identities when appropriate • Do not assume every patient is interested or engaging in sexual behaviors (some are asexual) or how they have sex. If unsure, ask based on a combination of "Do you have oral, anal, or vaginal sex" and "Do you have insertive,

(continued on next page)

Table 3 (continued)		
Category	**Action**	**Examples**
		receptive, or nonpenetrative sex" • Do not assume HIV status based on sexual orientation or gender identity. (People on antiretrovirals may be using them for pre-exposure prophylaxis)
Signage	Visibly demonstrate support, representation, and inclusion of sexual and gender minorities in clinical and research spaces	• Display signage of allyship in waiting rooms and examination rooms (posters, flyers, pride flags, and so forth) • Wear pronoun pins and allow patients to, as desired • Display patient bill of rights and contact information for the Patient Services Department • Have resources and pamphlets for patients with SGM in waiting and examination rooms • Share pronouns on video conferencing profiles and at team meetings during introductions • Offer options for gender-neutral facilities (eg, restrooms)
Public Support	Practice active allyship, role modeling, advocacy, direct feedback solicitation, and transparent hiring and promotional processes	• Correct team members who misgender patients or use other language that stigmatizes SGM people • Model appropriate use of pronouns and chosen names • Solicit feedback often from patients. Make response to feedback transparent and timely • Advocate for SGM patients' needs with leadership • Advocate for patient with SGM rights • Hire, mentor, develop, and promote SGM team members
Knowledge	Increase access to resources and training on community needs	• Attend DEI conferences, trainings, or workshops within your institution. If none exist, work with leadership to create one or find external ones • Work on implicit biases on an individual and institutional level. Patients should not be expected to teach providers about SGM identities or their health care

(continued on next page)

Table 3 (continued)		
Category	Action	Examples
		• Make active bystander training part of annual and onboarding training • Include training on SGM community as part of annual and onboarding training

Abbreviations: DEI, diversity, equity, and inclusion; EHR, electronic health record; HIV, human immunodeficiency virus; SGM, sexual and gender minority.
Data from Refs.[13,80–82,84–86,88]

marginalized communities in all segments of clinical and research practice has been termed community-based participatory action research, which can be used to mobilize collective action and create social innovations that benefit public health.[87]

GAPS IN CARE, KNOWLEDGE, AND THE LITERATURE

There are notable gaps in the literature describing FND phenotypes and treatments in SGM communities, as well as a need for affirming health-care options for patients with SGM as a whole. More community representation and iterative feedback is needed in the research and publication processes. Sexual orientation and gender identity data should be included in electronic health records and research registries. SGM health care should be included in the educational curricula within training programs and the examinations for licensing and credentialing. All patients should be treated with respect and dignity, including the appropriate use of pronouns and chosen names in clinical and research settings. Clinicians should endeavor to provide affirming and healing spaces for patients and begin to think of patients from a holistic, biopsychosocial, and intersectional perspective. This includes moving away from a deficits model of care toward one where a patient's strengths and agency are empowered to build resiliency against neuropsychiatric manifestations of systemic stressors and discrimination. Finally, more specific research is needed on FND in SGM communities.

SUMMARY

SGM community members may face unique minority stressors, which put them at risk for developing neuropsychiatric disorders, potentially including FND. FND and SGM identities are more prevalent in younger age demographics. In some patients, case reports suggest a potential temporal association between FND symptom onset and concealment of a SGM identity with symptom resolution through disclosing the identity and receiving affirming care. Larger cohorts of patients with FND suggest an increased prevalence of FND in the SGM population compared with the general population. Gaining a sense of agency, reframing threat assessment, and resiliency building are all protective factors that buffer against damaging neural changes in response to overwhelming stressors. More research is required to better characterize FND in SGM people.

Treatment approaches for FND in SGM communities should be biopsychosocial-focused, multidisciplinary, and involve local community agencies to help the patient build supports and find appropriate affirming services and resources. They should be informed by minority stress models and what is known regarding intersectionality.

Creating inclusive clinical and research environments is critical to the therapeutic alliance and healing process for SGM patients with FND.

Neurologists should potentially expect an increasing number of patients with SGM patients with FND to present to their clinics, given that a higher proportion of younger persons identify as members of these communities. More research and clinical support are required to better address the needs of SGM patients with FND.

CLINICS CARE POINTS

- We recommend neurologists working with SGM patients with FND learn nonpathologizing terminology relevant to these communities and create affirming environments in clinics and research settings.
- The clinical phenotypes of, and best treatments for, FND within the SGM community are unknown. Neurologists should continue to frame care using a biopsychosocial model that includes resiliency building, developing support systems, and gaining access to affirming care.
- Neurologists should not make diagnostic assumptions based on sex, sexual orientation, or gender. Rather, FND diagnoses should be based on physical examination signs and semiological features specific to the condition.
- Addressing intersectionality and social determinants of health is important to moderating the risk of developing and recovering from FND.

DISCLOSURES

Dr M.P. Lerario has served as expert witness for plaintiff for Weiss Law, PC. They are on the editorial board of *Neurology Clinical Practice* and the Vice-Chair of the LGBTQI Section of the American Academy of Neurology. Dr J.L. Waugh: None. Dr J. Turban reports receiving textbook royalties from Springer Nature and expert witness payments from The American Civil Liberties Union and Lambda Legal. He has received a pilot research award for general psychiatry residents from The American Academy of Child & Adolescent Psychiatry and Its Industry Donors (Arbor & Pfizer) and a research fellowship from The Sorensen Foundation. Dr N. Rosendale: Receives research funding from the American Academy of Neurology and NIH StrokeNet Fellowship. She receives royalties from McGraw Hill for authorship of an article in Current Medical Diagnosis and Treatment 2022 and 2023. Dr T. Maschi: None.

REFERENCES

1. Aybek S, Perez DL. Diagnosis and management of functional neurological disorder. BMJ 2022;o64. https://doi.org/10.1136/bmj.o64.
2. Gelauff J, Stone J, Edwards M, et al. The prognosis of functional (psychogenic) motor symptoms: a systematic review. J Neurol Neurosurg Psychiatr 2014;85(2): 220–6.
3. Stephen CD, Fung V, Lungu CI, et al. Assessment of emergency department and inpatient use and costs in adult and pediatric functional Neurological Disorders. JAMA Neurol 2021;78(1):88.
4. Stone J, Warlow C, Sharpe M. The symptom of functional weakness: a controlled study of 107 patients. Brain J Neurol 2010;133(Pt 5):1537–51.

5. Anderson KE, Gruber-Baldini AL, Vaughan CG, et al. Impact of psychogenic movement disorders versus Parkinson's on disability, quality of life, and psychopathology. Mov Disord 2007;22(15):2204–9.

6. Kozlowska K, Sawchuk T, Waugh JL, et al. Changing the culture of care for children and adolescents with functional neurological disorder. Epilepsy Behav Rep 2021;16:100486.

7. Jones JM. LGBT Identification in U.S. Ticks Up to 7.1%. *Gallup.* 2022;Politics. Available at: https://news.gallup.com/poll/389792/lgbt-identification-ticks-up. aspx. Accessed May 19, 2022.

8. Lidstone SC, Costa-Parke M, Robinson EJ, et al. Functional movement disorder gender, age and phenotype study: a systematic review and individual patient meta-analysis of 4905 cases. J Neurol Neurosurg Psychiatr 2022;93(6):609–16.

9. Kletenik I, Holden SK, Sillau SH, et al. Gender disparity and abuse in functional movement disorders: a multi-center case-control study. J Neurol 2022;269(6): 3258–63.

10. Morsy SK, Huepe-Artigas D, Kamal AM, et al. The relationship between psychosocial trauma type and conversion (functional neurological) disorder symptoms: a cross-sectional study. Australas Psychiatr 2021;29(3):261–5.

11. Konrad M, Kostev K. Increased prevalence of depression, anxiety, and adjustment and somatoform disorders in transsexual individuals. J Affect Disord 2020;274:482–5.

12. Lerario M, Galis A. The inclusion of historically oppressed genders in neurologic practice research. Neurol Clin Pract 2022;12(3):187–9.

13. Russell ST, Pollitt AM, Li G, et al. Chosen name use is linked to reduced depressive symptoms, suicidal ideation, and suicidal behavior among transgender youth. J Adolesc Health 2018;63(4):503–5.

14. Dolotina B, Turban JL. a multipronged, evidence-based approach to improving mental health among transgender and gender-diverse youth. JAMA Netw Open 2022;5(2):e220926.

15. Turban JL, de Vries ALC, Zucker KJ, et al. IACAPAP Textbook of Child and adolescent mental health. Vol transgender and gender non-conforming youth. Geneva, Switzerland: International Association for Child and Adolescent Psychiatry and Allied Professions; 2018.

16. Kletenik I, Sillau SH, Isfahani SA, et al. Gender as a risk factor for functional movement disorders: the role of sexual abuse. Mov Disord Clin Pract 2020;7(2): 177–81.

17. Baizabal-Carvallo JF, Jankovic J. Gender differences in functional movement disorders. Mov Disord Clin Pract 2020;7(2):182–7.

18. Ture HS, Tatlidil I, Kilicarslan E, et al. Gender-related differences in semiology of psychogenic non-epileptic seizures. Arch Neuropsychiatry 2019;56(3):178–81.

19. Alessi R, Valente KD. Psychogenic non-epileptic seizures at a tertiary care center in Brazil. Epilepsy Behav 2013;26(1):91–5.

20. Myers L, Trobliger R, Bortnik K, et al. Are there gender differences in those diagnosed with psychogenic nonepileptic seizures? Epilepsy Behav 2018;78:161–5.

21. Oto M, Conway P, McGonigal A, et al. Gender differences in psychogenic non-epileptic seizures. Seizure 2005;14(1):33–9.

22. Thomas AA, Preston J, Scott RC, et al. Diagnosis of probable psychogenic non-epileptic seizures in the outpatient clinic: Does gender matter? Epilepsy Behav 2013;29(2):295–7.

23. Korucuk M, Gazioglu S, Yildirim A, et al. Semiological characteristics of patients with psychogenic nonepileptic seizures: gender-related differences. Epilepsy Behav 2018;89:130–4.

24. Rosenbaum M. Psychogenic seizures. Psychosomatics 2000;41(2):147–9.

25. Holmes MD, Dodrill CB, Bachtler S, et al. Evidence that emotional maladjustment is worse in men than in women with psychogenic nonepileptic seizures. Epilepsy Behav 2001;2(6):568–73.

26. Del Bene VA, Arce Rentería M, Maiman M, et al. Increased odds and predictive rates of MMPI-2-RF scale elevations in patients with psychogenic non-epileptic seizures and observed sex differences. Epilepsy Behav 2017;72:43–50.

27. Gale SD, Hill SW, Pearson C. Seizure semiology in males with psychogenic non-epileptic seizures is associated with somatic complaints. Epilepsy Res 2015;115: 153–7.

28. Noe KH, Grade M, Stonnington CM, et al. Confirming psychogenic nonepileptic seizures with video-EEG: Sex matters. Epilepsy Behav 2012;23(3):220–3.

29. Kamble N, Prashantha DK, Jha M, et al. Gender and age determinants of psychogenic movement disorders: a clinical profile of 73 patients. Can J Neurol Sci J Can Sci Neurol 2016;43(2):268–77.

30. Asadi-Pooya AA, Emami M, Emami Y. Gender differences in manifestations of psychogenic non-epileptic seizures in Iran. J Neurol Sci 2013;332(1–2):66–8.

31. Say GN, Taşdemir HA, İnce H. Semiological and psychiatric characteristics of children with psychogenic nonepileptic seizures: gender-related differences. Seizure 2015;31:144–8.

32. Asadi-Pooya AA, Homayoun M. Psychogenic nonepileptic seizures: the sex ratio trajectory across the lifespan. Seizure 2020;75:63–5. https://doi.org/10.1016/j.seizure.2019.12.017.

33. Matin N, Young SS, Williams B, et al. Neuropsychiatric associations with gender, illness duration, work disability, and motor subtype in a U.S. functional neurological disorders clinic population. J Neuropsychiatry Clin Neurosci 2017;29(4): 375–82.

34. Garcin B, Villain N, Mesrati F, et al. Demographic and clinical characteristics of patients with functional motor disorders: the prospective salpêtrière cohort. Neurology 2021. https://doi.org/10.1101/2021.02.04.21251123.

35. Asadi-Pooya AA, Myers L, Valente K, et al. Sex differences in demographic and clinical characteristics of psychogenic nonepileptic seizures: a retrospective multicenter international study. Epilepsy Behav 2019;97:154–7.

36. Delgado C, Kurtis M, Martin B, et al. Clinical and demographic characteristics of patients with functional movement disorders: a consecutive cohort study from a specialized clinic. Acta Neurol Belg 2022;122(1):97–103.

37. Tinazzi M, Morgante F, Marcuzzo E, et al. Clinical correlates of functional motor disorders: an italian multicenter study. Mov Disord Clin Pract 2020;7(8):920–9.

38. Raper J, Currigan V, Fothergill S, et al. Long-term outcomes of functional neurological disorder in children. Arch Dis Child 2019;104(12):1155–60.

39. Goldstein LH, Robinson EJ, Mellers JDC, et al. Cognitive behavioural therapy for adults with dissociative seizures (CODES): a pragmatic, multicentre, randomised controlled trial. Lancet Psychiatr 2020;7(6):491–505.

40. Lagrand T, Tuitert I, Klamer M, et al. Functional or not functional; that's the question: can we predict the diagnosis functional movement disorder based on associated features? Eur J Neurol 2021;28(1):33–9.

41. Merode TV, De Krom MCTFM, Knottnerus JA. Gender-related differences in non-epileptic attacks: a study of patients' cases in the literature. Seizure 1997;6(4): 311–6.

42. Johnson KB, Harris C, Forstein M, et al. Adolescent conversion disorder and the importance of competence discussing sexual orientation. Clin Pediatr (Phila) 2010;49(5):491–4.

43. Basu AN. A case of conversion hysteria. Samiksa J Indian Psycho-Anal Soc. 1976;30(1):1–9.

44. Götestam KO, Coates TJ, Ekstrand M. Handedness, dyslexia and twinning in ho-mosexual men. Int J Neurosci 1992;63(3–4):179–86.

45. Myers L, Gray C, Roberts N, et al. Shame in the treatment of patients with psycho-genic nonepileptic seizures: the elephant in the room. Seizure 2022;94:176–82.

46. Sartaj D, Krishnan V, Rao R, et al. Mental illnesses and related vulnerabilities in the Hijra community: a cross-sectional study from India. Int J Soc Psychiatry 2021;67(3):290–7.

47. Boris JR, McClain ZBR, Bernadzikowski T. Clinical course of transgender adoles-cents with complicated postural orthostatic tachycardia syndrome undergoing hormonal therapy in gender transition: a case series. Transgender Health 2019; 4(1):331–4.

48. Schif A, Ravid S, Hafner H, et al. [Acute hemiplegia and hemianesthesia together with decreased tendon reflexes mimicking acute stroke representing a conver-sion disorder]. Harefuah 2010;149(1):29–32, 63, 62.

49. Orfanelli L, Borkowski WJ. Conversion disorder in a pediatric transgender patient. J Neurosci Nurs 2006;38(2):114–6.

50. Morabito G, Cosentini D, Tornese G, et al. Case report: somatic symptoms veiling gender dysphoria in an adolescent. Front Pediatr 2021;9:679004.

51. Williams AR. Transsexualism, 1 personality disorders, and spinal cord injury. J Gay Lesb Ment Health 2012;16(1):56–65.

52. Hendricks ML, Testa RJ. A conceptual framework for clinical work with trans-gender and gender nonconforming clients: an adaptation of the Minority Stress Model. Prof Psychol Res Pr 2012;43(5):460–7.

53. Brown JM, Naser SC, Brown Griffin C, et al. A multicultural, gender, and sexually diverse affirming school-based consultation framework. Psychol Sch 2022;59(1): 14–33.

54. Short AK, Baram TZ. Early-life adversity and neurological disease: age-old ques-tions and novel answers. Nat Rev Neurol 2019;15(11):657–69.

55. Gamarel KE, Reisner SL, Laurenceau JP, et al. Gender minority stress, mental health, and relationship quality: a dyadic investigation of transgender women and their cisgender male partners. J Fam Psychol JFP J Div Fam Psychol Am Psychol Assoc Div 2014;28(4):437–47.

56. Meyer IH. Prejudice, social stress, and mental health in lesbian, gay, and bisexual populations: conceptual issues and research evidence. Psychol Bull 2003; 129(5):674–97.

57. Brown TT, Partanen J, Chuong L, et al. Discrimination hurts: the effect of discrim-ination on the development of chronic pain. Soc Sci Med 2018;204:1–8.

58. Bockting WO, Miner MH, Swinburne Romine RE, et al. Stigma, mental health, and resilience in an online sample of the US transgender population. Am J Public Health 2013;103(5):943–51.

59. Dürrbaum T, Sattler FA. Minority stress and mental health in lesbian, gay male, and bisexual youths: a meta-analysis. J LGBT Youth 2020;17(3):298–314.

60. James S, Herman J, Rankin S, et al. The Report of the 2015 U.S. Transgender Survey. 2016. Available at: https://transequality.org/sites/default/files/docs/usts/USTS-Full-Report-Dec17.pdf. Accessed December 15, 2021.

61. Heise L, Greene ME, Opper N, et al. Gender inequality and restrictive gender norms: framing the challenges to health. Lancet Lond Engl 2019;393(10189):2440–54.

62. Meyer IH. Resilience in the study of minority stress and health of sexual and gender minorities. Psychol Sex Orientat Gend Divers 2015;2(3):209–13.

63. Streed CG, Beach LB, Caceres BA, et al. Assessing and addressing cardiovascular health in people who are transgender and gender diverse: a scientific statement from the american heart association. Circulation 2021;144(6):e136–48.

64. Haeder SF, Sylvester S, Callaghan T. Shared Stigma: The effect of LGBT status on attitudes about the opioid epidemic. World Med Health Pol 2021;13(3):414–35.

65. Keynejad RC, Frodl T, Kanaan R, et al. Stress and functional neurological disorders: mechanistic insights. J Neurol Neurosurg Psychiatr 2019;90(7):813–21.

66. Mustanski B, Andrews R, Puckett JA. The effects of cumulative victimization on mental health among lesbian, gay, bisexual, and transgender adolescents and young adults. Am J Public Health 2016;106(3):527–33.

67. Parent MC, Arriaga AS, Gobble T, et al. Stress and substance use among sexual and gender minority individuals across the lifespan. Neurobiol Stress 2019;10:100146.

68. Brewer R, Ramani SL, Khanna A, et al. A systematic review up to 2018 of HIV and associated factors among criminal justice-involved (CJI) black sexual and gender minority populations in the United States (US). J Racial Ethn Health Disparities 2021;9(4):1357–402.

69. Benotsch EG, Zimmerman R, Cathers L, et al. Non-medical use of prescription drugs, polysubstance use, and mental health in transgender adults. Drug Alcohol Depend 2013;132(1–2):391–4.

70. MacLachlan M, Khasnabis C, Mannan H. Inclusive health: inclusive health. Trop Med Int Health 2012;17(1):139–41. https://doi.org/10.1111/j.1365-3156.2011.02876.x.

71. World Professional Association of Transgender Health. Provider Directory Search. World Professional Association of Transgender Health. 2022. Available at: https://www.wpath.org/provider/search?provider_directory_search_form. Accessed June 30, 2022.

72. The Trevor Project. TrevorSpace. 2021. Available at: https://www.trevorspace.org/. Accessed August 5, 2022.

73. Gender Spectrum. Gender Spectrum. 2019. Available at: https://genderspectrum.org/resources. Accessed August 5, 2022.

74. Klee A, Chinman M, Kearney L. Peer specialist services: new frontiers and new roles. Psychol Serv 2019;16(3):353–9.

75. Heylens G, Verroken C, De Cock S, et al. Effects of different steps in gender reassignment therapy on psychopathology: a prospective study of persons with a gender identity disorder. J Sex Med 2014;11(1):119–26.

76. Matsuno E, Israel T. Psychological interventions promoting resilience among transgender individuals: transgender resilience intervention model (TRIM). Couns Psychol 2018;46(5):632–55.

77. Sloan CA, Berke DS, Shipherd JC. Utilizing a dialectical framework to inform conceptualization and treatment of clinical distress in transgender individuals. Prof Psychol Res Pr 2017;48(5):301–9.

78. Testa RJ, Habarth J, Peta J, et al. Development of the Gender Minority Stress and Resilience Measure. Psychol Sex Orientat Gend Divers 2015;2(1):65–77.

79. Swanbon T, Boyce L, Greenberg MA. Expressive writing reduces avoidance and somatic complaints in a community sample with constraints on expression. Br J Health Psychol 2008;13(1):53–6.

80. Kattari SK, Bakko M, Hecht HK, et al. Correlations between healthcare provider interactions and mental health among transgender and nonbinary adults. SSM - Popul Health 2020;10:100525.

81. Puckett JA, Cleary P, Rossman K, et al. Barriers to gender-affirming care for transgender and gender nonconforming individuals. Sex Res Soc Policy J NSRC SR SP 2018;15(1):48–59.

82. Bradford J, Reisner SL, Honnold JA, et al. Experiences of transgender-related discrimination and implications for health: results from the Virginia Transgender Health Initiative Study. Am J Public Health 2013;103(10):1820–9.

83. Turban JL, King D, Kobe J, et al. Access to gender-affirming hormones during adolescence and mental health outcomes among transgender adults. PLoS One 2022;17(1):e0261039.

84. Acosta W, Qayyum Z, Turban JL, et al. Identify, engage, understand: supporting transgender youth in an inpatient psychiatric hospital. Psychiatr Q 2019;90(3): 601–12.

85. Reisner SL, Radix A, Deutsch MB. Integrated and gender-affirming transgender clinical care and research. JAIDS J Acquir Immune Defic Syndr 2016;72(3): S235–42.

86. Turban J, Ferraiolo T, Martin A, et al. Ten things transgender and gender nonconforming youth want their doctors to know. J Am Acad Child Adolesc Psychiatry 2017;56(4):275–7.

87. Katz-Wise SL, Pullen Sansfaçon A, Bogart LM, et al. Lessons from a community-based participatory research study with transgender and gender nonconforming youth and their families. Action Res 2019;17(2):186–207.

88. Goldberg AE, Kuvalanka KA, Budge SL, et al. Health care experiences of transgender binary and nonbinary university students. Couns Psychol 2019;47(1): 59–97.

UNITED STATES POSTAL SERVICE® Statement of Ownership, Management, and Circulation
(All Periodicals Publications Except Requester Publications)

1. Publication Title	2. Publication Number	3. Filing Date
NEUROLOGIC CLINICS	000 – 712	9/18/2023

4. Issue Frequency	5. Number of Issues Published Annually	6. Annual Subscription Price
FEB, MAY, AUG, NOV	4	$353.00

7. Complete Mailing Address of Known Office of Publication (Not printer) (Street, city, county, state, and ZIP+4®)

ELSEVIER INC.
230 Park Avenue, Suite 800
New York, NY 10169

Contact Person: Malathi Samayan
Telephone (Include area code): 91-44-4299-4507

8. Complete Mailing Address of Headquarters or General Business Office of Publisher (Not printer)

ELSEVIER INC.
230 Park Avenue, Suite 800
New York, NY 10169

9. Full Names and Complete Mailing Addresses of Publisher, Editor, and Managing Editor (Do not leave blank)

Publisher (Name and complete mailing address)

Dolores Meloni, ELSEVIER INC.
1600 JOHN F KENNEDY BLVD. SUITE 1600
PHILADELPHIA, PA 19103-2899

Editor (Name and complete mailing address)

STACY EASTMAN, ELSEVIER INC.
1600 JOHN F KENNEDY BLVD. SUITE 1600
PHILADELPHIA, PA 19103-2899

Managing Editor (Name and complete mailing address)

PATRICK MANLEY, ELSEVIER INC.
1600 JOHN F KENNEDY BLVD. SUITE 1600
PHILADELPHIA, PA 19103-2899

10. Owner (Do not leave blank. If the publication is owned by a corporation, give the name and address of the corporation immediately followed by the names and addresses of all stockholders owning or holding 1 percent or more of the total amount of stock. If not owned by a corporation, give the names and addresses of the individual owners. If owned by a partnership or other unincorporated firm, give its name and address as well as those of each individual owner. If the publication is published by a nonprofit organization, give its name and address.)

Full Name	Complete Mailing Address
WHOLLY OWNED SUBSIDIARY OF REED/ELSEVIER, US HOLDINGS	1600 JOHN F KENNEDY BLVD. SUITE 1600 PHILADELPHIA, PA 19103-2899

11. Known Bondholders, Mortgagees, and Other Security Holders Owning or Holding 1 Percent or More of Total Amount of Bonds, Mortgages, or Other Securities. If none, check box. ☐ None

Full Name	Complete Mailing Address
N/A	

12. Tax Status (For completion by nonprofit organizations authorized to mail at nonprofit rates) (Check one)
The purpose, function, and nonprofit status of this organization and the exempt status for federal income tax purposes:

☒ Has Not Changed During Preceding 12 Months
☐ Has Changed During Preceding 12 Months (Publisher must submit explanation of change with this statement)

PS Form 3526, July 2014 [Page 1 of 4 (see instructions page 4)] PSN: 7530-01-000-9931 PRIVACY NOTICE: See our privacy policy on www.usps.com

13. Publication Title	14. Issue Date for Circulation Data Below
NEUROLOGIC CLINICS	AUGUST 2023

15. Extent and Nature of Circulation		Average No. Copies Each Issue During Preceding 12 Months	No. Copies of Single Issue Published Nearest to Filing Date
a. Total Number of Copies (Net press run)		168	159
b. Paid Circulation (By Mail and Outside the Mail)	(1) Mailed Outside-County Paid Subscriptions Stated on PS Form 3541 (Include paid distribution above nominal rate, advertiser's proof copies, and exchange copies)	100	87
	(2) Mailed In-County Paid Subscriptions Stated on PS Form 3541 (Include paid distribution above nominal rate, advertiser's proof copies, and exchange copies)	0	0
	(3) Paid Distribution Outside the Mails Including Sales Through Dealers and Carriers, Street Vendors, Counter Sales, and Other Paid Distribution Outside USPS®	51	57
	(4) Paid Distribution by Other Classes of Mail Through the USPS (e.g., First-Class Mail®)	12	14
c. Total Paid Distribution (Sum of 15b (1), (2), (3), and (4))		163	158
d. Free or Nominal Rate Distribution (By Mail and Outside the Mail)	(1) Free or Nominal Rate Outside-County Copies included on PS Form 3541	4	0
	(2) Free or Nominal Rate In-County Copies Included on PS Form 3541	0	0
	(3) Free or Nominal Rate Copies Mailed at Other Classes Through the USPS (e.g., First-Class Mail)	0	0
	(4) Free or Nominal Rate Distribution Outside the Mail (Carriers or other means)	1	1
e. Total Free or Nominal Rate Distribution (Sum of 15d (1), (2), (3) and (4))		5	1
f. Total Distribution (Sum of 15c and 15e)		168	159
g. Copies not Distributed (See Instructions to Publishers #4 (page #3))		0	0
h. Total (Sum of 15f and g)		168	159
i. Percent Paid (15c divided by 15f times 100)		96.73%	99.37%

* If you are claiming electronic copies, go to line 16 on page 3. If you are not claiming electronic copies, skip to line 17 on page 3.

16. Electronic Copy Circulation	Average No. Copies Each Issue During Preceding 12 Months	No. Copies of Single Issue Published Nearest to Filing Date
a. Paid Electronic Copies		
b. Total Paid Print Copies (Line 15c) + Paid Electronic Copies (Line 16a)		
c. Total Print Distribution (Line 15f) + Paid Electronic Copies (Line 16a)		
d. Percent Paid (Both Print & Electronic Copies) (16b divided by 16c × 100)		

☒ I certify that 80% of all my distributed copies (electronic and print) are paid above a nominal price.

17. Publication of Statement of Ownership

☒ If the publication is a general publication, publication of this statement is required. Will be printed in the NOVEMBER 2023 issue of this publication.   ☐ Publication not required.

18. Signature and Title of Editor, Publisher, Business Manager, or Owner

Malathi Samayan - Distribution Controller

Malathi Samayan   Date 9/18/2023

I certify that all information furnished on this form is true and complete. I understand that anyone who furnishes false or misleading information on this form or who omits material or information requested on the form may be subject to criminal sanctions (including fines and imprisonment) and/or civil sanctions (including civil penalties).

PS Form 3526, July 2014 (Page 3 of 4)   PRIVACY NOTICE: See our privacy policy on www.usps.com

Printed and bound by CPI Group (UK) Ltd, Croydon, CR0 4YY

03/10/2024

01040473-0002